The development
and integration of behaviour

The development and integration of behaviour

Essays in honour of Robert Hinde

Edited by

Patrick Bateson, FRS

*Professor of Ethology, University of Cambridge
and Provost of King's College, Cambridge*

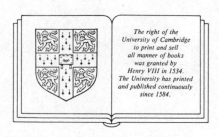

CAMBRIDGE UNIVERSITY PRESS

CAMBRIDGE

NEW YORK   PORT CHESTER

MELBOURNE   SYDNEY

Published by the Press Syndicate of the University of Cambridge
The Pitt Building, Trumpington Street, Cambridge CB2 1RP
40 West 20th Street, New York, NY 10011, USA
10 Stamford Road, Oakleigh, Melbourne 3166, Australia

First published 1991

Printed in Great Britain at the University Press, Cambridge

British Library cataloguing in publication data

The development and integration of behaviour: essays in honour of Robert Hinde.
I. Bateson, Patrick   II. Hinde, Robert
591. 51

Library of Congress cataloguing in publication data

The development and integration of behaviour: essays in honour of Robert
Hinde/edited by Patrick Bateson.
p.   cm.
Includes index.
1. Developmental psychobiology.   2. Developmental neurology.   3. Animal
behaviour.   4. Hinde, Robert A.   I. Hinde, Robert A.   II. Bateson, P. P. G.
QP363.5.D46 1991   90–49250   CIP
599′.051--dc20

ISBN 0 521 40356 1 hardback
ISBN 0 521 40709 5 paperback

UP

Contents

Contents

Contributors

R. J. Andrew, *School of Biological Sciences, University of Sussex, Falmer, Brighton, Sussex BN1 9QG, UK*

Patrick Bateson, *University of Cambridge, Sub-Department of Animal Behaviour, Madingley, Cambridge CB3 8AA, UK*

The Late John Bowlby

T. H. Clutton-Brock, *University of Cambridge, Department of Zoology, Large Animal Research Group, 34A Storeys Way, Cambridge CB3 0DT, UK*

Judy Dunn, *The Pennsylvania State University, College of Human Development, Henderson Human Development Building, University Park, Pennsylvania 16802, USA*

John C. Fentress, *Department of Psychology, Dalhousie University, Halifax, Nova Scotia B3H 4J1, Canada*

Jane Goodall, *Gombe Stream Reserve, Box 727, Dar es Salaam, Tanzania*

David A. Hamburg, *Carnegie Corporation of New York, 437 Madison Avenue, New York, NY 10022, USA*

Robert A. Hinde, *The Master's Lodge, St John's College, Cambridge CB2 1TP, UK*

Gabriel Horn, *University of Cambridge, Department of Zoology, Downing Street, Cambridge CB2 3EJ, UK*

J. B. Hutchison, *MRC Neuroendocrine Development and Behaviour Group, Institute of Animal Physiology and Genetics Research, Babraham, Cambridge CB2 4AT, UK*

Peter Marler, *Department of Zoology, Storer Hall, University of California at Davis, Davis, California 956163, USA*

Jay S. Rosenblatt, *Rutgers University, Institute of Animal Behaviour, 101 Warren Street, Newark, NJ 07102, USA*

Contributors

Thelma E. Rowell, *Department of Zoology, University of California, Berkeley, California 94720, USA*

Michael Rutter, *Institute of Psychiatry, De Crespigny Park, Denmark Hill, London SE5 8AF, UK*

Michael J. A. Simpson, *Development and Integration of Behaviour Unit, Madingley, Cambridge CB3 8AA, UK*

Joan Stevenson-Hinde, *University of Cambridge, Sub-Department of Animal Behaviour, Madingley, Cambridge CB3 8AA, UK*

The Late Niko Tinbergen

Marian Radke-Yarrow, *Laboratory of Developmental Psychology, National Institute of Mental Health, Building 15K, Bethesda, Maryland 20892, USA*

Preface

Although this book was planned as a celebration for Robert Hinde, a quick glance at the contents will reveal that it is no ordinary Festschrift. The person in whose honour the book was written is also a contributor. Since Robert Hinde is still highly active in research and is likely to remain so for a long time to come, the conventional commemorative volume seemed out of place. It seemed much more appropriate to involve him in the construction and editing of the book and to ask him to comment on the essays. The objective of the book has not been to dwell on the contributions that Robert Hinde has made, but rather to focus on the themes and organising principles that have emerged in the fields in which he has been active. The hope was that the book would be forward-looking in its survey of the fields for which he has done so much.

Robert Hinde has exerted an extraordinary influence on ethology, primatology and most recently on studies of human behavioural biology and development. He has always revelled in diversity, but none the less certain distinctive themes run through the whole book as they have through his own writing. The introductory chapter discusses the recurring themes of crossing and recrossing the boundaries between different levels of analysis and the need to study processes. The main part of the book starts with behavioural development studied in animals, moves on to the neural and endocrine aspects of behaviour and then to the social behaviour of non-human primates. The final transition from monkeys to humans, which Robert Hinde made in his own research, leads to a substantial section on the development of social behaviour in humans. The last scientific chapter picks up his own deep concern about aggression and the peculiarly human institution of war.

Even though this is first and foremost a book about the development and integration of behaviour, it carries the personal flavour of the man all the contributors wished to honour. Each of the authors has had long-standing relationships with Robert Hinde. Some were mentors, others were former students and four were the senior members of his Medical Research Council Unit which had the same name as this book. In the final section of the book, one of his teachers and old friends, Niko Tinbergen, wrote a brief memoir just before he died. Jane Goodall, who came to Cambridge to write up her first chimpanzee studies for a PhD under Robert Hinde's supervision in the early 1960s, also writes of her memories of him when he visited her camp in Africa.

The idea for this book originally came from Peter Marler with whom I was to have edited the book. However, the period in which most editing had to be done was also one when he was moving his house and laboratory from New York to California. He was not able to contribute in the way that he would have wished if he had been less busy. I am deeply grateful to him for his initiative, for his encouragement in the slow process of bringing the book together, and for contributing a chapter when he had so much else to do. The same gratitude must be extended to the other contributors, also extremely busy people, who were asked to think deeply as well as broadly about the subjects on which they work. Moreover, they had to do so in the knowledge that their contribution would be subject to public comment by a man who at the best of times and to the best of his friends is a formidable critic. Inevitably, some delivered more rapidly than others and I must thank the quicker writers for their patience and the slower ones for their persistence. Above all, I must thank the man in whose honour this book was written for agreeing to involve himself in its construction. I deeply appreciate the trouble he has taken both in helping with the editing, which he has done with his usual penetrating eye, and for his commentaries on the contributions.

Patrick Bateson
Cambridge, April 1990

I
Introduction

— 1 —

Levels and processes

Patrick Bateson

Behaviour is studied in many ways because people become absorbed in different types of problem. Some want to know, for instance, what a pattern of behaviour is for, while others want to know how it is controlled. Nevertheless, styles differ even when a problem is shared. The research of some people is driven by clear and explicit theories. Other people suppose that when enough information has been collected, the explanations for behaviour will stare them in the face. Some push a theory for all its worth until it overwhelms the opposition or collapses from weakness. Others, revelling in curiosity, enjoy the diversity of individuals and species. The opposition between these contrasting styles is easily overstated for they complement each other and, when those who work in different ways find a way of coming together, their union is often highly productive.

'Coming together' is perhaps a good way to describe the overall character of this book. One message, emerging strongly from it, is that ideas should flow in both directions between different levels of analysis. In that sense the stance differs sharply from a commonly held position that the people studying behaviour should pose problems for the neuroscientists who, having done their work, should pass on the project to the molecular biologists (e.g. Dudai, 1989). In the same vein, the study of social structure should not simply be reduced to the study of relationships. Both should be helped by the knowledge and the understanding obtained at the other level; likewise for the studies of social relationships and individuals' behaviour.

A second theme of the book is that, at all levels of analysis, scientists studying behaviour are faced with dynamical systems that have an awkward way of altering their characteristics when conditions change. The way to understand such systems is by studying them as processes, not by taking snapshots or by abstracting linear causal chains. In the study of behavioural

3

development, for instance, an approach, which now seems outmoded, was to make manipulations in early life and examine the long-term effects on adult behaviour. As the manipulations of the environment were combined with the use of strains of different genotype (e.g. Cooper & Zubek, 1958), the claim that differences are due solely to a particular aspect of experience or solely to genes was made less frequently than before. Nevertheless, even to the present day, influential voices are to be heard arguing that, if something is known about genetic and environmental variation, then it is possible to use standard statistical techniques to show how genes and the environment contribute to differences in a particular characteristic. The conclusion emerging from such thinking is that the genetic and environmental factors *add* together to produce their effects on behaviour (e.g. Loehlin, Willerman & Horn, 1988). However, even if the dynamics of development could be plausibly reduced in this way, major aspects of the interplay between the developing individual and its environment are easily missed by the analytical techniques used to derive such conclusions (Bateson, 1989; Wahlsten, 1990). The general point that recurs frequently in this book is that understanding is significantly improved when the processes involved in the development and integration of behaviour are studied directly. This places a spotlight on the behaviour of individuals.

The mood of a great many of the chapters in this book is a wish to understand how things are put together. Instead of explaining patterns of behaviour in terms of their parts or their origins, the drive is to understand the rules that make the processes work. The assumption is that getting to grips with the organisation of behaviour is the precursor to obtaining principles. At the very least, the questions that need answering are being formulated. In this introductory chapter I discuss briefly the contents of each essay in the scientific part of the book before returning to the themes that run through the whole book and the way they link to Robert Hinde's own interests.

Bateson and Marler

The chapters in Section II, which is about behavioural development in animals, deal primarily with two favourite and famous ethological examples, imprinting and song-learning in birds. In Chapter 2 my general concern is with how the undoubted complexities of development might be made more tractable by uncovering principles that make sense of that complexity. In order to illustrate how this might be done, I look at the particular case of imprinting. The features of the animal existing at the time when it normally starts to learn the characteristics of its close kin crucially affect the process by which an animal's social preferences develop in the way they do. Even though the hypothetical underlying rules for the developmental process are rather simple, what happens to the bird is not reducible to internal and external contributions that add together. An important conclusion is that as developmental processes are studied, the old nature/nurture dichotomies, which were always difficult to handle empirically, lose any usefulness that they might once seem to have had.

In Chapter 3 the interplay between the developing animal and its environment is disclosed in another way by Peter Marler who reviews the marked species differences found in the development of song in birds. Closely related species differ in how much they learn, the sounds which they are most likely to learn about and the sounds which they are most likely to make when they have been exposed to the same conditions. Songbirds also differ in when they learn most readily and in subsequent inventiveness in generating new patterns of song. Marler argues that all this evidence points strongly to the pervasive influences of genetic factors in generating those differences. Since he is dealing with learning, his examples also emphasise the importance of understanding the rules that underlie developmental processes. These rules have to develop, of course, and may well take on peculiar characteristics in special environmental conditions. Nevertheless, a crucial difference between different species will be those genes that influence the character of the features in any one set of circumstances. In essence, then, Marler exploits differences between species in getting at the way developmental processes work.

Fentress, Horn, Hutchison, Andrew and Rosenblatt

Section III deals with the neural and endocrine mechanisms underlying behaviour. In Chapter 4 John Fentress underscores the main themes of the book when he considers the rules of connection between behavioural and neural analysis. He regards what he calls the bi-directional perspective, looking up as well as looking down, as crucially important. This approach is now becoming an important part of neuroethology. Fentress recognises that the major problem facing scientists in this area is to put together properties that have been isolated for purposes of experiment and yet which must be interconnected in the free-running animal. He has led the way in showing how systems can sometimes operate autonomously and sometimes affect each other. The difficulty is, as he points out, that once a system has been abstracted, it is treated as though it cannot interact with another one. Even so, he is optimistic about the outcome of attempts to reassemble the integrated organism. The next chapters show why.

In Chapter 5 Gabriel Horn gives examples from imprinting in domestic chicks of how the interconnections between different levels of analysis are being made in practice. Problems of the organisation of behaviour, which had not even been thought of before the neural analysis of imprinting had

5

been carried out, are now being posed. The neural analysis has not only thrown light on the neural bases of recognition memory, but also has made possible the dissociation of the mechanisms involved in the initial preferences from the mechanisms involved in narrowing chicks' preferences to a familiar object. How do the development of predispositions and the specific effects of experience on preferences interact? How is mate choice affected by the lesions which have a highly specific effect on filial imprinting? Is it possible to dissociate the recognition memory aspect of imprinting from the operant and classical conditioning aspects which are known to accompany it? What are the functions of the memory systems storing representations of the imprinting object in different locations in the brain? All these questions have been or are now being studied at the behavioural level as a result of the research at the neural level.

Another example which further elaborates the general point made by Fentress about approaching problems at both the behavioural and neural levels is found in Chapter 6. John Hutchison links behavioural analysis of courtship with the biochemical techniques of neuroendocrinology, illustrating this interplay with the results of his own long-term work on birds and mammals. The male hormone testosterone is a precursor, broken into different metabolites by enzymes in brain cells. These metabolites affect behaviour differently. Whether or not a behaviour pattern is expressed depends on the brain enzymes, which in turn depend on the animal's state. Since the animal's state depends on environmental conditions, the advantages of bringing together expertise from different levels of analysis are obvious. Hutchison points out, furthermore, that the principles involved here are as important in development as in the control of adult behaviour.

The new knowledge about the various actions of testosterone on behaviour is also strikingly illustrated in Chapter 7 by Richard Andrew's account of his own studies of information processing and storage in domestic chicks. Surprisingly, the male hormone testosterone makes birds and mammals less distractable. The effect seems to be produced in two ways. Andrew suggests that the androgenic component of testosterone increases the persistence with which motor patterns are performed, while the oestrogenic component increases the time for which the representation of an event is held in working memory. The second, very interesting effect relates perhaps to increased span of attention found in humans with high circulating levels of testosterone. Andrew makes the general point that in science, surprising novel phenomena should be seized eagerly and studied with the best tools available. Further support for this stance is provided by the discovery of asymmetries in brain function of chicks at the behavioural level which Andrew reports and at the neural level which Horn reports in his chapter. No theorist, as far as I am aware, had anticipated these discoveries.

6

In Chapter 8 Jay Rosenblatt reviews the intensive research which has been conducted on the control of maternal state in rodents and then looks to the ways in which these ideas may be generalised to primates. Thanks in large part to Rosenblatt himself, rapid progress has been made in understanding the hormones and other neuroactive substances that stimulate the onset of maternal behaviour, the neural substrates on which these substances act and the stimulation from the young which maintains maternal behaviour. His own research on rodents is a fine example of working simultaneously at different levels. As in the case of the work described by John Hutchison, Rosenblatt shows how events external to the animal can trigger hormonal changes and modulate the effects of the hormones. Much less is known about primates, but it seems that, unlike rodents, hormones probably do not increase maternal responsiveness in the final stages of pregnancy. By contrast, primates are likely to be similar to rodents in the way that young animals can stimulate and maintain maternal behaviour. This comparison shows the extent to which more general principles of the organisation of behaviour are starting to emerge and where they are limited to a particular taxonomic group.

Clutton-Brock, Rowell and Simpson

Tim Clutton-Brock opens Section IV with a chapter on another aspect of the reproductive behaviour, the mating system. One of the consequences of the great growth of primate studies over the last 20 years has been that detailed knowledge is available now about a great array of species. This allows the comparative approach which Tim Clutton-Brock uses in his chapter. In Chapter 9 he examines the association between sex differences and the maximum number of mates that a male may have at any one time. He points out that the character of the mating system may have ramifying consequences for many other aspects of the biology of the species, partly because the conditions with which the two sexes have to cope are so different in those species in which a male may have many mates and the female only has one. Although Clutton-Brock is concerned first and foremost with functional issues, the extent of sex differences has an important developmental slant. A predisposition to behave in a particular way that differs from the other sex may be amplified or heavily damped by environmental conditions. This is particularly striking when the behaviour of the male depends on such factors as his body condition and the social environment. For instance, the Gelada baboon males may develop to twice the size of the females and defend harems against other males, or they may be the same size as females, look like females and never fight another male (Dunbar, 1984).

In Chapter 10 Thelma Rowell examines the emergence of ideas about social behaviour which have been strongly influenced by thinking on the different levels at which such behaviour may be analysed, namely individual interactions, social relations and social structure. Such work must start from treating animals as individuals, which has not been standard practice in those branches of biology that have been concerned with universals. She points out that a degree of complexity and continuity in the relationships of primates is now accepted in a way that would have been unthinkable thirty years ago. Even so, analysis at the highest level of social structure presents enormous practical difficulties of observation when studying animals in the field and she sees an as yet largely unbridged gap with the lower levels.

In Chapter 11 Michael Simpson argues that one individual may signal to another that it is likely to devote time, aid and resources to another when a variety of possible partners are available and when coordination between individuals is of mutual benefit in biological terms. He suggests that, when a non-human primate directs certain types of behaviour, such as grooming, selectively at a particular individual, such actions are the equivalents of 'promises or declarations of future commitment to a relationship' in humans. An individual signalling in this way benefits when its commitment enhances its value in the eyes of a potentially valuable partner and, thereby, helps to keep that partner. By selecting some human examples to illustrate his views about commitment in social behaviour, Simpson shows how such knowledge projected into other animals can provide valuable insight.

Bowlby, Stevenson-Hinde, Rutter, Dunn and Radke-Yarrow

The section on human behaviour begins with three studies of a specific problem, the long-term effects of the relationship between the mother and her child. John Bowlby saw the great potential of bringing the insights of psychoanalysis together with the concepts and methods of ethology, particularly when examining the lasting influences on social behaviour of the attachment of children to their mothers. In Chapter 12 Bowlby provides a lucid overview of where attachment theory now stands. His perspective on the field which he founded is very welcome. The ethological part of the theory was originally couched in terms of what was then thought to happen in the case of imprinting, namely an instantaneous, irreversible bond formed at a critical stage in development. Views of imprinting have changed a lot since then. The process is thought to be much more flexible and considerable attention is now paid to the additional steps which are involved when early experience leaves an impact on adult behaviour (e.g. ten Cate, 1989). Views of human developments have also changed a great deal.

In Chapter 13 Joan Stevenson-Hinde examines the relations between attachment and temperament. Typically they have been set in opposition, an unfortunate dichotomy reminiscent of other old debates in the study of development, so that temperament is seen as part of nature and attachment as part of nurture and the two sum together. Stevenson-Hinde rejects that approach. She argues that they are much more helpfully seen as separate systems and the child's behaviour represents the dynamic interplay between them. In this respect, her argument is very similar to that of Fentress and mine in earlier chapters.

The question of how the long-term effects on adult behaviour might be produced by the mother-child relationship is considered next. In Chapter 14 Michael Rutter takes a fresh look at the idea of maternal deprivation. In a comprehensive sweep of the modern literature, he examines the way in which the influence might be mediated. The linking processes involve the way children relate to people they encounter later in their development and, as a consequence, particular outcomes are only obtained in particular conditions. Rutter explicitly rejects the likening of this picture with the old one of imprinting in birds and, in my view, he is right to do so. This is not only because developmental concepts have been changing in both fields of research, but also because the nature of the mediating events and the influences on adult behaviour are turning out to be markedly different in the two cases. In birds, the early experience does lead to an internal representation of the familiar object which may control sexual behaviour at a later stage. In humans, Rutter suggests that the breakdown of the mother-child relationship in early life makes institutional rearing of the children more likely. This is often followed by a return in adolescence to a discordant family environment and escape from that to an ill-considered marriage, which then breaks down. In those circumstances, the young mother provides as inadequate a basis for a relationship for her own child as had been provided for her.

In Chapter 15 Judy Dunn examines the contributions to studies of child development that have come from ethological work on animals by Robert Hinde. At the methodological level she values highly the approach of observing directly the mutual influences on each other of children and mothers in their own world. At the conceptual level, she picks up the issue discussed by Rowell in the previous section and focuses on the framework that divides social behaviour into levels. She argues convincingly that no headway will be made in understanding the social development of individual children without an appreciation of the links between their individual characteristics, their relationships and the social norms of the wider group.

In Chapter 16 Marian Radke-Yarrow is concerned with the methods and conceptual apparatus needed in the study of child development. She points out that the perspective of the child influencing the world in which it develops as well as being affected by it is widely agreed upon by those working on development. However, the ways in which the data are collected have not been well adapted to studying the dynamics of developing relationships. While a mathematical crank can be turned in order to generate a picture of the causality, it is not at all difficult to think of subtle forms of interplay that would readily elude such statistical analysis. The fashioning of methods appropriate to the tasks is crucial. As a remedy she sees the need to characterise and measure carefully the environments in which children develop and the direct measurement of mutual influences. Like many others writing in this book, she emphasises the importance of studying the individual. She points out that, by doing so, access to the points of rapid change is much more likely – always an advantage when trying to understand the processes underlying development (see Hinde & Bateson, 1984). She also emphasises a point that recurs many times in the book, namely the need to draw together in collaboration people who have worked in different disciplines.

Hamburg

Section VI is devoted to a survey of the relations between behavioural knowledge and the problems created by humans' aggression towards other humans which culminates so disastrously in modern warfare. In Chapter 17 David Hamburg starts his analysis by dealing with non-human primates with a view to examining the precursors of human conflict. He emphasises that uncovering the likely course of evolution only provides a part of what is needed to have an understanding of human capacity to adapt to new conditions. Even so, by gaining a picture where humans came from, how they got there and how different present circumstances are from the ones in which the species evolved, the hope is that it may be able to modify the most dangerous aspects of human behaviour. The knowledge of the ways in which non-human primates respond to members of their own social group, as compared with members of other social groups, does give an important insight into human behaviour by pointing to the link between attachment and aggression. Dehumanisation of the adversary plays an important role in justifying violent behaviour that is rarely, if ever, considered against members of one's own group. The next step is to understand the conditions when such behaviour is likely to be expressed so that thought can be given to controlling those conditions. Violent behaviour is particularly likely to come to the fore when individuals perceive a conflict of vital interest between their own group and others, an unacceptable difference in privileges and status, or differences in attitudes that threaten their own self-respect.

Hamburg emphasises that in making progress in a matter that should concern everybody, collaboration between different disciplines is crucial.

Hamburg's emphasis on collaboration draws attention to a third theme that runs throughout the book. The emphasis on different levels and on studying dynamics require more knowledge and expertise than any one person can usually command. The obvious conclusion is that links must be made between different disciplines and specialists have to learn to work with others who speak what seems to be at first mutually incomprehensible scientific languages.

Changes in approach

The contents of this book invite comparison with *Growing Points in Ethology*, a collection of essays edited by Robert Hinde and myself 15 years ago (Bateson & Hinde, 1976). The two books have ten authors in common and both emerge from the same stable. The wits of the time nicknamed rather cruelly the earlier book as 'Groaning Points' or 'Growing Pains' because many chapters made them work harder than they would have liked. *Growing Points* was published just after E. O. Wilson (1975) produced his great book on sociobiology. The appeal of evolutionary theory, in which sociobiology was embedded, was that it seemed to make a complicated subject manageable. However, after 15 years in which concerns for the function and evolution of behaviour have been dominant in studies of animal behaviour, the major practitioners are beginning to appreciate the need for knowledge of the mechanisms (e.g. Clutton-Brock, 1990). In this sense they are rediscovering the wisdom of the founding fathers of ethology who saw the value of keeping both the 'how' and 'why' questions in play at the same time.

In what sense has research on the mechanisms of behaviour pulled the field together? It would be nice to say that a thorough understanding of rules underlying the development and integration of behaviour has been achieved. If that were the case the life of the student wrestling with a formidable literature would be made a great deal easier. The size of this book suggests that such a happy state has not yet been reached – the book might have been a lot thinner if it had! Even so, I think that at the least the questions that must be answered in order to provide a sense of coherence are much more clearly formulated than they were.

Apart from this trend, four differences between the two books stand out – at least to my eye: the growth of neuroethology, a reduction in the space given to functional approaches to behaviour, a new readiness to take subjective insights into human behaviour and apply them along with the objective approaches to animals, and a big increase in the proportion of

11

chapters devoted to child development. Of course, these differences represent changes that have taken place in the stable from which the books come as much as, or even more than, they do general trends in the study of behaviour. In particular, the much larger section on child development in this book reflects the extent to which Robert Hinde has been moving his own research in this direction in the last 15 years. It is worth looking at each of the other three features a little more closely.

Neuroethology

Niko Tinbergen (1951) wrote that it was the ethologists' job to carry the analysis of behaviour down the level of the physiologist. Despite Tinbergen's encouragement, the links between the subjects remained relatively tenuous for many years. The ethologists became increasingly preoccupied with ecology and evolutionary biology and, for their part, the majority of the neurobiologists remained profoundly uninterested in the output of the whole nervous system. Not a single essay in *Growing Points* was concerned with the neural analysis of behaviour. This was partly because the problems had proved much more difficult than some of the earlier advocates of 'neuroethology' had imagined and partly because many of the people working with whole animals felt that a specifically behavioural analysis was a proper goal in its own right. As Robert Hinde and I noted at the time, the recognition that questions can be posed properly at each level should not be taken to imply that, once holes are found for pigeons, they should no longer coo to each other. Our point was not only that behavioural analysis could lead to analysis of neural events, but also that neurobiology should become fruitful in suggesting directions for behavioural studies. The need for providing links between levels has remained as strong as ever and now finally the need is being met. Quite suddenly, previously intractable problems seem to be solvable and, at last, the behavioural and neural levels of analysis are being brought together in exciting ways.

Function and evolution

The trends towards studies of function and behavioural ecology, which had been strongly fostered by ethologists, became the slogans of the new sociobiology movement of the 1970s. Imaginations were captured by the new ideas from evolutionary biology and by the ways in which behavioural biology had been attractively married to population biology. The majority of aspiring graduate students wanted to work on a problem in sociobiology or behavioural ecology. The drawback to the subject as a whole was that large chunks of behavioural biology, which had been central concerns of ethology, were deemed to be irrelevant or uninteresting. Few students wanted to work on how behaviour develops or on how it is controlled. Gradually it has become apparent that this neglect of an important part of the biology of behaviour was a serious mistake (e.g. Barlow, 1989; Dawkins, 1989). This is because what animals actually do is so important in stimulating (as well as constraining) ideas about the function and evolution of behaviour. That having been said, the stimulus works both ways as many chapters in this book testify.

Projections from humans to animals

Projections from animals to humans have been common enough and subject to much and well-known criticism, even though its judicious use has an important place in thinking about ourselves (e.g. Hinde, 1987). The anthropomorphism, rampant in writing about animal minds in the early part of this century, led to the behaviourist reaction and projections the other way have, until comparatively recently, been covert and generally regarded as illicit. The so-called cognitive revolution altered all that. Even so, people who study behaviour, like other scientists, are in the business of using empirical evidence to change the way they think. For that reason, mentalistic explanations for behaviour should be translatable into terms that can be categorised and measured. The difficulty about using words that carry an unwarranted baggage of meaning is that they are liable to beg the question of how the process produces its outcome. Concepts referring to unseen mechanisms tend to acquire additional meanings that are not suggested by the evidence they are intended to explain. For these reasons, considerable ambiguity and misunderstanding can arise when words like 'choice', 'attempt', 'feeling' and 'intention' are treated as though they referred to events that can be directly observed. On the other hand, emphasis on the dangers of anthropomorphism undoubtedly constrained research. A scientist who never treats an animal as though it were a human is liable to miss much of the richness and complexity of its behaviour. If an animal is only thought of as a piece of clockwork machinery, then some of its most interesting attributes are likely to be overlooked.

The growing interest in animal awareness is encouraging ever more sophisticated studies of animal cognition (e.g. Mackintosh, 1987; Byrne & Whiten, 1988). The change in approach has raised much more sharply focused questions about to what extent is the projection into animals of human feelings and intentions merely a useful means to understand animal behaviour and to what extent is the goal to provide an account of their imputed feelings or intentions. Thinking of behavioural outcomes as the goals of animal intentions has undoubtedly helped many people studying behaviour to deal with the complex processes that control the animal's behaviour. Maybe it is because humans spend so much time planning their own lives that they find it easier to think about complex dynamical systems in this way. Genuine benefits, in terms of uncovering the factors that influence them, flow from projecting human intentions and feelings into the animals. This is not inconsistent, however, with a return to the full rigour of using operational or ostensive definitions when the time is ripe. Nor does attributing the power of thought to an animal, in order to do more imaginative science, mean that, when efforts are crowned with success, proof has been obtained that the animal thinks. This point lies at the heart of the difference between the heuristic and the truth value of the attribution.

As so often proves to be the case, a balance is involved between different types of cost in the use of language. Foregoing the use of empathy, intentional language and the associated concepts has real disadvantages in terms of uncovering the influences on an animal's behaviour. Attributing reality to explanatory terms with hidden connotations also leads to trouble. Pragmatic usage of language would minimise the costs of clumsiness and, at the same time, minimise the costs of confusion.

Conclusion

The common themes running through this book are, unsurprisingly, related to the approach of the person whom the authors of this book all honour. The message in so many of Robert Hinde's writings is that, even though the move in every subject is towards greater and greater specialisation and towards reducing large problems to smaller ones at lower levels of analysis, satisfying explanations are rarely going to come from one method or a single theoretical framework. Getting to grips with the development and control of behaviour requires scientists to 'cross and recross' (a favourite Hinde phrase) the boundaries between different levels. This is a major theme of the book as, indeed, it has been in Robert Hinde's writings. Another important theme in the book is the need to study processes in individuals; this too has recurred throughout Robert Hinde's writings.

To mount such arguments is not, of course, to present a theory or a set of scientific principles. Rather it is to provide an approach which is a precondition for constructing a sensible theory or deriving a coherent principle. Is this simply a glimpse of an obvious truth in which everyone believes? Evidently not, since many powerful voices have urged the behavioural and social sciences to model themselves on the success stories of classical physics or molecular biology. The obvious attraction of producing simple, easily understood explanations has meant that crucial distinctions have been fudged in the name of being straightforward and analysis has been focused on single factors in the name of clarity. This has been particularly obvious in studies of development. However, as Robert Hinde has frequently warned, little progress is made in the end if the straightforwardness and clarity are illusions. Nobody likes to think that their pet principles are constrained. Indeed, a common feature of bolder writers is to make a virtue of this dislike and drive their explanations all over the place as though these were the attractive and necessary simplifications for which everybody craves.

Being complicated for its own sake has no merit either, but explanations are worthless if they do not bear some relation to real phenomena. Understanding how the parts relate to each other is a precondition to understanding process and understanding process is the precursor to uncovering principles. Inevitably, tension still exists between ideas that emphasise differences and celebrate complexity and those that unify and simplify. But given that there is no royal road, the old 1960s slogan, 'Make love, not war' is worth remembering. Those who grapple with the development and integration of behaviour should value the search for coherence as well as the skills, based on experience with free-running systems.

Acknowledgements

I am grateful to Judy Dunn, Robert Hinde, Gabriel Horn, John Hutchison, Alex Kacelnik, Michael Simpson and Joan Stevenson-Hinde for their comments on a draft of this manuscript.

References

Barlow, G. W. (1989). Has sociobiology killed ethology or revitalized it? In *Perspectives in Ethology, Vol 8. Whither Ethology?*, ed. P. P. G. Bateson and P. H. Klopfer, pp. 1–45. New York: Plenum Press.

Bateson, P. (1989). Additive models may mislead. *International Journal of Behavioral Development*, **12**, 407–11.

Bateson, P. P. G. & Hinde, R. A. (ed.) (1976). *Growing Points in Ethology*. Cambridge: Cambridge University Press.

Byrne, R. & Whiten, A. (1988). *Machiavellian Intelligence: Social Expertise and the Evolution of Intellect in Monkeys, Apes, and Humans*. Oxford: Clarendon Press.

Clutton-Brock, T. H. (1990). *The Evolution of Parental Care*. Princeton, NJ: Princeton University Press.

Cooper, R. M. & Zubek, J. P. (1958). Effects of enriched and restricted early environments on the learning ability of bright and dull rats. *Canadian Journal of Psychology*, **12**, 159–64.

Dawkins, M. S. (1989). The future of ethology: how many legs are we standing on? In *Perspectives in Ethology, Vol. 8. Whither Ethology?*, ed. P. P. G. Bateson and P. H. Klopfer, pp. 47–54. New York: Plenum Press.

Dudai, Y. (1989). *The Neurobiology of Memory*. Oxford: Oxford University Press.

Dunbar, R. I. M. (1984). *Reproductive Decisions*. Princeton, NJ: Princeton University Press.

Hinde, R. A. (1987). *Individuals, Relationships and Culture*. Cambridge: Cambridge University Press.

Hinde, R. A. & Bateson, P. (1984). Discontinuities versus continuities in behavioural development and the neglect of process. *International Journal of Behavioral Development*, **7**, 129–43.

Loehlin, J. C., Willerman, L. & Horn, J. M. (1988). Human behavior genetics. *Annual Review of Psychology*, **39**, 101–33.

Mackintosh, N. (1987). Animal minds. In *Mindwaves*, ed. C. Blakemore and S. Greenfield, pp. 111–20. Oxford: Blackwells.

ten Cate, C. (1989). Behavioral development: toward understanding processes. In *Perspectives in Ethology, Vol. 8. Whither Ethology?*, ed. P. P. G. Bateson and P. H. Klopfer, pp. 243–69. New York: Plenum Press.

Tinbergen, N. (1951). *The Study of Instinct*. Oxford: Clarendon Press.

Wahlsten, D. (1990). Insensitivity of the analysis of variance to heredity–environment interaction. *Behavioral and Brain Sciences*, **13**, 109–61.

Wilson, E. O. (1975). *Sociobiology*. Cambridge, Mass: Harvard University Press.

II
The development of behaviour

—2—
Are there principles of behavioural development?

Patrick Bateson

Introduction

Behavioural development has been treated by ethologists as a Cinderella subject for many years – interesting and beautiful, yet widely ignored. Understanding what happens has seemed incredibly difficult and the prospects for coherent explanations of the type found in, say, evolutionary biology did not seem rosy. Certainly, after sociobiology and behavioural ecology became fashionable in the 1970s, biology students voted with their feet and preferred to study aspects of behaviour which they thought they would be better able to understand.

The particular approach to the Cinderella subject, which Robert Hinde founded and fostered and in which I have been involved, used to provoke some teasing. Members of the Oxford Animal Behaviour Group, for example, used to mock: 'At Madingley, never use a simple explanation when a more complicated one will do instead.' However, behind the seemingly trivial Cambridge refrain that behavioural development *is* complicated, lie three crucial points. First, questions that are put in too general a form are rarely helpful. Second, many influences do combine to generate the differences that are observed between adults. Third, armchair theorising about the dynamics of behavioural development is extremely unlikely to be successful in our present state of knowledge. Possibly over-arching explanations for development may never be produced because the numerous influences on adult behaviour can combine in such profuse ways. However, I am optimistic that regularities can be found. In this chapter I am going to argue that Robert Hinde's general approach, easily accused of over-emphasising complexity, has been essential in bringing genuine understanding to the subject. The approach has brought us to the point where principles have started to emerge.

19

Conceptual clarity

Anybody who has been a student of Robert Hinde or had a paper criticised by him will be aware of how quick he is to pounce on poor reasoning. He particularly dislikes sloppy generalisation. The mistake is easily made. When writing, most of us some of the time will slip from answering one question to addressing another. Unless the reader concentrates very carefully, the mistake goes unnoticed – except by a person like Robert Hinde who seems not to blink when he reads. In studies of development, evidence that some functional patterns of behaviour are expressed without obvious opportunities to copy or practice the patterns has been used to justify two categories of behaviour, namely 'genetic' and 'learned' (see Dudai, 1989, for a recent example). Indeed, the treatment of different types of problem as though they were the same has been rife in the subject (Johnston, 1988).

In his critique of dichotomies used in the study of behaviour he noted that classifications into two categories had been used for quite different purposes (Hinde, 1969). Traditionally, dichotomies were applied to behaviour, but they were also applied to development as in the distinction between maturation and experience. Konrad Lorenz (1965) made an interesting and useful break with this tradition when he proposed that behaviour should be classified in terms of whether or not the patterns had been adapted to their present use during the course of the individual's lifetime. It made sense to argue that a behaviour pattern obtained its functional fit to the environment by means of Darwinian evolution or by a process of associative learning. However, the categories are not mutually exclusive since a behaviour pattern (such as pecking in young gulls) that owed some of its general adaptive character to Darwinian evolution may be fine-tuned by associative learning to local environmental conditions. Furthermore, in complex animals we can recognise three sources of adaptation, not two, since culturally transmitted behaviour may also be adaptive (Bateson, 1983). So, the solution to separating corn from sand by winnowing the mixture in water was discovered by one clever Japanese macaque and then was evidently copied by others (Kawai, 1965).

Although critical of the excessive simplification in thought produced by dichotomies, Robert Hinde (1969) suggested that recognising two sources of *difference* had promise as an analytical tool. For instance, he wrote:

... if we subject two individuals or groups of individuals which differ genetically to identical conditions, then any differences in behaviour which appear must ultimately be due to the genetic difference　　　　　　　　　　　　　　(Hinde, 1969, p. 11).

Conversely, behavioural variation found between genetically identical individuals must be attributed to their differences in experience. Of course, differences between individuals may arise from interactions between genes and experience. Particular genes may be expressed only in special environmental conditions, as in the temperature-sensitive mutants (e.g. Wu *et al.*, 1978); identical twins may actively seek different roles from each other (see Plomin, DeFries & Fulker, 1988); and so forth. Even so, the broad critique of dichotomies of behaviour was surely correct and, as far as I know, has never been contested. It is often ignored and sometimes excites despair. Here, for example, is the wry parenthetic comment on Robert Hinde's point about sources of difference by Konrad Lorenz's biographer: 'If the reader finds this difficult to follow, pity the poor biologist who must live among all these landmines!' (Nisbet, 1976, p. 143).

Most careful thinkers would follow Hinde and argue that if the term 'innate' is to be used for anything, it is for those behavioural differences between individuals that arise from genetic differences. Even so, the punning continues and many other usages are still to be found in the modern scientific literatures as well as in colloquial speech. At least six meanings are attached to the term: present at birth; a behavioural difference caused by a genetic difference; adapted over the course of evolution; unchanging throughout development; shared by all members of a species; and not learned. 'Instinctive' is less commonly used in the modern technical literature, but, when it is used, is deployed in similar ways to innate. However, a further and special meaning is also attached to instinct, namely a distinctly organised system of behaviour driven from within. The important issue in relation to conceptual clarity is whether one of the connotations of innateness or instinct necessarily applies to a given activity when another has been demonstrated. Consider the following questions which might be applied to that pattern of behaviour:

1. Does the activity appear at a particular stage in development?
2. Are individual differences in the activity due to genetic differences?
3. Was the activity adapted to its present function by the Darwinian process of evolution?
4. Once present, are the frequency and form of the activity unchanged by learning?
5. Is the activity shared by all members of the species?
6. Does the activity develop without previous opportunities for learning?
7. Does the activity have the characteristics of an organised behavioural system?

A categorical answer to any one of the above questions is liable to trigger an academic dispute. The practical difficulties in demonstrating, for instance, that a piece of behaviour is not learned are immense. Evidence that genetic relatives resemble each other behaviourally is open to the non-trivial

21

objection that they are liable to share common experiences. Even so, I am concerned here with the underlying logic – or the lack of it. What would be implied if some of the answers to the questions were 'No'? Would that disqualify the behaviour pattern from being termed innate or instinctive? I imagine not. The trouble commonly arises from the human tendency to generalise too much. If one plausible 'Yes' is obtained, six others are implied. When that is done, the reasoning is clearly at fault. For instance, if a behaviour pattern develops without obvious practice or example, the activity may subsequently be modified by learning. The modification of pecking at their parents' bills in young gulls provides a classic example (e.g. Hailman, 1967).

Barlow (1989) has recently complained that, while these points are well taken, an impression has been left that all behaviour patterns develop in the same way. He observed that behaviour patterns can be arranged along a spectrum from those that are well-buffered against change to those that are extremely labile. Modal action patterns of many species show scarcely any noteworthy variation within and among individuals (Barlow, 1977). This is a point that Robert Hinde has also repeatedly made himself, noting at the same time that well-buffered patterns of behaviour may have been labile at an earlier stage in development (Hinde, 1982, p. 87). I think the major conclusion to draw from the debate is that conceptual clarity is never a fault. Say what you mean (even if it uses a bit more space) rather than unintentionally confuse your reader by employing a word such as innate that carries so many different connotations.

Many influences and the study of process

Robert Hinde has consistently championed the view that when we deal with the development and the control of behaviour we should recognise the multitude of factors that influence the outcome. Such a view was consistent with his opposition to crude dichotomies. The alternative to a misleadingly over-simplified dichotomy of behaviour is to place the emphasis on the development of individuals as an interplay between them and their environment. The current state of each individual influences which genes are expressed, and also the social and physical world about it. Individuals are then seen as choosing and changing the conditions to which they are exposed. The interplay required for the development of an individual is not between heredity and environment. It is between the individual and environment. This does not mean that the contributions of genetic and environmental sources of variation to behavioural development can never be analysed separately. Nor does it mean that individuals' transactions with their environments modify their patterns of behaviour in all respects throughout their lives. Many examples of behaviour are greatly influenced by certain sorts of experience at particular stages of development, in so-called sensitive periods, but are much less affected by similar experience at other stages. Emphasis on the interplay between developing individuals and their environments means unequivocally that we have to abandon thinking about causation as a single, straight arrow.

The growing acceptance of the inadequacies of the causal arrow approach to development has brought about a subtle change. Instead of asking whether behaviour is caused by genes or the environment, the question becomes: 'How much?' In more sophisticated form it is stated as: 'How much of the variation in a character is due to variation in a particular factor?' When individual differences in behaviour can be attributed to variation in genetic and environmental sources, the nature/nurture controversy appears to be resolved by a neat rephrasing of that misleading old question about where behaviour comes from. I have argued elsewhere that this approach, when coupled with techniques like Analysis of Variance, can seduce us into accepting almost unthinkingly that the various influences add together (Bateson, 1987a, 1989). This arises in part because of the way the questions are formulated ('What percentage of the variation is accounted for by variation in a given factor?'). The additive approach has been helped along because Analysis of Variance is so insensitive to statistical interactions (Wahlsten, 1990) and empirical scientists have not been offered techniques to deal with the results generated by complex dynamical systems. Even so a useful corrective to simple-minded explanation is to list the factors known to influence the outcome of a developmental process.

In the area in which I have worked extensively, the results of imprinting experiments depended greatly on the conditions that were used (Bateson, 1966). Many authors reported, for instance, that the character of the stimuli used, both for training and testing the chicks, greatly affected the outcome (e.g. Smith, 1962). An early study suggested that the stimulus value of an object might change with age (Gray, 1961). Recently, substantial support for this view came from studies in which chicks had either been trained with a flashing, rotating light or with a rotating stuffed jungle fowl and then given a choice between them (Horn & McCable, 1984; Bolhuis, Johnson & Horn, 1985). The artificial and naturalistic stimuli were matched for their effectiveness in eliciting approach from 1-day-old domestic chicks by varying the rate of rotation of the object. Despite the matching, the stuffed jungle fowl became more attractive than the box in untrained birds by the second day after hatching. The shift towards a stronger fowl bias was also apparent in birds that were imprinted with either a fowl or a box. Finally, the developmental process that led to a strengthening preference for the fowl could be facilitated by accentuating both visual and non-visual experience.

23

Subsequent work has suggested that features of the jungle fowl that make it especially attractive as the predisposition emerges are located around the head. However, they are not specific to jungle fowl since a stuffed rotating Gadwall duck and a polecat were equally attractive (Johnson & Horn, 1988).

The development of the chick's predispositions to respond more strongly to some stimuli than to others already looks complicated. However, the problems for explanation do not end here. The results of an imprinting experiment depend greatly on the conditions that were used. Konrad Lorenz had clearly realised that the stage of the bird's development at which the object was first presented would greatly affect what happened. He also knew that the characteristics of the object were important, although perhaps he did not realise quite how important. Other features of the process were less compatible with the classical image of imprinting. For instance, the length of time for which the object was first presented made an enormous difference: the longer the bird was exposed, the stronger the effects. The bird's experience prior to first presentation of the object and its experience after the first presentation also made a big difference. The precise character of the stimulus presentation is important; for example, whether the exposure is continuous, at fixed intervals or unpredictably intermittent (Bolhuis & Johnson, 1988). The less continuous and the more unpredictable the timing, the more strongly the bird responds. The importance of arousing or potentiating stimuli, such as the natural maternal calls of the mother, has been stressed by Gottlieb (1971) for many years. In Japanese quail, the posture of the mother has a powerful motivating effect on the response of the chicks to her (ten Cate, 1989).

When an area of research gets to this point, the commonly used metaphors (such as 'imprinting') and the verbal models tend to be inadequate or simply misleading. We need to have some idea of the process that brings everything together. The question is: how do we get there?

How should process be studied?

If many factors affect the outcome of a developmental process, what should be done about it? The chances are that all the different influences will not add together and, if they do not, small changes in certain factors may sometimes make big differences to the outcome and large changes in others will have no effect whatsoever. This will not seem strange to people in the physical sciences. Indeed, many mathematical techniques have been developed to deal analytically with the complexities of dynamical systems such as catastrophe theory and 'chaos' – the modern mathematical treatment of dynamical systems.

In looking back through Robert Hinde's work, I was struck by the way he

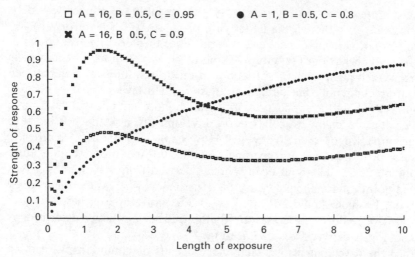

Figure 1. Hypothetical changes in the mobbing response of a chaffinch to an owl as a function of exposure to the owl. In order to generate the results shown here the product of two equations are multiplied together (y_i. y_d). The equation for the hypothetical incremental process relating to general state is: $y_i = 1 + A(B^t)$ and that for the decremental process relating to the specific characteristics of the owl is: $y_d = 1 - C^t$, where A, B and C are constants and t is the length of exposure to the owl.

has consistently been sensitive to the non-linear relationships between a factor affecting behaviour and the behavioural outcome. For instance, in his classic study of habituation of the mobbing response by the chaffinch, he noted that even an apparently simple procedure of exposing an animal to an unchanging stuffed owl can have seemingly complex results because such treatment has more than one effect (reviewed in Hinde, 1970). To explain such a result at least two processes must be postulated. Figure 1 shows the results of multiplying the outcome of a decremental and an incremental process. The decremental might be a specific one that reduces the effectiveness of the familiar object. The incremental process might be a general one that influences the animal's alertness or, in subjective terms, its sense of unease. The equations used by Robert Hinde do, indeed, simulate the empirical results he had obtained, even though the outcome is highly sensitive to the parameter values of the two equations – as is shown in Figure 1. One of the most intriguing empirical results was the way in which the response to an initially less effective stimulus (a stuffed dog) could be enhanced by exposure to one that was initially more effective (a stuffed owl). If the stimulus value of the familiar object declines as the result of repeated exposure, but the alarmed state of the bird increases, then the resulting dynamics would be complicated, even though the underlying processes are straightforward.

Non-linear mathematics are comforting, since they describe what most of us who study behaviour find intuitively plausible – even though we may have sometimes felt slightly ashamed that our intuition about the relation between two variables did not come out as a straight line. However, even if we become enthusiastic about the application of the much more complicated descriptive mathematics of 'chaos' to behavioural development, how much is likely to be encompassed by such treatment? How can we distinguish empirically between processes that are genuinely stochastic and those that produce chaotic outcomes deterministically? Ideas derived from 'chaos' imply that the end points of development have no consistency, whereas in practice they often do. Fashion should not blind us to alternative approaches. Negative and positive feedback processes are dynamical but are better described by methodologies derived from engineering.

When the development of a character depends on conditions, as it often does, the mechanisms are often highly constrained. The astonishing way in which sex is determined in some reptiles by the temperature to which they were exposed during embryonic life provides a good example (e.g. Bull, 1980). One explanation for what happens is that the animals are equipped with something akin to the rules used in computer programming, namely IF the ambient temperature is below 30 °C THEN develop into a female, IF it is above 30 °C THEN develop into a male. Of course, the all-or-nothing character of these IF...THEN...rules might be misleading in many cases and the relations could be continuous. If a graded set of behaviour patterns is produced in response to a graded set of conditions, we are back to other formulations.

None of the methods imported from other disciplines tell us how the mechanisms work and they can all be misleading in their different ways. Their benefit is that they provide routes to the solution of complex problems by keeping in play simultaneously a set of interacting variables. In the sense that they help us to deal with complex processes, they are a bit like metaphors. Admittedly, they provide insight for some people and none for others (as is the case with metaphors). However, when they lead to formalisation and simulation, the sharpening up of thought can be highly beneficial and the outcomes often surprise us. I will give an example from imprinting in which, as I have already indicated, we know that many factors are involved and operate in different ways.

A model of imprinting

For a long while it was thought that, in the case of filial imprinting, movement was critical to the young bird. By degrees it became plain that colour, contrast and configuration were all important. In an attempt to put this in a word I used to argue that the most effective objects in imprinting experiments are the most conspicuous ones (Bateson, 1966). It never seemed quite right, but I certainly believed that the flashing rotating box, modified from an ambulance light, that we used in a lot of our experiments was a super-normal stimulus (e.g. Bateson & Reese, 1969; Bateson & Seaburne-May, 1972; Bateson & Wainwright, 1972). A breakthrough came when Horn & McCabe (1984) were led by the reanalysis of old data to the conclusion that features in the jungle fowl, the ancestral form of the domestic fowl, were particularly attractive to chicks. The preference for aspects of naturalistic stimuli had been missed because, under laboratory conditions, the detectors take longer to develop in chicks than do the ones driven by my ambulance light. Even though the predisposition is less specific than at first it seemed (Johnson & Horn, 1988), it looks as though such a head–neck feature detector, along with others responding to movement, colour and contrast, feed into those bits of the brain that establish representations of the object to which the bird has been socialised (see Bateson, 1990a).

What about the core of the imprinting process, namely the plastic change in the brain that leads to selective response to a particular object? Is the result of imprinting simply a privileged form of recognition? As a result of seeing an object with the right kind of features at the right stage of development, a representation is formed of that object and the representation controls first filial behaviour and later sexual behaviour. Is that all there is to it? For a variety of reasons I think that imprinting involves another type of plasticity in the nervous system, namely connecting up the representation of the familiar object exclusively to the system controlling filial behaviour and, much later in development, to the one controlling sexual behaviour (Bateson, 1981, 1987b). I shall not review all the evidence here, but one compelling strand is taming. When a bird is well-imprinted and then exposed to another object, at first the bird withdraws showing every sign of great alarm. By degrees this alarm habituates and the bird becomes tame. However, tame birds do not express any social behaviour towards the object that is by now very familiar. They evidently recognise it, but that is all. It seems, therefore, that at least two stages are involved in imprinting. One involves recognition and one involves the control of social behaviour by the representation of the familiar object. From this consideration emerges a three-stage model involving Analysis, Recognition and Execution (see Figure 2). The first step involves detection of features in a stimulus presented to a young bird.

27

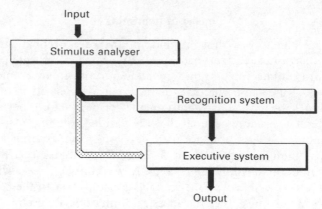

Figure 2. A flow diagram of the stages from input to output involved in filial responses to a mother hen or a substitute imprinting object. In domestic chicks the stimulus analyser is thought to continue developing until the second day after hatching. Plasticity resulting from imprinting occurs both in the recognition system and at the limited access to the executive system controlling filial behaviour. Finally the direct input to the executive system from the stimulus analyser may degenerate or become inhibited with increasing use of the recognition system (from Bateson, 1987b).

Aspects of the stimulus which the bird is predisposed to find attractive are picked out by particular detectors at this level of processing. The second step involves comparison between what has already been experienced and the current input. Of course, before imprinting has taken place, no comparison is involved. Once it has occurred, recognition of what is familiar and what is novel is crucial. Finally, the third stage involves control of the various motor patterns involved in executing filial behaviour. In the case of the tame bird, the assumption is that a representation is formed, but this representation has no way of gaining access to the executive system.

The Analysis–Recognition–Execution model presents a rather passive view of the animal's role in its own development. Birds that have been taken out of a dark incubator do not simply wait patiently for an object to come their way. They actively search for something that has the right features. What is more, they will rapidly learn to perform simple tasks which bring them into contact with objects that have such features. They can learn to press a pedal that turns on flashing, rotating light with astonishing speed (Bateson & Reese, 1969). The conspicuous object acts as a reward and reinforces the action of pressing the pedal.

The active aspect of the young bird's behaviour can be built into the suggested explanations for imprinting by supposing that as a bird comes into

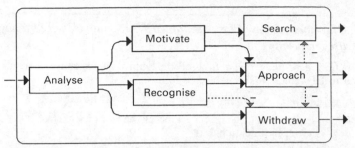

Figure 3. A scheme of how a chick's social behaviour is controlled (from Bateson, 1990b). The chick is thought to search for objects with certain features when it is in a particular motivational state. Some of the features of the objects for which it may search further enhance its motivational state. The effective objects also elicit approach behaviour which simultaneously inhibits search and any tendency to withdraw. Output from the recognition system also inhibits withdrawal directly. As a bird becomes increasingly familiar with an object, the representation of that object gains increasing access to the executive system and displaces direct control by the analysis system. As a consequence the chick may withdraw from novel objects until it has become familiar with them.

the right motivational state at a particular stage in development, the executive system which controls searching is activated. The searching may bring the animal into contact with an object that has the right features such as one with head and neck. The conspicuous object, through the feature detectors in the analysing system, drives the executive system controlling approach. Simultaneously, searching is inhibited, but possibly the last searching actions to have been performed are strengthened as inhibition occurs. As a result, when the bird is lost it is more likely to do what it did last time. At this initial stage in imprinting, the recognition system is addressed, but nothing has yet been stored there. I imagine that stimulation also has some positive effect on motivational state since birds rapidly get more ready to approach when they are exposed to a conspicuous object for the first time (e.g. Horn, Rose & Bateson, 1973; Bateson & Jaeckel, 1974). When the bird is well-imprinted, a familiar object matches its representation in the recognition system which by now exclusively controls approach movements. Finally, when a bird encounters a strange object, this fails to match the representation of the familiar object and therefore the withdrawal executive system comes into operation. The whole model is shown in Figure 3.

A scheme like this takes the familiar three-layered model of neural processing, grafts on only a few extra features and the model bird is transformed from being a stimulus–response machine to something that

---

Box 1. *The equations used for withdrawal from or approach to a novel object after imprinting in chicks*

The function describing the output of the approach executive system, o_a, is assumed to be sigmoid and obtained as follows.

$$o_a = 1 - \exp\left(i_n . K_e (\exp(-i_n) - 1)\right) \quad \ldots\ldots\ldots\ldots\ldots \text{Equation 1}$$

where K_e is a constant influencing the shape of the response curve.
      i_n is given by Equation 2.

The input to the executive system is given as follows:

$$i_n = a_n . m(g_n . c_f + (1 - c_f)) \quad \ldots\ldots\ldots\ldots\ldots\ldots \text{Equation 2}$$

where a_n is the stimulus value of the novel object. It is a characteristic of the organism based on a prior predisposition.
      m is the current motivational state of the bird affecting its readiness to approach
      g_n is given by Equation 3.
      c_f is given by Equation 4.

The shape of the generalisation gradient is assumed to be bell-shaped. Progressing from novel to familiar.

$$g_n = 1 - \exp\left(K_g . s_n (\exp -s_n) - 1)\right) \quad \ldots\ldots\ldots\ldots \text{Equation 3}$$

where s_n is the proportion of features in the familiar shared by the novel.
      K_g is a parameter influencing the shape of the generalisation gradient.

The extent to which output from the representation of the familiar object has captured access to the executive system is given as follows:

$$c_f = 1 - \exp\left(-a_f . m . t . K_c\right) \quad \ldots\ldots\ldots\ldots\ldots \text{Equation 4}$$

where a_f is the stimulus value of the familiar, imprinting object. It is subject to exactly the same assumptions as the stimulus value of novel objects.
      t is the length of exposure to the imprinting object.
      K_c is a constant affecting the rate of capture of the executive system by an output from the recognition system.

Withdrawal from a novel object will occur when $a_n . K_w > o_a$ where K_w is a constant influencing the output of the withdrawal executive system, o_w. As the bird became familiar with a novel object, o_w wanes.

(exp refers to an exponent of the natural logarithm, e. Most programming languages and many scientific calculators have a command for obtaining a given value. e^{-t} starts at 1 when t is 0 and drops towards 0 quickly at first and then more slowly as t increases.)

---

actively engages its environment. Another aspect to the activity relates to working for slight novelty. If the same thing is presented continuously, after a while the incoming pathway will tend to adapt, a form of short-term habituation. This may then lift the inhibition on searching and some evidence clearly indicates that, after up to 30 minutes of exposure to an imprinting object, chicks are ready to work for something a bit different from it (Jackson & Bateson, 1974).

An advantage of separating imprinting into sub-processes is that it becomes much easier to distinguish those aspects that give it its special flavour from those that are likely to be much more general (Bateson, 1990a). Some of the characteristics of imprinting are undoubtedly due to the naïve animal searching for and responding selectively to particular stimuli. At least two types of plastic change seem to be involved in imprinting. The first change is likely to be the process used in most forms of recognition, namely establishing an internal representation of the familiar object. The second is a pre-emptive capturing by that representation of the systems controlling filial behaviour and, much later in development, sexual behaviour. This is likely to generate the phenomenon of a sensitive period.

The model shown in Figure 3 is readily formalised (Bateson, 1990b). An important feature of the equations is that some crucial variables and parameters are multiplied together rather than added. As with the chaffinch mobbing example, the justification for doing this, when dealing, for example, with the interaction between the attractiveness of an object and the bird's motivational state, is that if either has a zero value, nothing happens. If the model were additive, an unmotivated bird would learn the characteristics of things and motivated birds would appear to learn in the absence of anything to learn about. The equations for the model are given in Box 1.

The parameters described as 'features of the organism' refer in the real animal to properties of its nervous system which also have to develop. These features may or may not be affected by relatively small changes in the conditions of development or by variation in genotype. If and when they can be estimated, they should not be treated as though they were similar to gravitational constants. When external conditions affect the parameters that are regarded as features of the organism, the developmental effect would be relatively non-specific, an issue that has been frequently considered in the literature on behavioural development (e.g. Lehrman, 1970; Bateson, 1976a).

An example of what the model does when a novel object has a higher stimulus value than the familiar object is shown in Figure 4. It was deliberately chosen because of its relevance to those studies in which the stimuli were initially unequal in attractiveness, or became so as the animal developed – as with the jungle fowl and the rotating box. If the same parameter values are used, while varying the length of exposure, the growing preference for a familiar rotating box when compared with a novel stuffed fowl can be simulated. The result is shown in the lower curve in Figure 4. The simulation which produced the lower curve was based on the assumption that the stimulus value of the novel object was fully developed. In the case

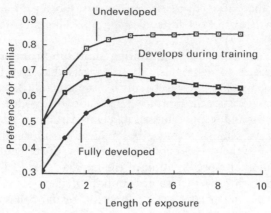

Figure 4. Simulations of changes in the preference for rotating box in a choice between the box and an unfamiliar jungle fowl. The top curve shows the development of the preference as a function of length of exposure to the box when the predisposition to prefer a jungle fowl has not yet developed. The bottom curve shows what happens after the predisposition has already developed. The middle curve shows what happens when the preference for the jungle fowl starts to emerge during the course of the tests as a non-specific result of exposure to the box. The values entered into the equations shown in Box 1 are $a_f = 0\cdot5$, $a_n = 0\cdot5–1\cdot0$, $s_n = 0\cdot3$, $m = 1$, $K_c = 2$, $K_g = 6$, $K_e = 2$.

of the jungle fowl the stimulus value has not usually developed fully immediately after imprinting on the first day, at least when the birds are reared in the dark. If the stimulus value of the novel object is the same as that of the familiar one, then the upper curve is obtained. Perhaps the most interesting case is the middle one where the training has a specific effect on preference for the familiar and also a non-specific effect on the development of the predisposition of the fowl. In the simulation, the constant affecting the rate of development of the predisposition is a quarter that affecting the development of the preference. In all cases a bird's preference in a test is affected both by how strongly it is attached to the familiar object and by the stimulus value of the novel object relative to that of the familiar.

Another example of experience having both specific and non-specific effects is provided by simulations of the so-called sensitive period for imprinting. At the onset of the sensitive period for imprinting the motivational state rises from 0. Once chicks are ready to be affected by particular types of stimulation from the environment, they are also liable to be affected by the conditions around them, irrespective of how sub-optimal those conditions might be. In the model, then, the rate of increase of the

---

Box 2. *A method for calculating the change in motivational state at the onset of the sensitive period*

$$m_t = m_{t-\partial} + (1 - m_{t-\partial})(1 - \exp(-a_c . K_m . \partial))$$

where m_t is the motivational state at time t.

$m_{t-\partial}$ is the motivational state at the previous step.

a_c is the stimulus value of the conditions in which the chick is kept.

∂ is the time interval of each successive step.

K_m is a parameter affecting the rate of increase of the motivational state concerned with filial behaviour.

---

motivational state depends on the character of the stimulation. The process is fast if the birds are kept with members of their own species in the light (conditions that have high stimulus value); it is much slower if they are kept in isolation and slower still if they are kept in a patternless environment (low stimulus value) (see Bateson & Wainwright, 1972). The equation is given in Box 2.

As with the chaffinch example simple rules can produce complex results. For instance, if the quality of the bird's experience affects its motivational state, the response to a novel object can be enhanced. However, in this case, the restricting effects of imprinting are such that the curve turns over and eventually novel objects are avoided (see Figure 5).

As already noted, an important feature of the model is that it does not depend on the effects of predispositions and the specific effects of experience adding together. This is obvious where the response to the familiar depends on multiplying the familiar object's stimulus value (due to a predisposition) by the additive combination of the initial responsiveness and the effect of imprinting on the bird. I could not find a sensible alternative that was not multiplicative in this respect because such a version would have meant that some kind of response would be given in a vacuum. Furthermore, the effects of experience are not likely to be linear. Note, though, that the response is a product of the whole system. The subsystem concerned with generating a predisposed tendency to respond to some objects more strongly than to others may be located in a different place from the subsystem concerned with plasticity. This, indeed, appears to be the case and the two subsystems also seem to develop in different ways (Horn, 1985 and Chapter 5).

The case for some degree of formalisation is that an explicit working model brings with it mental discipline and may expose weaknesses in a verbal argument that are all too easily missed. It can also serve several other valuable functions. It can show how we are easily misled by the dynamics of development into supposing that the processes are so complicated that they are beyond comprehension. From the standpoint of empirical research, it

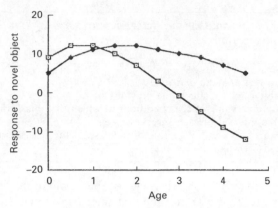

Figure 5. Hypothetical changes in responsiveness to a novel object as a result of increasing age. When the exposure conditions have a higher stimulus value (open squares, $a_c = 0.4$) the development of withdrawal from novelty is quicker than when their stimulus value is lower (solid dots, $a_c = 0.2$). However, in both cases the effect of the exposure conditions is initially to *increase* responsiveness to the novel object. The values entered into the equations shown in Boxes 1 and 2 are $a_n = 1$, $K_w = 0.2$, $\delta = 0.5$, $K_m = 0.5$.

can suggest profitable new lines of enquiry. Finally, it bears directly on the general arguments about the interplay between internal and external factors. I suspect that the major advantages are to the people doing experiments on behaviour rather than to the neuroscientists. However, as far as linking to other levels of analysis is concerned, the models point to the parameters that are features of the organism as opposed to ones that might be manipulated externally by experiment such as the constant affecting the rate at which plastic changes occur. These hypothetical features of the organism, if real, must have some correspondence to underlying neural mechanisms.

I have dwelt on a particular theoretical approach to a particular developmental problem at length not simply because it is close to my heart. I believe it illustrates the interplay that is needed between theory and practice. If the theories of process pay no attention to the real world, they quickly go astray. I also believe it begins to show one way in which we shall start to understand behavioural development.

What about principles?

What have been the consequences of Robert Hinde's demands for rigorous thought, the acceptance of many influences and the study of process? Can we point to one of those general, unifying ideas that serves to reduce what needs to be known? Put that way the question sounds intimidatingly lofty. I suspect that nobody could provide a current idea as an example of a general principle of behavioural development without somebody else snorting with impatience: 'Not nearly grand enough!' or, attacking from the other side, Robert Hinde himself saying: 'That's so general, it's vacuous.' Even so, what is the equivalent to the classic principles of genetics inferred from studies of whole organisms such as particulate inheritance? To answer a question like that, we need to be clear at what level explanation is sought. My guess is that the unifying principles that emerge will be the ones of operation rather than the ones of detailed mechanism. The outcome matters, not the way in which it is achieved.

Richard Dawkins (1976) adopted an attractive approach when he wrote:

If a computer is doing something clever and lifelike, say playing chess, and we ask how it is doing it, we do not want to hear about transistors, we accept them... We need *software explanations* of behaviour. I do not mean that animals necessarily work like computers. They may be very different. But just as the lowest level of explanation is not always the most appropriate for a computer, no more is it for an animal. Animals and computers are both so complex that something on the level of software explanation must be appropriate for both of them.

Rules like 'store a representation of the input and then compare output against it' have been very important in obtaining understanding of song-learning (Marler, 1976). Modifications of Miller, Galanter & Pribram's (1960) Test-Operate-Test-Exit rule in which the preferred value changes with age have considerable value, explaining the dynamic but ordered way in which developmental processes can home in on a particular adult end-point (see Bateson, 1976b; Chalmers, 1987). The conditional IF... THEN rules are useful in understanding individual differences (Caro & Bateson, 1986). The competitive exclusion rule explains the dynamics of sensitive periods (Bateson, 1987b). In their different ways all these ideas when applied to development at the right level may provide some of the useful ways to reduce the complexity. While they may show us how the job might be done, are we wholly satisfied? I suspect that many biologists want to be told *why* the job needs to be done. In other words, they want to be given a functional account.

Robert Hinde himself noted how much ethology has been helped by considering the function of a behaviour pattern, even when the primary concern is with mechanism (see Hinde, 1982). To give one example from development, the functional approach provides a way of thinking about the difference in timing between sexual imprinting and filial imprinting. The suggestion is that an animal should not tune its reference point for mating preferences too early in development lest it obtain information about the juvenile appearance of its siblings that could not be used effectively when the time comes to choose a mate. On the other side, it must not tune its mating preferences too late in development after the family group has broken up and it is likely to be exposed to non-kin. Indeed, the evidence suggests that birds delay sexual imprinting until their siblings have moulted into adult plumage (see Bateson, 1979). In this way the bird is able to use its experience of close kin so that it chooses a mate that is genetically a bit different from itself, but not too different. If the two types of imprinting are treated as part of the same general process, the difference seems to be of no importance and is quickly forgotten about. However, with attention focused on the problem, we can attempt to analyse the mechanisms responsible for the difference in timing. The point is, then, that the functional approach can frame and stimulate research on the processes of development.

In the previous section, I gave an example of how some understanding of imprinting may be obtained with quite simple ideas. The proposed mechanism performs its functional role by restricting responsiveness to close kin under natural conditions. It shows how it is necessary to postulate features of the organism that have developed prior to the stage in which one is interested. But it also shows how subsequent development depends on current conditions external to the organism. The nature of the process is straightforward, but it is emphatically not additive. Finally, the example draws attention to the advantage of separating analytically motivational state, stimulus analysis, the capacity for plastic change and the executive control of behaviour. All these ideas are well established in the ethological literature and whether or not one would want to call them principles is a moot point. Be that as it may, the example of imprinting shows how the old either/or oppositions applied to behaviour simply evaporate when knowledge starts to advance. However, the emphasis on process, which many others have argued for (e.g. Oyama, 1985; Johnston, 1988), draws attention to the predispositions and the rules for development. Since these were almost certainly fine-tuned to the conditions in which the animals evolved, species differences in patterns of development should be expected (see Marler, Chapter 3).

Conclusion

I have argued that three themes in Robert Hinde's writings have given, at the very least, all those working on behavioural development pause for thought. He has insisted on conceptual clarity when formulating the problems that are to be tackled, awareness of the large number of influences which affect the outcome of development, and the importance of studying process when attempting to understand what happens. Many people have found this a hard mental regime to accept. As a result, distinctions were fudged in the name of being straightforward and analysis was focused on single factors in the name of clarity. However, the straightforwardness and clarity were illusory. Those who incorporated the three themes of Robert Hinde's thinking into their work may have had a difficult time of it, but are now coming out of a long tunnel and the approach is starting to pay off.

While we do not have all the concepts that we need to explain what happens in behavioural development, we are in a much better position than we were. I have tried to show how the work on imprinting, which generated so much perplexity a few years ago, now looks promising. When critics say: 'You make the whole process of development sound so complicated', it is possible to reply: 'No, the explanatory devices are really rather simple.' Importantly, they enable combinations of conditions to be explored systematically, which would take a long time with live animals. Furthermore, in the process of such explorations, surprises are frequently encountered which then propose experiments with real animals or re-examination of data not previously analysed. The ideas that give us some genuine understanding of what is going on do more than reduce complexity. They make functional sense.

A sceptic will doubtless argue that my optimism is self-serving. I am simply trying to peddle my ideas in the guise of celebrating a close friend and former teacher. Maybe, but much is happening. Ethologists are willing once again to consider mechanism. Neurobiologists are beginning to look up to more complex levels of organisation and listen to what ethologists have to tell them (see Fentress, Chapter 4). Of course, this might reflect nothing more than a change in fashion or delayed reaction to the sociobiology boom. However, it may also reflect, as I believe to be the case, that Cinderella has finally arrived at the ball.

Acknowledgements

As with so much of my earlier work Robert Hinde provided penetrating comments on this chapter. I am very grateful to him, to Joan Stevenson-Hinde and to Nick Thompson for their help.

References

Barlow, G. W. (1977). Modal action patterns. In *How Animals Communicate*, ed. T. A. Sebeok, pp. 98–134. Bloomington: Indiana University Press.

Barlow, G. W. (1989). Has sociobiology killed ethology or revitalized it? In *Perspectives in Ethology, Vol. 8. Whither Ethology?*, ed. P. P. G. Bateson and P. H. Klopfer, pp. 1–45. New York: Plenum Press.

Bateson, P. P. G. (1966). The characteristics and context of imprinting. *Biological Reviews*, **41**, 177–220.

Bateson, P. P. G. (1976a). Specificity and the origins of behaviour. *Advances in the Study of Behaviour*, **6**, 1–20.

Bateson, P. P. G. (1976b). Rules and reciprocity in behavioural development. In *Growing Points in Ethology*, ed. P. P. G. Bateson and R. A. Hinde, pp. 401–421. Cambridge: Cambridge University Press.

Bateson, P. (1979). How do sensitive periods arise and what are they for? *Animal Behaviour*, **27**, 470–86.

Bateson, P. (1981). Control of sensitivity to the environment during development. In *Behavioural Development*, ed. K. Immelmann, G. W. Barlow, L. Petrinovich and M. Main, pp. 432–53. Cambridge: Cambridge University Press.

Bateson, P. (1983). Rules for changing the rules. In *Evolution from Molecules to Men*, ed. D. S. Bendall, pp. 483–507. Cambridge: Cambridge University Press.

Bateson, P. (1987a). Biological approaches to the study of behavioural development. *International Journal of Behavioural Development*, **10**, 1–22.

Bateson, P. (1987b). Imprinting as a process of competitive exclusion. In *Imprinting and Cortical Plasticity*, ed. J. P. Rauschecker and P. Marler, pp. 151–68. New York: Wiley.

Bateson, P. (1989). Additive models may mislead. *International Journal of Behavioural Development*, **12**, 407–11.

Bateson, P. (1990a). Is imprinting such a special case? *Philosophical Transactions of the Royal Society*, B, **329**, 125–31.

Bateson, P. (1990b). Making sense of behavioural development in the chick. In *Neural and Behavioural Plasticity: The Use of the Domestic Chick as a Model*, ed. R. J. Andrew. Oxford: Oxford University Press (in press).

Bateson, P. P. G. & Jaeckel, J. B. (1974). Imprinting: correlations between activities of chicks during training and testing. *Animal Behaviour*, **22**, 899–906.

Bateson, P. P. G. & Reese, E. P. (1969). The reinforcing properties of conspicuous stimuli in the imprinting situation. *Animal Behaviour*, **17**, 692–9.

Bateson, P. P. G. & Seaburne-May, G. (1973). Effects of prior exposure to light on chicks' behaviour in the imprinting situation. *Animal Behaviour*, **21**, 720–5.

Bateson, P. P. G. & Wainwright, A. A. P. (1972). The effects of prior exposure to light on the imprinting process in domestic chicks. *Behaviour*, **42**, 279–90.

Bolhuis, J. J. & Johnson, M. H. (1988). Effects of response-contingency and stimulus presentation schedule on imprinting in the chick (*Gallus gallus domesticus*). *Journal of Comparative Psychology*, **102**, 61–5.

Bolhuis, J. J., Johnson, M. H. & Horn, G. (1985). Interaction between acquired preferences and developing predispositions in an imprinting situation. *Animal Behaviour*, **33**, 1000–6.

Bull, J. J. (1980). Sex determination in reptiles. *Quarterly Review of Biology*, **55**, 3–21.

Caro, T. M. & Bateson, P. (1986). Organisation and ontogeny of alternative tactics. *Animal Behaviour*, **34**, 1483–99.

Chalmers, N. R. (1987). Developmental pathways in behaviour. *Animal Behaviour*, **35**, 659–74.

Dawkins, R. (1976). Hierarchical organisation: a candidate principle for ethology. In *Growing Points in Ethology*, ed. P. P. G. Bateson and R. A. Hinde, pp. 7–54. Cambridge: Cambridge University Press.

Dudai, Y. (1989). *The Neurobiology of Memory*. Oxford: Oxford University Press.

Gottlieb, G. (1971). *Development of Species Identification in Birds*. Chicago: University of Chicago Press.

Gray, P. H. (1961). The releasers of imprinting: differential reactions to color as a function of maturation. *Journal of Comparative and Physiological Psychology*, **54**, 597–601.

Hailman, J. P. (1967). The ontogeny of an instinct. The pecking response in chicks of the laughing gull (*Larus atricilla* L.) and related species. *Behaviour Supplement*, **15**, 1–159.

Hinde, R. A. (1969). Dichotomies in the study of development. In *Genetic and Environmental Influences on Behaviour*, ed. J. M. Thoday and A. S. Parkes. Edinburgh: Oliver & Boyd.

Hinde, R. A. (1970). Behavioural habituation. In *Short-term Changes in Neural Activity and Behaviour*, ed. G. Horn and R. A. Hinde, pp. 3–40. Cambridge: Cambridge University Press.

Hinde, R. A. (1982). *Ethology*. Oxford: Oxford University Press.

Horn, G. (1985). *Memory, Imprinting, and the Brain*. Oxford: Clarendon Press.

Horn, G. & McCabe, B. J. (1984). Predispositions and preferences. Effects on imprinting of lesions to the chick brain. *Animal Behaviour*, **32**, 288–92.

Horn, G., Rose, S. P. R. & Bateson, P. P. G. (1973). Experience and plasticity in the central nervous system. *Science*, **181**, 506–14.

Jackson, P. S. & Bateson, P. P. G. (1974). Imprinting and exploration of slight novelty in chicks. *Nature*, **251**, 609–10.

Johnson, M. H. & Horn, G. (1988). Development of filial preferences in dark-reared chicks. *Animal Behaviour*, **36**, 675–83.

Johnston, T. D. (1988). Developmental explanation and the ontogeny of birdsong: Nature/nurture redux. *Behavioural and Brain Sciences*, **11**, 617–63.

Kawai, M. (1965). Newly-acquired pre-cultural behavior of the natural troop of Japanese monkeys on Koshima islet. *Primates*, **6**, 1–30.

Lehrman, D. S. (1970). Semantic and conceptual issues in the nature–nurture problem. In *Development and Evolution of Behavior*, ed. L. R. Aronson, E. Tobach, D. S. Lehrman and J. S. Rosenblatt, pp. 17–52. San Francisco: Freeman.

Lorenz, K. (1965). *Evolution and Modification of Behavior*. Chicago: University of Chicago Press.

Marler, P. (1976). Sensory templates in species-specific behavior. In *Simpler Networks and Behavior*, ed. J. C. Fentress, pp. 314–29. Sunderland, Mass.: Sinauer.

Miller, G. A., Galanter, E. & Pribram, K. H. (1960). *Plans and the Structure of Behavior*. New York: Holt.

Nisbett, A. (1976). *Konrad Lorenz*. London: Dent.

Oyama, S. (1985). *The Ontogeny of Information*. Cambridge: Cambridge University Press.

Plomin, R., DeFries, J. C. & Fulker, D. W. (1988). *Nature and Nurture during Infancy and Early Childhood*. Cambridge: Cambridge University Press.

Smith, F. V. (1962). Perceptual aspects of imprinting. *Symposium of the Zoological Society of London*, **8**, 193–8.

ten Cate, C. (1989). Stimulus movement, hen behaviour and filial imprinting in Japanese Quail (*Coturnix coturnix japonica*). *Ethology*, **82**, 287–306.

Wahlsten, D. (1990). Insensitivity of the analysis of variance to heredity–environment interaction. *Behavioral and Brain Sciences*, **13**, 109–61.

Wu, C. S., Ganetzi, B., Jan, Y. N. & Benzer, S. (1978). A *Drosophila* mutant with a temperature sensitive block in nerve-conduction. *Proceedings of the National Academy of Sciences of the USA*, **75**, 4047–51.

—3—
Differences in behavioural development in closely related species: birdsong

Peter Marler

When animals assess others as prospective mates or rivals, the processes involved have a powerful influence on the evolution of associated behavioural, morphological, and physiological traits (Stamps, 1990). Studies of the proximate mechanisms underlying such behaviour, of a kind long championed by Robert Hinde, are thus directly relevant to the investigation of ultimate factors that shape the evolution of behaviour.

The same applies to assessment mechanisms by which others are chosen as models for the experiential moulding of personal phenotypes by social inheritance, as in the selection of tutors for song-learning in birds (e.g. Payne, 1985; Clayton, 1989). The potential impact upon evolutionary processes is greatest when the favoured models are parents, but non-trivial consequences may also ensue if social inheritance influences the channels for acquisition of traits from individuals which are not immediate kin. Any heritable predisposition that biases the cultural transmission of behaviour in animals is thus germane to theories about how that behaviour, and other traits correlated with it, will evolve (Boyd & Richerson, 1985). This will be the case whatever the means by which the predispositions are inherited.

A large corpus of information accumulated by ethologists (e.g. Hinde, 1970, 1982, 1983; Hinde & Tinbergen, 1958) thus assumes a direct bearing on studies of behavioural evolution. Such information is especially relevant when, as is so often the case with Hinde's work, there is a focus on developmental processes and the constraints imposed on them, particularly when those constraints can be identified as 'local' in nature (i.e. those confined to particular taxa (see Maynard Smith *et al.*, 1985). While the term 'constraints', for a variety of reasons (cf. Gould & Marler, 1984; Stearns, 1986; Gould, 1989), will not be used in this chapter, comparative studies of

41

behavioural development provide a rich potential source of information on 'constraints' on the forces of natural selection.

A recurrent theme in Robert Hinde's many trenchant and penetrating critiques of research on behavioural development is the paucity of in-depth, longitudinal studies of the ontogeny of behaviour, covering a significant portion of the life span, and of a kind designed to illuminate the nature of developmental and genetic influences on evolutionary adaptation. Few such studies encompass the range of biologically relevant environmental factors necessary for a full understanding of the developmental process. Another significant area of neglect to which Hinde draws attention is the study of differences in behaviour in individuals, populations, and species, and their ontogeny, Hinde's own pioneering work on development, especially of non-human primates, being a prominent exception (Hinde 1983; Hinde & Stevenson-Hinde, 1986). The paucity of comparative analyses of individual differences in behaviour and their ontogenetic basis both within and between species is especially regrettable in view of the insights that such studies can throw on genetic contributions to the ontogeny of behaviour and the potential for adaptive change. As I hope to establish in this review, research on the ontogeny of birdsong and other aspects of avian vocal behaviour fulfils some of these requirements (Hinde, 1969; Kroodsma & Miller, 1982; Marler, 1984).

The basic developmental issues at stake are clear enough. 'The characteristics of the organism come from only two sources: the zygote and the environment of the developing individual' (Hinde 1970, p. 427; cf. Pringle, 1951; Lorenz, 1965). Yet, despite the theoretical emphasis of ethologists on inherited contributions to behaviour we know far more about environmental influences than we do about the role of genetic factors in behavioural ontogeny. Furthermore, when causes of developmental differences are in dispute, the benefit of the doubt is generally given to environmental rather than to genetic factors. Both for practical reasons and because of lingering inhibitions about the propriety of invoking genetic contributions to behavioural development, even ethologists have sadly neglected the genetic component in the ontogenetic equation both in their research and in their thinking. Instead the lead has been taken by geneticists, exploiting the dramatic conceptual and methodological advances in molecular biology (e.g. Hirsch, 1967; Benzer, 1973; Gould, 1974; Hall, Greenspan & Harris, 1982).

Even today, as we begin to reap the benefits of the revolution in molecular genetics, there is widespread scepticism among behavioural biologists about the prospects of significant insights into genetic contributions to behavioural development being derived from comparative studies (Hinde, 1970). I believe this scepticism to be seriously misplaced, placing the whole enterprise of ethological research on behavioural development in jeopardy. Comparative experiments in particular, properly designed, offer unique insights into the major contributions of genetic factors to the development of behaviour.

The purpose of this paper is to review certain aspects of research on song development in birds, with an emphasis on studies of species differences, the results of which point to pervasive contributions from genetic factors in the social transmission of such differences.

A text from Hinde is the inspiration for the approach that has been adopted.

Given two organisms that differ in behavior, we can ask if the differences can be traced to a genetic difference or if it is due to environmental factors. It is in the study of differences that quantitative methods are most likely to be fertile, and a dichotomy of differences *is useful where other types of dichotomy . . . are not. Evidence that a difference in behavior is to be ascribed to genetic differences must come ultimately from the rearing of animals, known to differ genetically, in similar environments.*

(Hinde, 1970, pp. 430–1).

The relevance of this viewpoint to the interpretation of species differences in singing behaviour is explored, as a step towards countering what I view as sterile and scientifically crippling inhibitions about acknowledging genetic contributions to behavioural development. In asserting his position on this topic, Hinde is at pains to counter the mistaken practice of dichotomising behaviour into 'innate' and 'learned' components (Hinde, 1970, p. 433). Such dichotomising is not merely unfruitful but logically incorrect. Yet it is still a common lay view. Behaviour is often viewed as either learned or instinctive, but is rarely if ever both. According to this common view, lower animals display instincts, but with the exception of a few very basic drives, our own species displays instincts rarely. Rather we are presumed to illustrate what can be achieved by the emancipation from instinctive control (Gould & Marler, 1987).

As Hinde documents with typical lucidity, the antithesis is false. All behaviour develops out of genomic–environmental interactions. Even the most extreme case of purely arbitrary, culturally transmitted behaviour is the result of the operation of genetic mechanisms. Such genetic mechanisms may be generalised, or highly specialised in function ('universal' or 'local' in the terminology of Maynard Smith *et al.*, 1985) but without them there would be no organism to develop. Without them, learning could not occur.

One focal question thus becomes, how do genetic mechanisms make learning possible? How do they provide appropriate substrates for the pervasive ontogenetic plasticity that so many behaviour patterns display, opening the way for social transmission of behavioural traits, and for the striking variations in the behaviour of individuals, populations and species

43

that result? By focusing on differences in song development in birds reared in identical environments, in this case, individuals that are members of different species, we are forced to confront the extent to which members of even very closely related species differ in their modes of interaction with the same environments. The plan of this chapter is to use birdsong to demonstrate that this is a logical and productive approach, even with behaviour that is perhaps the best illustration available to us from the animal kingdom of culturally transmitted behaviour (cf. Cavalli-Sforza & Feldman, 1981; Mundinger, 1982; Boyd & Richerson, 1985).

I intend to show that species differ in the ways in which they approach the task of vocal imitation, and that even aspects of song development that ensure the existence of individuality in singing behaviour, essentially creative in nature and thus relatively free of specific, immediate environmental determinants, vary, not only between individuals, but also between species. My aim is to show that we cannot begin to understand individualized processes of song invention and improvisation without taking account of variations in the nature of the physiological mechanisms employed in the process of developing song.

The motor development of oscine birdsong

A pattern of motor ontogeny recurs in all oscine songbirds that have been studied. This pattern appears to be unique to birds in which natural song patterns are learned by social transmission and in which normal song fails to develop in birds reared in isolation from their species song. Swamp and song sparrows, which have been studied intensively in this regard, serve as examples.

There are three major stages in the maturation of singing behaviour: subsong, plastic song and crystallised song. In young male swamp sparrows, for example, the first efforts at singing, subsong, occur in two phases, one from about 20 to 70 days of age and another from 120 to 170 days of age, with an intervening period in midwinter when no singing occurs. Then at about 170 days, in the first spring of life, a progression through plastic song to mature singing proceeds rapidly. Full song continues for about 100 days and then ceases for the fall and winter, to resume the following spring, prefaced by a short period of plastic song. This cycle continues for the rest of the male swamp sparrow's life, with the same patterns of mature song recurring year after year.

Subsong

In contrast to oscine songbirds, species in which song develops normally in isolation lack subsong. Their first efforts at singing behaviour are immediately identifiable as immature versions of what will ultimately emerge

44

as the normal crystallised song (e.g. the alder flycatcher: Kroodsma, 1984). These early stages may be noisy and fragmented, but there is a direct maturational progression to full song.

In songbirds the process of motor development is quite different. It is discontinuous, with a kind of metamorphosis intervening between subsong and later stages of song development. Subsong is remarkably lacking in organised structure. The jumbled and erratic temporal organisation and noisy spectral structure of the subsong of swamp and song sparrows is typical. Only when the transition to plastic song occurs do the first clear signs of mature syllabic and syntactical structure appear, and imitations become detectable for the first time.

Despite the amorphous nature of subsong, close scrutiny reveals some species differences, even in the very earliest efforts. In the mature song of song and swamp sparrows, among many other differences in acoustic structure, there is a species difference in mean note duration. Notes are, on average, shorter in swamp than in song sparrow song. This contrast can also be detected in the earliest subsong. As mentioned later, auditory feedback plays a major role in several aspects of song development. Auditory mechanisms are also implicated in this early species contrast in subsong structure, which is absent in the subsong of males deafened prior to the onset of any singing behaviour. The subsong of deaf male swamp and song sparrows appears to be indistinguishable. In a sense we can regard it as a common point of departure for the motor development of song in members of these two closely related species. What insights can we gain into the causes of subsequent divergence in their developmental trajectories that might throw light on the potential for evolutionary change?

The functional significance of subsong remains a mystery. It is believed to be involved in the development of the motor skills of singing, and also in honing the ability to guide the voice by the ear, which is a prerequisite for vocal imitation, but irrelevant for species in which learning from others plays no role in song development. It may be functionally advantageous to proceed with motor development in steps, completing one stage, and establishing a set of sensorimotor routines which serve as a stepping-stone to subsequent stages. Establishing the basic motor skill that underlies production of the tonal sounds of birdsong, evidence of which begins to emerge in late subsong, is one such step, perhaps facilitated by practice gained in coordinating actions on two sides of the syrinx during subsong (Nottebohm, 1972; Nowicki & Marler, 1988). This in turn prepares the young bird to embark on the next, more challenging stage, of learning to produce song imitations from memory.

Plastic song

As plastic song emerges, rehearsal of previously memorised song patterns begins and production of syllables in trilled sequences commences. In contrast with mature song, plastic songs incorporate several trilled syllables in the same string. Normal song syntax, consisting of a single trill of the same repeated syllable only emerges late in swamp sparrow ontogeny, at the time of song crystallisation.

As the time for crystallisation approaches, significant numbers of plastic song themes are discarded. Extensive overproduction of song types occurs during plastic song in swamp sparrows, so much so that a five-fold reduction in repertoire size may occur before crystallisation is completed. Social factors that may influence the choice of themes retained in the mature song repertoire will be considered later. It is clear from the process of overproduction that much more is memorised than is present in the final products of motor song development, with a potential influence on song perception later in life.

Crystallised song

In swamp sparrows the process of song crystallisation is completed in a period of a few days. One sign of crystallisation is the emergence of songs consisting of a single string of one syllable type, replacing the multi-syllable strings that prevail in plastic song. Another sign is a drastic decrease in the variability of song duration. A period of about 3 months follows in which crystallised song is produced in the absence of earlier developmental stages.

Crystallised song patterns are characterised by the relative stereotypy of the acoustic patterns produced, in morphology, duration, and in the rhythm of delivery. A distinctive pattern for progressing through song repertoires emerges at this time. A mature male swamp sparrow has a repertoire of 1–6 song types, averaging about three. These are delivered in a definite programme. A swamp sparrow works through its repertoire by delivering a bout of fifty or so repetitions of one song type before changing to another. This basic programme, shared with many other sparrow species, illustrates what is termed 'ultimate variety' as opposed to the 'immediate variety' with which some other birds, such as thrushes, deliver their song repertoires: they produce different song types consecutively, without repetitions. There is much variability in these programmatic rules for repertoire delivery, varying between species and individuals, illustrating another dimension of singing in which significant variation can occur.

Song crystallisation is a typical event in oscine song development. In swamp sparrows there is no further potential for major change in the song repertoire, once crystallisation has taken place. This is not to say that adult singing behaviour is completely stereotyped and unchanging. There is still a significant degree of variation, and shifts may occur in the preference for different items in the repertoire and some may be dropped altogether. In species with more complex songs, such as the song sparrow, the potential for microvariation may be extensive, although of a very different degree and nature than that occurring in plastic song (S. Nowicki *et al.*, unpublished data). This microvariation is partly stochastic, and partly a concomitant of changing circumstances, including hormonal state and patterns of social stimulation. In other species, within-individual song repertoire variations are more striking, with distinct song themes for use in sexual and aggressive situations, for example (e.g. Lien, 1978; Kroodsma, 1986).

There is ample room for individual variation in the timing of development of swamp sparrow song, the significance of which remains unclear. A male that begins subsong earlier than his fellows in the spring also tends to be ahead with the transitions to plastic and crystallised song (Marler & Peters, 1982 a). In other words, late-developing birds do not catch up. On the other hand the duration of the swamp sparrow subsong and sub-plastic song periods combined is negatively correlated with the duration of the plastic song period. Thus there are hints of a possible compensatory relationship between these two stages.

A search for possible correlations between age and development also revealed a negative relationship between hatching date and the age of onset of the major stages of song development. Thus the earlier in the season in which a bird was hatched, the later the age at which subsong or sub-plastic song, plastic song, and full song began. The differences became amplified in the process, so that one bird hatched 24 days before another started spring subsong or sub-plastic songs 65 days later than the other. The functional significance of this correlate of hatching time is not understood.

The transition from plastic song to crystallised song is associated with a distinctive hormonal milieu. Study of motor development in male swamp sparrows castrated at 20 days of age revealed an unexpected propensity to produce both subsong and early stages of plastic song even though there was no testosterone in the blood plasma. These castrates failed to crystallise their song patterns, however. Testosterone therapy resulted in almost immediate production of crystallised song, maintained until the exogenous sources of testosterone were removed (Marler *et al.*, 1988). There are probable associated changes in neural organisation accompanying crystallisation, although thus far investigations have failed to reveal them (Nordeen, Marler & Nordeen, 1989).

Motor development in comparative perspective

The patterns of motor development described for the swamp sparrow recur in other emberizine finches, with the precise timing and duration of the different developmental stages varying from individual to individual and, in greater degree, from species to species. In other songbirds the variations are more radical. The subsong period can be brief or extended. Overproduction during plastic song is more extreme in some species than in others. The first themes crystallised may dominate a male's song repertoire for the rest of his life, or song structure may change from year to year or even within a season. Mature song continues for much of the year in adults of some species and is restricted to a few weeks in others.

Despite these many variations in patterns of song development and production from species to species, the same basic themes tend to recur. Stages of song development may be largely separated in time, or they may interdigitate, so that one song theme may occur as plastic song at a time when other themes are already crystallised. The species-specificity of patterns of motor development is statistical rather than absolute. Some variation is attributable to genomic differences, and some to differences in the environments in which individuals develop. In male song sparrows, for example, plastic song consistently begins several weeks earlier than in swamp sparrows kept in identical conditions in individual isolation in the laboratory (P. Marler & S. Peters, unpublished data). Temporal programmes for the motor development of song are susceptible to environmental influence. Variation in photoperiod affects hormonal cycles of testis growth and regression, thus influencing the timing of many aspects of reproductive behaviour, including song. Effects of early to late-season hatching have already been alluded to.

Social factors affect temporal programmes for development. Young male white-crowned sparrows exposed to the singing of adults pass through all stages of song development up to crystallisation significantly earlier than males raised in the laboratory and deprived of such stimulation (DeWolfe, Baptista & Petrinovich, 1989). Kroodsma (1974) recorded acceleration of song development in Bewick's wren as a consequence of song stimulation by adult males. Thus patterns of song development display variation, some of which is attributable to environmental influences. The extent of such variation is a consequence of interaction between environmental and genetic factors. To overlook contributions of the latter is to omit a vital component of the ontogenetic equation.

Species differences in songs developed in isolation

The environmental factor with the most dramatic effects on song ontogeny is auditory stimulation by the songs of others. The impact is most readily demonstrated by deprivation of song stimulation during ontogeny. If the motor development of song is studied in male song and swamp sparrows reared from the egg in the laboratory, in complete isolation from adult song of their species, their singing is abnormal. Many species differences in their singing behaviour nevertheless emerge. Even in the earliest subsong there is a difference in note duration, as already mentioned. With time this contrast is supplemented by many others until, by the time songs crystallise, there are many species-specific differences, in a dozen or more song characteristics (Marler & Sherman, 1985).

Abnormal song repertoires

There are many ways to view the songs of birds raised in social isolation. One could focus on individual differences, which are considerable, but before these can be interpreted, more general trends must be examined. Their singing behaviour has obvious abnormalities. Comparisons with normal songs of their species reveal many differences. Song repertoire sizes, for example, are significantly reduced in isolates, to about half normal size. Thus repertoire sizes are rendered aberrant by raising in isolation.

On the other hand, we can take a comparative viewpoint, and ask whether the species differences in repertoire size found in nature persists in isolates. Repertoire sizes average about three times larger in wild song sparrows than in swamp sparrows. Those of isolates differ in the same direction, and to about the same degree. Thus, despite the obvious impact of development in isolation on song repertoire size, the fact that rearing conditions were identical serves to reveal a genetic contribution to species differences in song repertoire size.

Abnormal song phonology

No ethologist would hesitate to identify isolate sparrow songs as abnormal. In song and swamp sparrows the abnormality is most evident to our ears in song phonology, by which I refer to the number, timing and acoustic structure of the notes from which songs are constructed. The number of notes per song is reduced to about one-third of the normal value in both species. The reduction is evident both in the overall note number per song, and also in the composition of subunits within the song.

A general distinction is made between trills and note complexes in song sparrow song. Note complexes are unrepeated note sequences, and trills consist of identical consecutive repetitions of note clusters called syllables. In natural song sparrow song, the number of notes in a trilled syllable averages 2–3. In isolates, trill syllables typically consist of a single note. Similarly in swamp sparrow song, which consists of one single trill, the number of notes per syllable is reduced from an average of about three to a single note in isolates.

Note duration, on the other hand, tends to be abnormally long in songs of isolation-reared males, the increase ranging from three-fold in swamp sparrow isolates to five-fold in song sparrow isolates. Internote intervals are also longer in isolates. Thus an isolate song gives the overall impression of being simpler than normal, with few components, and a slower tempo. In these respects the resulting motor pattern is clearly outside the normative range for the species.

Species differences in song phonology

The fact that development is so abnormal in sparrows raised in isolation, with a high degree of intraspecific variation, does not by any means imply that species differences are eliminated. In all of these phonological features that develop abnormally in isolation, an interspecies comparison of isolate songs and of those of males singing in nature reveals species differences in the normal direction.

Species do not always differ to the same degree in normal and isolate song, however. Note duration, for example, is 60 % longer in normal song sparrow than in normal swamp sparrow songs, whereas in isolates the species difference increases to more than 200 %. Similarly with the number of notes per song, there are about 25 % more in normal swamp sparrow than in song sparrow songs, whereas in isolates the difference, in the same direction, increases to about 50 % more in swamp than song sparrows, telling us something about the relative potential for evolutionary change in this trait in these two species. With other measures, such as the duration of internote intervals and the number of notes in a trilled syllable, the species differences are very similar in normal and isolate song.

Song syntax

In contrast with the many abnormalities in the phonology of isolate songs, an unexpectedly large number of syntactical features are similar in isolate and natural songs of a given species. In song and swamp sparrows these include the number of trills per song, the total number of trilled syllables, and the number of syllables in a trill. Song duration is also similar in normal and isolate songs of these species.

In all of these song features, the direction and degree of the difference between the two species is similar in isolate and natural song. The same trend occurs in the number of segments per song, which is not significantly different in natural and isolate song sparrow songs, but shows an increase in isolated swamp sparrows over the wild condition as a result of an increase in the number of two- and three-segmented songs. Even in this case, however, there are still more segments in an isolate song sparrow than in isolate swamp sparrow songs, as occurs in nature.

Thus the list of syntactical features that are developmentally conservative, resisting change in the face of isolation from stimulation by normal song of their species, is a long one. This conservatism implies a strong genetic contribution to their development but the same is true of song traits that are developmentally more labile, and more sensitive to effects of song stimulation.

Species differences in natural and isolate song

This comparison of natural and isolate song in two species reveals that, irrespective of whether a trait develops normally or abnormally in isolation, every feature studied shows a species difference in the same direction as in the natural song. Since these birds were raised under identical conditions we can infer that the differences are genetically based. The implication is just as clear and unequivocal when the trait is plastic and develops abnormally in isolation, as when the trait is resistant to variation in the face of environmental change, bringing to mind once more Hinde's comments on the meaninglessness of dichotomising features into those which are innate and those which are acquired. It would be equally illogical, however, to conclude that the natural singing behaviour of these birds develops independently of environmental influences. There is ample evidence to the contrary, not least in the many features that develop abnormally in isolation.

The abnormality of isolate songs proves to be attributable mainly to drastic changes, in both species, in three aspects of the structure of isolate song. First, there are fewer notes per song, less than half as many as in songs of wild birds. Second, the duration of notes and of internote intervals show a several-fold increase, so that the overall tempo is abnormally slow. Third, the number of notes per syllable is decreased, in most cases to a single note, hence the impression of simplicity to our ears, by comparison with the more elaborate sounds of natural song.

Species differences in isolation effects

Despite the many trends in common in isolate songs of the two species, there are some interesting contrasts. In the song sparrow the number of trills per song was not significantly different in normal and isolate songs. In isolation-reared swamp sparrows, however, the number of trills increased significantly compared with those in nature. The resistance to environmentally induced change in overall normal song syntax appears to be less in the swamp sparrow than in the song sparrow.

Other evidence along these lines was also found when birds of both species were exposed in infancy to identical sets of synthetic two-part songs, each consisting of two trills. Male swamp sparrows showed a significant increase in the number of two-trill songs. Two-parted songs also occur at a low rate in nature as well (Marler & Peters, 1980). Evidently song sparrows are inherently less prone to diversion from the species-specific pattern of overall song structure than swamp sparrows, indicating another contrast in the potential for evolutionary change. As will be seen later, however, these trends are probabilistic rather than absolute, and under certain conditions song sparrows can be induced to produce quite abnormal song syntax.

Species song differences in the absence of auditory feedback

Deprivation of social stimulation during ontogeny has drastic effects on song development, but we have seen that many species differences nevertheless develop in males raised in isolation from song. Two obvious mechanisms for imposing genetic influences on the ontogeny of song motor patterns are (i) by endogenously generated motor commands from the central nervous system, and (ii) by auditory song templates to which a bird would match its own voice in the course of development. We know from the pioneering work of Konishi (1964, 1965a, b) that auditory templates play a major role in the control of song development. He showed that the songs of deaf birds develop much more abnormally than those of males raised in isolation with their hearing intact. There is controversy, however, about the role of endogenous motor programmes, and about the precise extent to which species differences are lacking in the songs of deaf birds.

In the white-crowned sparrow, males deafened early in life developed a noisy, unstructured song, lacking most of the structural features present in songs of males raised in isolation with their hearing intact, other than duration and frequency range (Marler & Tamura, 1964; Konishi, 1965b). The songs of early-deafened white-crowned sparrows were so amorphous that it was tempting to conclude that all significant species-specific characteristics were lacking. It will be recalled that the early subsong of deaf swamp and song sparrows appears to lack any consistent species differences (Marler *et al.*, unpublished data).

Are songs of deaf birds structureless?

Extending study of the effects of deafening to other birds, Konishi found some species whose songs were as formless as those of early deafened white-crowned sparrows (Konishi, 1964, 1965a, b). In other species, however, such as the Oregon junco and the black-headed grosbeak, more normal song traits were present after early deafening (Konishi, 1964, 1965b). This suggested that some birds can realise a significant degree of species-specific song structure without auditory feedback.

Nottebohm (1966, 1968) countered with the proposal that apparent species differences in the singing of deaf birds might be attributable to experimental variation in the amount of pre-deafening song experience. His experiments on effects of deafening of chaffinches at various stages of development indicated that, after a certain stage, the birds retained song structure achieved prior to deafening. On this basis he predicted that deafening of different songbirds at comparable developmental stages would yield results corresponding with those he obtained. Male chaffinches produced what he interpreted as a virtually structureless song after early deafening (Nottebohm, 1966, 1968).

What do we find if we take two species whose song development in social isolation has been well studied, raise them under identical conditions of isolation, deafen them at the same developmental stage, prior to any song production and subject their songs to a quantitative comparison? If their songs are indistinguishable this would argue against a significant role for central motor programmes that differ genetically from species to species.

The variability of deaf songs masks species differences

Quantitative study of songs developed by early-deafened male song and swamp sparrows makes it clear why the issue of song species-specificity has been controversial. In some deaf songs the loss of species-specificity is almost complete. Yet, despite the crude, noisy and variable phonology always present in songs of early-deafened birds, others display definite signs of species-specificity. Some deaf song sparrow songs are clearly multi-segmental, and some deaf swamp sparrow songs are unquestionably simply trills.

Quantitative analysis confirms both the great variability and the persistence of species differences in songs of deaf birds. Measurements of the number of segments in a song show that the variation is much greater in deaf than in natural and isolate songs. In natural songs the distributions are non-overlapping, whereas in songs of deaf birds the variance is great and the overlap very extensive. Nevertheless, the mean number of segments per song is greater for deaf song sparrows than for swamp sparrows, although this difference tends to be masked by the extraordinary variability, both between song types and between individuals. Species differences in the normal direction also occurred in song duration, frequency and in repertoire size. Deaf song sparrows have larger repertoires than deaf swamp sparrows, as occurs in nature.

To this extent, then, an element of species-specificity is present in songs of early-deafened birds. Many fewer features display species differences, however, than is the case with songs of birds raised in isolation with their hearing intact. In particular, none of the species contrasts in phonology, present consistently in the songs of isolates with their hearing intact, are discernible in deaf birds' songs, including number of notes per song, note duration, and the number of trilled syllables per song.

Species differences in auditory templates and central motor programmes

The effects of deafening on song imply the involvement in development of auditory mechanisms that birds use to monitor their own vocalisations. These have been conceptualised as 'auditory song templates' (Konishi, 1964, 1965a, b; Marler, 1976; Marler & Sherman, 1983). As long as the auditory feedback loop is intact, birds produce songs with many features that differ from species to species. With the loop broken, the ability to monitor self-produced sounds is disrupted. Under this condition, songs are produced that are exceedingly variable from individual to individual, and even from song to song within an individual's repertoire. In some songs, interspecies differences are virtually lacking. In others there is a degree of specific distinctiveness. In all cases songs of deaf birds lack certain species contrasts that, in intact birds raised in isolation, develop normally. Auditory templates are thus implicated in the genesis of many species differences in song structure.

The species differences that develop without auditory feedback suggest the existence of central motor programmes that differ genetically from species to species. Perhaps the greatest degree of deprivation from auditory feedback was achieved in an experiment with canaries (Marler *et al.*, 1973; Marler &

Waser, 1977). Young males were hatched and reared in high-level white noise, sufficient to mask their own voices and those of their parents. At independence the young were removed from the noise and immediately deafened. Despite the virtually total occlusion of the auditory pathway both for sound stimuli and for vocal feedback, a significant number of species-specific features developed in the songs of these deaf canaries, especially those of a syntactical nature. This was particularly evident in the syntactical structure of their song, which displayed features recurring in the songs of related cardueline finches as well (Güttinger 1979, 1981; Güttinger, Wolfgramm & Thimm, 1978). Similarly in cardinals, red-winged blackbirds and zebra finches, songs of early-deafened males all have some degree of species-specific syntax, despite the gross abnormality of their phonology (Dittus & Lemon, 1970; Marler *et al.*, 1972; Price, 1979).

Thus some birds with learned songs possess the ability to generate motor programmes that differ from species to species. Such central motor programmes for singing behaviour represent another vehicle, in addition to auditory song templates, by which genetic influences can be exerted on the process of song development.

Song-learning preferences

What is necessary to ensure normality in the songs of sparrows raised in the laboratory? For some species, access to a live, singing tutor is necessary. In song and swamp sparrows, it suffices to play tape recordings of normal song to them at a certain stage of development. They then produce songs that not only qualify as normal, but also incorporate many specific details of the songs they have learned. What happens if we present a young bird with an array of polyspecific songs or tutors to learn from? Are they equipotential as stimuli, or are some preferred over others? If there are preferences, do species differ in the songs they favour, or is a song that is a strong learning stimulus for one, also strong for others?

This question was addressed by bringing young male swamp and song sparrows into the laboratory, rearing them under identical conditions and exposing them to tape recordings with equal numbers of normal swamp sparrow and song sparrow songs. Unlike some birds, these two sparrows learn readily from tape recordings, and the imitations are sufficiently precise that they are readily ascribable to particular models among those experienced.

The experiment was repeated under two conditions. First, birds were taken as nestlings from the field at an age of 3–10 days, reared by hand in the laboratory, and then given the opportunity to learn from tape recordings. In a second experiment, eggs were taken from wild nests of the same two species, early in incubation, hatched in the laboratory under canaries, and then raised by hand with no opportunity at all to hear adult song of their species. The contrasting design served to explore the hypothesis posited by Johnston (1988) that auditory experience of conspecific song in the egg, and during the first few days of nestling life, as occurs in nature, exerts an influence on the choice of models for song learning.

Species-specific learning preferences

The results were similar in the two experiments. Both species displayed a significant preference for acquiring and producing songs of their own species. The design was balanced in the sense that exactly the same training tapes were played to the two species, while they were housed in individual isolation, after independence. The results show that the songs that were strong learning stimuli for one species were weak stimuli for the other, and vice versa.

We conclude that both swamp and song sparrows display a preference in favour of songs of their own species when given a choice. It is interesting to note that the preference was weaker in song sparrows than in swamp sparrows, both as nestling-reared and as egg-reared subjects. A similar bias is evident from measures of heart rate change in 3-week-old song and swamp sparrows in response to song (Dooling & Searcy, 1980). Again, the discrimination in favour of conspecific song was stronger in swamp sparrows than in song sparrows.

In some songbirds social interaction with live tutors plays a significant role in song learning, and in certain species it can be a prerequisite for learning to take place (Pepperberg, 1988). In areas where the two sparrow species live within earshot of one another song sparrows never learn swamp sparrow song, so far as we can determine. It may that the song sparrow is another case in which the opportunity for social interaction with live tutors influences the choice of models for song learning. If this proves to be so, we may conclude that social interaction further reinforces a bias in favour of conspecific song that is manifest with sounds of song alone.

Given the ease with which songs can be synthesised by digital techniques, the fact that a preference in favour of conspecific song can be sustained solely by auditory stimulation with tape-recorded song in both song and swamp sparrows, makes it possible to investigate the nature of the acoustic features on which preferences are based.

The acoustic basis of learning preferences

The use of learning stimuli consisting of synthetic songs in which different acoustic features have been independently and systematically varied reveals that the learning preference of male swamp sparrows is based on syllable phonology (Marler & Peters, 1989). Given access to synthetic songs in a variety of syntactical patterns, and made up of either swamp sparrow syllables or song sparrow syllables, male swamp sparrows unerringly favour those with conspecific syllables. They display this preference irrespective of the syntactical patterns in which the syllables are presented. The syllables are usually recast into normal swamp sparrow syntax, whether or not this pattern was present in the songs to which they were exposed. Thus in choosing models for learning, the syllable is the primary, salient focus for a swamp sparrow.

The situation in song sparrows is different. In this species conspecific learning preferences are based both on syllabic structure, and also on song syntax. Several syntactical features are involved, including the number of segments, and their internal phrase structure – whether syllables are trilled, or unrepeated, as in a note complex – and such attributes as the tempo in which they are delivered. There is no evidence that male swamp sparrows refer to any of these syntactical features in choosing models for song learning.

These experiments show that swamp and song sparrows differ in the features upon which song-learning preferences are based. The design of the experiments permits us to conclude that the species difference in learning preferences is genetically based. But the intrusion of genetic influences does not by any means imply that the parameters of song responsiveness in these two sparrows are fixed and immutable. Quite to the contrary, the patterns of responsiveness that differ from species to species are employed, not to develop a fixed behaviour, but as the basis for a learning process. Having focused attention on the particular set of exemplars that satisfy certain criteria, male sparrows then learn those exemplars, and reproduce them, often in specific detail, including the local dialect that they represent.

Song dialects

A frequent consequence of the dependence of mature song structure on stimulation by song characteristics of the place in which a male songbird finds himself is the emergence of dialects. These vary greatly in scale, from hundreds of birds living in extensive geographical areas to a dozen males in a very restricted locality (Lemon, 1975; Baker & Cunningham, 1985). In the swamp sparrow geographical song variants are defined by the patterning of notes within a syllable, with local rules for the ordering of note types. Population differences are a result of differences in what they hear when they are young. A New York bird exposed to Minnesota songs in its youth will learn the Minnesota dialect, and vice versa. Both males and females prove to be responsive to these dialect variations. New York birds are more responsive to the New York pattern of note ordering than to the note sequences that are typical in Minnesota (Balaban, 1988a, b, c). Thus the fact that male swamp sparrows are genetically predisposed to favour songs of their own species does not in any way compromise their acquisition of responsiveness to local dialects by social transmission.

The capacity to learn heterospecific songs

Having established the existence of learning preferences, it is important to add that such biases as they possess are not completely binding. If conspecific songs are withheld, and only heterospecific songs are provided as models, these sparrows will learn non-preferred songs. Heterospecific imitation has been shown to occur in other sparrow species, especially the white-crowned sparrow (review in Baptista, 1988). With tape-recorded songs alone, this species displays a preference for learning those of its own species (Marler & Tamura, 1964; Marler, 1970), but a high rate of heterospecific song learning can be achieved by imposing interaction with a live tutor of another species at close quarters (Baptista & Petrinovich, 1984, 1986).

Thus the process of choosing models for song learning is determined probabilistically and is not absolute. Genetically biased preferences can be overridden. In the usual course of events, however, tutors and songs displaying conspecific attributes will be available as the most potent sources of stimulation for the young male, permitting conspecific preferences to be exercised. As a consequence, certain probabilistic trajectories to the learning process will be established, with features that differ from species to species. Do the results of behavioural experiments indicate how one might model the physiological mechanisms underlying such learning preferences?

Parallel processing in song learning

There is ample experimental evidence that birds can hear the songs of other species perfectly well (Dooling, 1980, 1982; Okanoya & Dooling, 1988). They can be taught to discriminate between heterospecific songs, and to distinguish between songs of different individuals, although they discriminate less precisely between songs of other species than between those of their own (Okanoya & Dooling, 1988). Thus sensory processing of conspecific and heterospecific songs appears to be equivalent. Yet, some influence song development and others do not.

These sparrows behave as though any song presented as a stimulus is processed normally, but if it is heterospecific, in the usual course of events, it is then either lost from memory, or remembered, but withheld from influence on the development of the motor patterns of song. It may have an effect on song development in certain circumstances, if conspecific song stimuli are also present in temporal contiguity, or if the exposure is unusually massive, continuing day after day, or if it is associated with strong arousal, as when male white-crowned sparrows learn from a singing male song sparrow with which they are caged in close proximity (Baptista & Petrinovich, 1984, 1986).

Conspecific songs as 'enabling signals'

If conspecific stimuli are presented at a time when males are receptive, even with as few as 20 exposures (e.g. Hultsch & Todt, 1989), birds behave as though they suddenly become attentive, and a brief time window is opened during which the stimulus cluster being processed at the time becomes more salient and memorable, and more likely to be used subsequently as a basis for the motor development of song. The most obvious way in which to model this behaviour is in terms of parallel neural processing. Viewed in this fashion, certain auditory circuits are construed as responsible for general auditory processing, and other circuits, operating in parallel, as committed to the identification of stimuli especially worthy of the attention of the general processing machinery.

According to this interpretation, responsiveness to cues that are equivalent to the sign stimuli of Lorenz and Tinbergen, may function both as behavioural triggers and also as cues for learning, serving as what we might think of as 'enabling signals'. Enabling signals are viewed as stimuli, which may be environmental (Marler, 1987) or physiological (Cooper, 1987; Rauschecker, 1987), whose presence increases the probability of learning stimuli that are otherwise unlikely to be committed to memory. Such enabling functions may be served by many of the 'releasers' of classical ethology, and may be the primary function for many of them (Marler, Zoloth & Dooling, 1980, 1981; Gould & Marler, 1984, 1987). The notion that sign stimuli have enabling effects on learning demonstrates once more the futility of any dichotomy into innate and learned behaviours, and illustrates the insights that can be derived from a comparative, experimental approach to behavioural development.

Environmental shaping of the crystallisation process

One of the most intricate environmental effects on song development concerns the overproduction of plastic songs, and the factors that determine which are retained and which are set aside in the process of crystallisation. In swamp sparrows this attrition process occurs months after the sensitive period for song acquisition is completed.

For a male swamp sparrow developing song in individual isolation it is difficult to predict which of its many plastic songs will be crystallised. Those retained are not necessarily the first developed nor given most often in early plastic song. The choice is not a random one, however (Marler & Peters, 1982b). For example, swamp sparrows that have acquired some song sparrow elements from synthetic songs in which swamp and song sparrow material was intermingled, are more likely to reject heterospecific than conspecific components during the attrition process.

There are many opportunities for experience to interact with development to influence the final outcome. The transition from plastic song to full song takes place at a time when a young male swamp sparrow is striving to establish his first territory, and is actively engaged in countersinging with neighbouring residents. There is often a premium in songbirds on countersinging against rivals with similar themes if they are available. Indications are that stimulation by the songs of rivals during the attrition process favours the retention, from the overproduced repertoire, of those themes that most closely match those of neighbours.

Nice (1943) described such a process in male song sparrows. Young males establishing territories reply to rivals with similar songs, even though many of these are subsequently dropped from the repertoire. She concluded that 'each young song sparrow has a large fund of potential songs, as is clear from listening to the rambling warblings of juveniles'. She suggested that what might appear to be a process of imitation occurring during early territorial establishment is actually 'a calling forth of songs already in the potential repertoire, most of them being later lost through disuse' (Nice, 1943, p. 139).

The behaviour described by Nice in song sparrows corresponds to the overproduction and attrition that occurs in swamp sparrows. The implication is that stimulation by rival songs results in song matching, not as a consequence of acquisition of new themes, but rather by influencing the process of retention from an excess of themes that are invented, or acquired earlier in life. Reinforcement is evidently provided by the heightened reactions of rivals to those themes in the plastic song repertoire that most closely match their own.

A loss of overproduced songs prior to crystallisation has been noted in other songbirds, such as the red-winged blackbird and the white-crowned sparrow (Marler *et al.*, 1972). Once again, song stimulation at this time appears to have an effect on which are retained. DeWolfe *et al.* (1989) have described such a process in detail, with settling fledglings tending to use themes matching those of neighbours during countersinging bouts, using songs drawn from a repertoire acquired earlier and developed during plastic song overproduction.

Perhaps the most remarkable illustration of the impact of environmental stimulation, not on song acquisition, but on the process of selection from an overproduced plastic song repertoire, comes from the work of King & West (1988) on the brown-headed cowbird. Overproduction in plastic song has been documented in cowbirds, and again a selective process is involved in the choice of which songs are retained and crystallised. In this case, however, the stimulation originates not from countersinging males, but from females. Certain plastic songs elicit a distinctive 'wing stroke' response from females, which evidently reinforces production of that particular song type. Subsequent playback tests to females comparing the salience of these 'wing stroke' songs with other songs demonstrated that the former were in fact the most potent in eliciting solicitation for copulation from adult females during the breeding season (West & King, 1988). Thus male–female interactions play a tutorial role during song ontogeny not by an influence on song acquisition, but rather by selective effects on retention and rejection of songs acquired earlier in life.

The fact that environmental factors can influence not only which songs are acquired and reproduced, but also which are discarded in the formation of an adult repertoire, serves as a further reminder of the diverse ways in which experience can affect the process of song development.

Species differences in inventiveness

Individual variation appears to be a universal phenomenon in oscine birdsongs, providing an ample basis for natural selection to operate on, assuming that it has a heritable basis. Individual differences have been thoroughly documented in scores of cases, and are often conspicuous, even to the untutored human ear. In every species studied songs have proved to serve as markers for personal identity, and are used to identify neighbours and distinguish them from strangers (Falls, 1982). This is true even of species with a high degree of conformity to local population norms, when local dialects are very marked (Falls, 1982). Even when neighbours have song types in common, they are rarely, if ever, absolutely identical, either because of invention or errors in the copying process, or perhaps because there is, by design, a tendency to depart from the original models in certain respects.

Thus the tendency to concentrate on processes of imitation in research on song learning, although appropriate enough as a research strategy, may lead to the neglect of other kinds of process, often inventive in nature, that also contribute to the process of song development.

Frequently, learned models are not reproduced in their entirety, although this can occur. More typically, models are broken down into phrases, syllables and even into notes, and these components are then recombined to create new patterns, by a process of re-editing. Laboratory-reared song sparrows often use components of two songs presented as tape recordings to create novel song patterns.

Such re-editing of song components, which appears to occur commonly in nature (e.g. the mistle thrush: Marler, 1959), involves the division of learned songs into segments, and implies that birds are capable of partitioning acquired songs and processing the component parts separately.

Component-partitioning of learned songs

There are other indications that the perceptual processing of different song segments can be partitioned. A case of partitioning occurs in rufous-sided towhees, whose song consists of a simple, unspecific tone followed by a more complex trill. Towhees appear to use the tone as an alerting signal and the trill for species identification (Richards, 1981). When brown-headed cowbirds and red-winged blackbirds are given the task of classifying conspecific songs into categories, they base their classifications on different song segments from when they perform an equivalent task with songs of another species (Sinnott, 1984). This suggests that particular predispositions are brought to bear on the perceptual processing of conspecific songs, distinct from those that operate on acoustic stimuli in general. Discrimination tests in the laboratory with isolated song segments show that these two species do equally well with introductory sections of their own and the other species. Required to discriminate between terminal portions of song, however, which are the most highly species-specific, each does better with conspecific than with heterospecific songs (Dooling, 1982).

A case of partitioning of different note types within the song repertoire of a species has also been described. Each syllable of a swamp sparrow song is composed of between two and five separate notes. Analysis of a large sample recorded throughout the species range revealed that notes can be sorted into six note-types, with some intergradation between them (Marler & Pickert, 1984; Clark, Marler & Beeman, 1987). Two note types in particular, types I and VI, play distinct roles in the construction of syllables in different populations. In New York songs, type I notes most commonly occur in the initial position in three-note syllables and type VI notes in the terminal position. In songs from northern Minnesota, the note-order rule is reversed. Type VI notes predominate in first position and type I in terminal position. These population differences in note usage prove to be salient to male swamp sparrows in field playback tests, and to females in laboratory experiments (Balaban, 1988a, b). New York birds of both sexes respond more strongly to songs with New York syntax than to songs with the same notes rearranged into Minnesota syntax.

A difference in duration appears to be the main factor differentiating between type I and type VI notes. By carefully selecting pairs of notes varying in duration, some falling within a category, and other pairs falling astride a boundary, and incorporating these into songs played to wild territorial males, it has been shown that these note series are processed categorically (Nelson & Marler, 1989).

As has been demonstrated with the processing of certain speech sounds by human subjects (Liberman *et al.*, 1957; Harnad, 1987), the perceptual processing of the duration of notes in swamp sparrow song is categorical rather than continuous, with boundary placement where the incidence of intermediates in produced songs is minimal. The universal occurrence of these note types in all swamp sparrow songs, and the responsiveness of naïve male swamp sparrows to the distinctive characteristics of swamp sparrow phonology when acquiring song during the sensitive period, both suggest that this case of categorical perception reflects the operation of developmentally conservative, species-specific auditory mechanisms, likely to vary from species to species. The potential for categorical perceptual processing may be another attribute of auditory song template mechanisms, engaged both in the acquisition process, when young males commit songs to memory and in adulthood, in the perceptual processing of songs of other males.

As an alternative to the hypothesis that songs are partitioned by perceptual processes during acquisition, recombination may be primarily a motor phenomenon. New approaches are needed to resolve these alternatives, both to explore the perceptual processing of songs prior to production, and also for analysis of the earliest efforts to reproduce vocal imitations and inventions, during the transition from subsong to plastic song (e.g. Clark *et al.*, 1987).

Re-editing of song components can occur both within a given song model, and also between models. Such between-exemplar re-editing can take place, both with songs acquired at the same time, and at different times. In a study of sensitive periods for acquisition of song by male song sparrows from tape recordings, one male created new songs by combining syllables and phrases that were acquired more than 100 days apart (Marler & Peters, 1989).

Analyses of plastic song production in captive sparrows suggest that recombinations of phrases drawn from different models sometimes first appear surprisingly early in the process of song development, without any obvious signs of preceding experimentation by trial and error. Thus it seems conceivable that some active processing is taking place during periods of song acquisition and storage. It may be that, prior to any production, memorized songs are subjected to some degree of breakdown and reassemblage, especially at the level of phrases and syllables. Given the differences between songbirds in the predisposition to recombine components of learned songs, it may be that bird species differ even in the very processes by which learned songs are committed to memory.

Species differences in invention and improvisation

If the rules for parsing acquired songs into components and recombining them are species-specific, there is also species variation in the faithfulness with which a bird adheres to the structure of a given learned model. Some, like swamp and song sparrows, are relatively conservative. They recast syllables often, but adhere to the basic structure of the re-edited syllables, which makes them good subjects for learning studies.

Other species, such as the red-winged blackbird, are compulsive improvisers. During plastic song, a male red-wing submits acquired themes to continuous experimentation and embroidery during development, transforming them to such a degree that the originals become barely recognizable (Marler *et al.*, 1972).

Even more intriguing is the evidence that improvisation and invention may be applied consistently more to some segments of song than to others, which tend to be left as pure, unadulterated imitations. Thus a species like the white-crowned sparrow, in which birds in a given locality adhere closely to a given dialect, nevertheless has song segments or features that are less constrained to conform to acquired models during development, and are more free for individual improvisation. The corn bunting appears to be a very similar case (McGregor & Thompson, 1988). Thus cues for personal identification arising from improvisation may be encoded in one song segment or feature, cues for the local dialect in another, and cues for species recognition in yet another set, the arrangement varying from species to species (Marler, 1960).

It seems clear that there are deep-rooted species differences in the focus, nature and rate of these creative activities, ultimately only attributable to variations in the structure and operation of underlying neural mechanisms. Yet it is also the case that the nature and pace of invention and improvisation must be influenced by environmental stimulation, especially of a social nature. Once more we are reminded, as Hinde has cautioned so often, of the futility of any simple dichotomy into innate and learned behaviours. Even creative processes such as song invention and improvisation have a heritable basis, and are thus subject to influence by genetic factors in the course of ontogeny, with the potential to vary widely from species to species.

Conclusions

This review of species differences in mechanisms of behavioural development makes it clear that, of the proximate factors bearing on song development, some are 'universal' and others are 'local', in the sense of Maynard Smith and his colleagues (Maynard Smith *et al.*, 1985). So called 'local constraints' can be taxonomically so restricted that they differ even between closely related species. An appreciation of the nature and causal basis of these proximate factors, their potential plasticity, and the factors enhancing or imposing limitations on this plasticity, would seem to be crucial to any effort to understand the impact of evolutionary forces on the behaviour concerned. In varying degrees, the same must be true of all kinds of behaviour, although the high level of variation in birdsong, between individuals, populations, and species, and the strong dependence upon social transmission as a means of inheritance, brings these considerations especially to the fore.

As Stamps (1990) has indicated, further progress in understanding behavioural evolution is likely to become increasingly dependent on an understanding of the proximate mechanisms responsible for the ontogeny of the particular behaviour, in the particular species under study. As the need for a more integrated view of the importance of both proximate and ultimate factors on behaviour evolution becomes more widely appreciated, it will become clear that the work of Robert Hinde is a mine of information bearing directly on such problems. This will be the case, whether the behaviour under study is aggressive, sexual, parental, or communicative, whether the topic is learning, imprinting, habituation, or the establishment of social relationships and the emergence of human attachments, whether the focus is upon the development of behaviour in birds, non-human primates or our own species (Hinde, 1956, 1959, 1961, 1965, 1969, 1972a, b, 1974, 1979, 1982). As Hinde (1981) has anticipated, the potential exists for highly productive and dynamic synergism between research on the proximate and the ultimate causes of behaviour. We can look forward to the insights to be provided by activities of a new generation of researchers, equally well versed in evolutionary theory and in the causal mechanisms underlying behaviour. Hinde's encyclopedic documentation of proximate mechanisms underlying behavioural development will be a priceless resource in this enterprise.

References

Baker, M. C. & Cunningham, M. A. (1985). The biology of birdsong dialects. *Behavioral and Brain Sciences*, **8**, 85–133.

Balaban, E. (1988a). Bird song syntax: learned intraspecific variation is meaningful. *Proceedings of the National Academy of Sciences (USA)*, **85**, 3657–60.

Balaban, E. (1988b). Cultural and genetic variation in swamp sparrows (*Melospiza georgiana*): I. Song variation, genetic variation and their relationship. *Behaviour*, **105**, 250–91.

Balaban, E. (1988c). Cultural and genetic variation in swamp sparrows (*Melospiza georgiana*): II. Behavioral salience of geographic song variants. *Behaviour*, **105**, 292–322.

Baptista, L. F. (1988). Song learning in white-crowned sparrows (*Zonotrichia leucophrys*): sensitive phases and stimulus filtering revisited. *Proceedings of the International 100. DO-G Meeting, Current Topics in Avian Biology*, Bonn.

Baptista, L. F. & Petrinovich, L. (1984). Social interaction, sensitive phases and the song template hypothesis in the white-crowned sparrow. *Animal Behaviour*, **32**, 172–81.

Baptista, L. F. & Petrinovich, L. (1986). Song development in the white-crowned sparrow: social factors and sex differences. *Animal Behaviour*, **34**, 1359–71.

Benzer, S. (1973). Genetic dissection of behavior. *Scientific American*, **229**, 24–37.

Boyd, R. & Richerson, P. R. (1985). *Culture and the Evolutionary Process*. Chicago: University of Chicago Press.

Cavalli-Sforza, L. L. & Feldman, M. W. (1981). *Cultural Transmission and Evolution: A Quantitative Approach*. Princeton, NJ: Princeton University Press.

Clark, C. W., Marler, P. & Beeman, K. (1987). Quantitative analysis of animal vocal phonology: an application to swamp sparrow song. *Ethology*, **76**, 101–15.

Clayton, N. S. (1989). Song, sex and sensitive phases in the behavioral development of birds. *Trends in Evolution and Ecology*, **4**, 82–4.

Cooper, (1987). Cortical plasticity: theoretical analysis, experimental results. In *Imprinting and Cortical Plasticity: Comparative Aspects of Sensitive Periods*, ed. J. P. Rauschecker and P. Marler, pp. 177–92. New York: John Wiley.

DeWolfe, B. B., Baptista, L. F. & Petrinovich, L. (1989). Song development and territory establishment in Nuttall's white-crowned sparrows. *Condor*, **91**, 397–407.

Dittus, W. P. J. & Lemon, R. E. (1970). Auditory feedback in the singing of cardinals. *Ibis*, **112**, 544–8.

Dooling, R. J. (1980). Behavior and psychophysics of hearing in birds. In *Comparative Studies of Hearing in Vertebrates*, ed. A. N. Popper and R. R. Fay, pp. 261–88. Berlin: Springer-Verlag.

Dooling, R. J. (1982). Auditory perception in birds. In *Acoustic Communication in Birds, Vol. 1*, ed. D. E. Kroodsma and E. H. Miller, pp. 95–130. New York: Academic Press.

Dooling, R. J. & Searcy, M. H. (1980). Early perceptual selectivity in the swamp sparrow. *Developmental Psychobiology*, **13**, 499–506.

Falls, J. B. (1982). Individual recognition by sounds in birds. In *Acoustic Communication in Birds, Vol. 2*, ed. E. Kroodsma and E. H. Miller, pp. 237–78. New York: Academic Press.

Gould, J. L. (1974). Genetics and molecular ethology. *Zeitschrift für Tierpsychologie*, **36**, 267–92.

Gould, J. L. & Marler, P. (1984). Ethology and the natural history of learning. In *The*

Biology of Learning, ed. P. Marler and H. S. Terrace, pp. 47–74. New York: Springer-Verlag.

Gould, J. L. & Marler, P. (1987). Learning by instinct. *Scientific American*, **256**, 74–85.

Gould, S. J. (1989). A developmental constraint in Cerion, with comments on the definition and interpretation of constraint in evolution. *Evolution*, **43**, 516–39.

Güttinger, H. R. (1979). The integration of learnt and genetically programmed behaviour: a study of hierarchical organization in songs of canaries, greenfinches and their hybrids. *Zeitschrift für Tierpsychologie*, **49**, 285–303.

Güttinger, H. R. (1981). Self-differentiation of song organization rules by deaf canaries. *Zeitschrift für Tierpsychologie*, **56**, 323–40.

Güttinger, H. R., Wolfgramm, J. & Thimm, F. (1978). The relationship between species specific song program and individual learning in songbirds: A study of individual variation in songs of canaries, greenfinches, and hybrids between the two species. *Behavior*, **65**, 241–62.

Hall, J. C., Greenspan, R. J. & Harris, W. A. (1982). *Genetic Neurobiology*. Cambridge, Mass.: MIT Press.

Harnad, S. (1987). *Categorical Perception*. New York: Cambridge University Press.

Hinde, R. A. (1956). The biological significance of the territories of birds. *Ibis*, **98**, 340–69.

Hinde, R. A. (1959). Behaviour and speciation in birds and lower vertebrates. *Biological Review*, **34**, 85–128.

Hinde, R. A. (1961). The establishment of parent–offspring relations in birds, with some mammalian analogies. In *Current Problems in Animal Behaviour*, ed. W. H. Thorpe and O. L. Zangwill, Cambridge: Cambridge University Press.

Hinde, R. A. (1965). Interaction of internal and external factors in integration of canary reproduction. In *Sex and Behavior*, ed. F. A. Beach. New York: Wiley.

Hinde, R. A. (1969). *Bird Vocalizations*. Cambridge: Cambridge University Press.

Hinde, R. A. (1970). *Animal Behaviour: A Synthesis of Ethology and Comparative Psychology*. New York: McGraw-Hill.

Hinde, R. A. (1972a). Aggression. In *Biology and the Human Social Sciences*, ed. J. W. S. Pringle. Oxford: Clarendon Press.

Hinde, R. A. (ed.) (1972b). *Non-verbal Communication*. Cambridge: Cambridge University Press.

Hinde, R. A. (1974). *The Biological Bases of Human Social Behaviour*. New York: McGraw-Hill.

Hinde, R. A. (1979). *Towards Understanding Relationships*. London: Academic Press.

Hinde, R. A. (1981). Animal signals: ethological and games theory approaches are not incompatible. *Animal Behaviour*, **29**: 535–42.

Hinde, R. A. (1982). *Ethology: Its Nature and Relations with Other Sciences*. Oxford: Oxford University Press.

Hinde, R. A. (1983). *Primate Social Relationships*. Sunderland, Mass.: Sinauer.

Hinde, R. A. & Stevenson-Hinde, J. (1986). Relating childhood relationships to individual characteristics. In *Relationships and Development*, ed. W. W. Hartup and Z. Rubin, pp. 27–50. Hillsdale, NJ: Erlbaum.

Hinde, R. A. & Tinbergen, N. (1958). The comparative study of species-specific behavior. In *Behavior and Evolution*, ed. A. Roe & G. G. Simpson. New Haven, Conn.: Yale University Press.

Hirsch, J. (1967). *Behavior-Genetic Analysis*. New York: McGraw-Hill.

Hultsch, H. & Todt, D. (1988). Song acquisition and acquisition constraints in the nightingale, *Luscinia megarhynchos*. *Naturwissenschaften*, **76**, 83–5.

Johnston, T. D. (1988). Developmental explanation and the ontogeny of birdsong: nature/nurture redux. *Behavioural and Brain Sciences*, **11**, 631–75.

King, A. P. & West, J. J. (1988). Searching for the functional origins of song in eastern brown-headed cowbirds, *Molothrus ater ater*. *Animal Behaviour*, **36**, 1575–88.

Konishi, M. (1964). Effects of deafening on song development in two species of juncos. *Condor*, **66**, 85–102.

Konishi, M. (1965a). The role of auditory feedback in the control of vocalization in the white-crowned sparrow. *Zeitschrift für Tierpsychologie*, **22**, 770–83.

Konishi, M. (1965b). Effects of deafening on song development in American robins and black-headed grosbeaks. *Zeitschrift für Tierpsychologie*, **22**, 584–99.

Kroodsma, D. E. (1974). Song learning, dialects, and dispersal in the Bewick's Wren. *Zeitschrift für Tierpsychologie*, **35**, 352–80.

Kroodsma, D. E. (1984). Songs of the alder flycatcher (*Empidonax alnorum*) and willow flycatcher (*Empidonax traillii*) are innate. *Auk*, **101**, 13–24.

Kroodsma, D. E. (1986). Song types and their uses: development flexibility of the male blue-winged warbler. *Ethology*, **79**, 235–47.

Kroodsma, D. E. & Miller, E. H. (1982). *Acoustic Communication in Birds*. New York: Academic Press.

Lemon, R. E. (1975). How birds develop song dialects. *Condor*, **77**, 385–406.

Liberman, A. M., Harris, K. S., Hoffman, H. S. & Griffith, B. C. (1957). The discrimination of speech sounds within and across phoneme boundaries. *Journal of Experimental Psychology*, **54**, 358–68.

Lien, M. R. (1978). Song variation in a population of chestnut-sided warblers (*Dendroica pennsylvanica*): its nature and suggested significance. *Canadian Journal of Zoology*, **56**, 1266–83.

Lorenz, K. (1965). *Evolution and Modification of Behaviour*. Chicago: University of Chicago Press.

Marler, P. (1959). Developments in the study of animal communication. In *Darwin's Biological Work*, ed. P. R. Bell, pp. 150–206, 329–35. Cambridge: Cambridge University Press.

Marler, P. (1960). Bird songs and mate selection. In *Animal Sounds and Communication*, ed. W. N. Tavolga, pp. 348–67. A.I.B.S. Symposium Proceedings.

Marler, P. (1970). A comparative approach to vocal learning: Song development in white-crowned sparrows. *Journal of Comparative and Physiological Psychology Monographs*, **71**, 1–25.

Marler, P. (1976). Sensory templates in species-specific behavior. In *Simpler Networks and Behavior*, ed. J. Fentress, pp. 314–29. Sunderland, Mass.: Sinauer.

Marler, P. (1984). Song learning: innate species differences in the learning process. In *The Biology of Learning*, ed. P. Marler and H. S. Terrace, pp. 289–309. New York: Springer-Verlag.

Marler, P. (1987). Sensitive periods and the role of specific and general sensory stimulation in birdsong learning. In *Imprinting and Cortical Plasticity*, ed. J. P. Rauschecker and P. Marler, pp. 99–135. New York: Wiley.

Marler, P., Dooling, R. J. & Zoloth, S. (1980). Comparative perspectives on ethology and perceptual development. In *The Comparative Method in Psychology: Ethological, Developmental and Cross-cultural Viewpoints*, ed. M. Bornstein, pp. 189–230. Hillsdale, NJ: Erlbaum.

Marler, P., Konishi, M., Lutjen, A. & Waser, M. S. (1973). Effects of continuous noise on avian bearing and vocal development. *Proceedings of the National Academy of Science (USA)*, **70**, 1293–396.

Marler, P., Mundinger, P., Waser, M. S. & Lutjen, A. (1972). Effects of acoustical stimulation and deprivation on song development in red-winged blackbirds (*Agelaius phoeniceus*). *Animal Behaviour*, **20**, 586–606.

Marler, P. & Peters, S. (1980). Birdsong and speech: Evidence for special processing. In *Perspective on the Study of Speech*, ed. P. Eimas and J. Miller, pp. 75–112. Hillsdale, NJ: Erlbaum.

Marler, P. & Peters, S. (1982a). Structural changes in song ontogeny in the swamp sparrow *Melospiza georgiana*. *Auk*, **99**, 446–58.

Marler, P. & Peters, S. (1982b). Developmental overproduction and selective attrition: new processes in the epigenesis of birdsong. *Developmental Psychobiology*, **15**, 369–78.

Marler, P. & Peters, S. (1989). Species differences in auditory responsiveness in early vocal learning. In *The Comparative Psychology of Audition: Perceiving Complex Sounds*, ed. R. Dooling & S. Hulse, pp. 243–73. Hillsdale, NJ: Erlbaum.

Marler, P., Peters, S., Ball, G. F., Dufty, A. M. Jr, Wingfield, J. C. (1988). The role of sex steroids in the acquisition and production of birdsong. *Nature*, **336**, 770–2.

Marler, P. & Pickert, R. (1984). Species-universal microstructure in the learned song of the swamp sparrow (*Melospiza georgiana*). *Animal Behavior*, **32**, 673–89.

Marler, P. & Sherman, V. (1983). Song structure without auditory feedback: Emendations of the auditory template hypothesis. *Journal of Neuroscience*, **3**, 517–31.

Marler, P. & Sherman, V. (1985). Innate differences in singing behaviour in sparrows reared in isolation from adult conspecific song. *Animal Behavior*, **33**, 57–71.

Marler, P. & Tamura, M. (1964). Culturally transmitted patterns of vocal behavior in sparrows. *Science*, **146**, 1483–6.

Marler, P. & Waser, M. S. (1977). The role of auditory feedback in canary song development. *Journal of Comparative and Physiological Psychology*, **91**, 8–16.

Maynard-Smith, J., Burian, R., Kauffman, S., Alberch, P., Campbell, J., Goodwin, B., Lande, R., Raup, D. & Wolpert, L. (1985). Developmental constraint and evolution. *Quarterly Review of Biology*, **60**, 265–87.

McGregor, P. K. & Thompson, D. B. A. (1988). Constancy and change in local dialects of the Corn Bunting. *Ornis Scandinavica*, **19**, 153–9.

Mundinger, P. C. (1982). Microgeographic and macrogeographic variation in acquired vocalizations in birds. In *Acoustic Communication of Birds, Vol. 2*, ed. D. E. Kroodsma and E. H. Miller, pp. 147–208. New York: Academic Press.

Nelson, D. A. & Marler, P. (1989). Categorical perception of a natural stimulus continuum: birdsong. *Science*, **244**, 976–8.

Nice, M. M. (1943). Studies in the life history of the song sparrow II. The behavior of the song sparrow and other passerines. *Transcripts of the Linnaeus Society, NY*, **6**, 1–238.

Nordeen, K. W., Marler, P. & Nordeen, E. J. (1989). Addition of song-related neurons in swamp sparrows coincides with memorization, not production of learned songs. *Journal of Neurobiology*, **20**, 651–61.

Nottebohm, F. (1966). The role of sensory feedback in the development of avian vocalizations. Ph.D. thesis, University of California, Berkeley

Nottebohm, F. (1968). Auditory experience and song development in the chaffinch (*Fringilla coelebs*). *Ibis*, **110**, 549–68.

Nottebohm, F. (1972). Neural lateralization of vocal control in a passerine bird. II. Subsong, calls and a theory of vocal learning. *Journal of Experimental Zoology* (1979), 35–49.

Nowicki, S. & Marler, P. (1988). How do birds sing? *Music Perception*, **5**, 391–426.

Okanoya, K. & Dooling, R. J. (1988a). Obtaining acoustic similarity measures from animals: A method for species comparisons. *Journal of the Acoustic Society of America*, **83**, 1690–3.

Payne, R. B. (1985). Behavioral continuity and change in local song population of village indigobirds *Vidua chalybeata*. *Zeitschrift für Tierpsychologie*, **70**, 1–44.

Pepperberg, I. M. (1988). The importance of social interaction and observation in the acquisition of communicative competence: possible parallels between avian and human learning. In *Social Learning: A Comparative Approach*, ed. T. T. Zentall and B. G. Galef, Jr, pp. 279–99. Hillsdale, NJ: Erlbaum.

Price, P. H. (1979). Developmental determinants of structure in zebra finch song. *Journal of Comparative and Physiological Psychology*, **93**, 260–77.

Pringle, J. W. S. (1951). On the parallel between learning and evolution. *Behaviour*, **3**, 174–215.

Rauschecker, J. P. (1987). What signals are responsible for synaptic changes in cortical plasticity? In *Imprinting and Cortical Plasticity: Comparative Aspects of Sensitive Periods*, ed. J. P. Rauschecker and P. Marler, pp. 193–220. New York: John Wiley.

Richards, D. (1981). Alerting and message components in songs of rufous-sided towhees. *Behaviour*, **76**, 223–49.

Sinnott, J. M. (1984). Modes of perceiving and processing information in birdsong. In *Categorical Perception*, ed. S. Harnad. New York: Cambridge University Press.

Stamps, J. A. (1990). Why evolutionary issues are reviving interest in proximate behavioral mechanisms. *American Zoologist* (in press).

Stearns, S. C. (1986). Natural selection and fitness; adaptation and constraint. In *Patterns and Processes in the History of Life*, ed. D. M. Raup and D. Jablonski, pp. 23–44. New York: Springer-Verlag.

West, M. J. & King, A. P. (1988). Female visual displays affect the development of male song in the cowbird. *Nature*, **334**, 244–6.

Commentary

— 1 —

Pat Bateson may have acted improperly in inviting me to comment on the chapters in this volume, but I am delighted that he has done so for at least three reasons. For one thing, the rose-tinted spectacles through which the contributors sometimes perceive my bumbling efforts require a corrective lens. Another is that it provides me with an opportunity to make clear the debts that, in various ways, I owe to them. And third, I have been fortunate in that my most active research years coincided with four decades of exciting growth in the behavioural sciences, and this is an opportunity to hint at some of the interweaving influences that have operated amongst a loosely defined group of colleagues.

Developmental issues enter into nearly all the chapters in this book, but the chapters by Pat Bateson and Peter Marler focus specifically on the problems of development. And both stem indirectly from the work of my own mentor, W. H. Thorpe (see Hinde, 1987). As the result of his work on insects, Bill Thorpe (1956) saw that understanding the relations between 'learning and instinct' was one of the crucial problems for the student of behaviour. Believing that birds with their stereotyped movement patterns and considerable learning capacities were ideal subjects for this enterprise, he established the 'Ornithological Field Station' (later Sub-Department of Animal Behaviour) at Madingley. I was fortunate to be involved in its beginnings. In the early years, Bill Thorpe initiated three main programmes of work. Studies of why some birds can learn to pull up food on the end of a piece of string, while others cannot, were taken up and extended by Vince (1961). The problem of imprinting, initiated by the writings of Konrad Lorenz, was tackled by Thorpe with moorhens and coots. What Bill really liked to do was to have moorhens follow him across the field in Lorenzian fashion. My role was to start some experiments, but they were almost unbelievably crude. I did a little work with chickens, but when Pat Bateson took over he carried out some really carefully designed experiments which met world-wide standards in control and conceptual sophistication (e.g. Bateson, 1964). From there he has extended his work in three directions: in collaboration with Horn and others to neurophysiological studies (see Chapter 5), to studies of mate choice and to computer modelling, as here. But his central concern has been the nature of development and how the processes involved could be conceptualised. This has been really to my benefit, because we have now been exchanging ideas for about thirty years. In addition, for 23 years he carried the administrative load of the Sub-Department while I got on with what interested me as the Honorary Director of the Medical Research Council Unit within his laboratory.

The third line of research that Thorpe initiated, and the one into which he put most of his energies, was song-learning. I used to have to cycle out to Madingley before dawn to help hand-rear chaffinches for him, but otherwise I played a minor part in that work. Very early on Peter Marler, already a PhD in Botany, came to do a PhD in Animal Behaviour. He studied the field behaviour of chaffinches while I studied them in aviaries and, both of us still insecure in our careers, we used to have fierce arguments on such important topics as whether the 'lop-sided wings-drooped posture' was or was not a suitable name for a particular courtship posture. Peter Marler then became involved in the song-learning work and, as his chapter demonstrates, he has pursued it with unqualified success ever since. His work, in turn, had led to important advances in neurophysiology and other fields (Nottebohm, e.g. 1980; Konishi, e.g. 1987).

No two chapters could demonstrate more convincingly the apparent complexity of behavioural development. Such is the progress that has been made, that it is now almost unbelievable that twenty-five years ago it was necessary to warn of the dangers of a simple dichotomy of behaviour – though, as Bateson emphasises (Chapter 2), it is still easy to fall into bad ways. And even the dichotomy of sources of differences, which both Bateson and Marler agree has been methodologically fertile, must be handled with care. Bateson cites the way in which identical twins reared together come to differ from each other more than do identical twins reared apart. Apparently, although each has virtually the same environment which includes a genetically identical twin, they seek out ways to differentiate themselves from each other. Presumably this builds on small differences produced by differential parental treatment or chance environmental perturbations. Another example comes from the apparent existence of innovation in song development, as described by Marler. Thorpe (1961) had earlier shown that groups of chaffinches reared together but in isolation from chaffinch song produced song patterns similar amongst group members but differing between groups. That is perhaps not so surprising: the individuals would have differed genetically both within and between groups, and song development was not channelled by an input of the species-characteristic song. But consider a thought experiment: if we could rear genetically identical individuals in identical acoustically isolated environments, would they 'invent' different song patterns? In the past, we would have said no – and if they did, fall back on saying that the environments can't have been absolutely identical, *really*.

In any case, Marler's chapter brings up again an issue raised in Section II – the importance of individual differences. Here, however, he is able to use the nature of the differences *between* individuals to produce generalisations about development *across* individuals.

Both chapters raise a further issue that is central to the ethological approach – the need both to separate questions of causation, development, function and evolution, and to recognise their interfertility. As has often been said, it was unfortunate that E. O. Wilson's *Sociobiology* (1975) downgraded causal and developmental questions. The power of his approach and the questions it raised diverted ethologists from these problems – but it is now becoming apparent that the functional problems posed by Wilson and Trivers cannot be solved without causal and developmental understanding. Here Bateson emphasises how functional considerations can assist developmental analysis, and Marler how causal analysis can contribute to evolutionary studies.

All in all, it is an exciting time for developmental studies. Animal research is producing new insights into the interaction between genetic and environmental factors in development, and human twin and adoption studies are contributing to the same issues from a different direction (e.g. Plomin & de Fries, 1983; Scarr & Kidd, 1983). Animal studies are throwing light on the nature of, diversity of and constraints on learning processes, and of the diversity of factors operating. Studies of human learning are also emphasising the diversity of learning processes (Rozin, 1976), and the manner in which both learning and cognitive processes are influenced by circumstances (Donaldson 1978; Carraher, Carraher & Schliemann, 1985). Both animal and human studies are emphasising the role of social factors in development (Vygotsky, 1934; Bowlby, 1969). The value and limitations of the concept of sensitive periods have been studied in a wide range of species (Bateson & Hinde, 1987). Modelling techniques are being used to aid in understanding the interactions between the diverse factors operating in development (Bateson, Chapter 2). And we may hope soon to see an integration between the understanding of continuities and discontinuities in development reached by both animal and human studies (Hinde & Bateson, 1984; Rutter, 1985), and incorporation of recent work on 'risk' and 'protective' factors and on 'turning points' in development (e.g. Garmezy & Rutter, 1983; Rutter, 1988 and Chapter 14) into an overall understanding of behavioural development.

References

Bateson, P. (1964). Effects of similarity between rearing and testing conditions on childs' following and avoidance responses. *Journal of Comparative and Physiological Psychology*, **57**, 100–3.

Bateson, P. & Hinde, R. A. (1987). Developmental changes in sensitivity to experience. In *Sensitive Periods in Development*, ed. M. H. Bornstein. Hillsdale, NJ: Erlbaum.

Bowlby, J. (1969). *Attachment and Loss, Vol. 1. Attachment.* London: Hogarth.

Carraher, T. N., Carraher, D. W. & Schliemann, A. D. (1985). Mathematics in the streets and in the schools. *British Journal of Developmental Psychology*, **3**, 21–9.

Donaldson, M. (1978). *Children's Minds.* London: Fontana.

Garmezy, N. & Rutter, M. (ed.) (1983). *Stress, Coping and Development in Children.* New York: McGraw Hill.

Hinde, R. A. (1987). William Homan Thorpe. *Biographical Memoirs of Fellows of the Royal Society, 33.*

Hinde, R. A. & Bateson, P. (1984). Discontinuities versus continuities in behavioural development and the neglect of process. *International Journal of Behavioural Development*, **7**, 129–43.

Konishi, M. (1987). Developmental plasticity in the auditory system. In *Imprinting and Cortical Plasticity*, ed. J. P. Rauscheker and J. Marler. New York: Wiley.

Nottebohm, F. (1980). Brain pathways for vocal learning in birds: a review of the first 10 years. *Progress of Psychobiology and Physiological Psychology*, **9**, 85–124.

Plomin, R. & de Fries, B. C. (1983). The Colorado adoption project. *Child Development*, **54**, 276–89.

Rozin, P. (1976). The evolution of intelligence and access to the cognitive unconscious. In *Progress in Psychobiology and Physiological Psychology*, 6, ed. J. R. Sprague and A. N. Epstein. New York: Academic Press.

Rutter, M. (1985). Continuities and discontinuities from infancy. In *Handbook of Life and Development*, ed. J. Osofsky. New York: Wiley.

Rutter, M. (ed.) (1988). *Studies of Psychosocial Risk.* Cambridge: Cambridge University Press.

Scarr, S. & Kidd, K. K. (1983). Developmental behaviour genetics. In *Mussen Handbook of Child Psychology, Vol. II*, ed. J. J. Campos and M. M. Haith. New York: Wiley.

Thorpe, W. H. (1956). *Learning and Instinct in Animals.* London: Methuen.

Thorpe, W. H. (1961). *Bird Song.* Cambridge: Cambridge University Press.

Vince, M. A. (1961). Development changes in learning capacity. In *Current Problems in Animal Behaviour*, ed. O. L. Zangwill and W. H. Thorpe. Cambridge: Cambridge University Press.

Vygotsky, L. S. (1934). *Thought and Language.* Cambridge, Mass: MIT Press.

Wilson, E. O. (1975). *Sociobiology.* Cambridge, Mass: Harvard University Press.

R.A.H.

III
Neural and endocrine aspects of behaviour

—4—

Analytical ethology and synthetic neuroscience

John C. Fentress

Overview

As Robert Hinde has often reminded us, appreciation for diversity is the hall-mark of ethological research. This diversity is reflected not only in patterns of behavioural organisation for different species, but also in different classes of action, levels and time frames of organisation, and contexts of expression. The search for generalisations based explicitly upon this diversity is a risky but also an exciting and important challenge. Perhaps the most fundamental issue is how we, as investigators, choose to divide our observations into manageable properties in conjunction with our search for the rules by which these properties are connected in space and in time. There are no universally acceptable guidelines. One approach is to employ complementary descriptive, analytical, and synthetic perspectives, and to compare the pictures that these perspectives reveal. In this way transformations in our databases can be related explicitly to the measures we make (Fentress, 1990a).

In addition to a sensitivity towards species (and individual) diversity, two complementary temporal perspectives have marked Robert Hinde's personal research on the development and integration of behaviour. Within these perspectives Robert Hinde has sought to clarify changes in profiles and principles that occur when one crosses time frames as well as levels of organisation. He has taught many of us that our empirical and conceptual divisions in patterns of behaviour are often best treated as heuristics for deeper understanding, not truth in themselves (Fentress, 1990a).

Robert Hinde has always been a champion of hard data, but he has also recognised the overriding importance of focusing upon difficult issues:

...the temptation to pursue a line of research just because it yields hard data, even though those data are trivial and unlikely to lead anywhere new, must be resisted

(Hinde, 1979, p. 6).

Clearly, the search for links between ethology and neuroscience has much to gain from sensitivities to these issues. The reverberating balance between analysis and synthesis that has marked Robert Hinde's own career is an important guide.

I use the term synthetic neuroscience in this context. Analytical ethology is the complement, stressing as it does the need to refine our observations of behaviour into ever finer units, without losing touch with the broader contexts within which these abstracted units are expressed. The issue is not just how we divide behaviour into finer and finer units for analysis, but also how we evaluate the collaborative expression among these abstracted units – at whatever level they are defined initially.

In this essay I shall explore diverse and multilevelled data as they may contribute to the search for recurrent *themes* of organisation. The abstraction of themes is the precursor to the establishment of principles. The fundamental theme is that of dynamic balance among intrinsic and extrinsic properties *however* we define any given behavioural or neural system. In the study of behaviour as well as neuroscience the investigator must typically deal with interlocking *networks* of organisational processes, rather than being satisfied with simple linear conceptualisations. Viewed in this way, the theme of interactive/self-organising systems (ISO; cf. Fentress, 1976a) exhibits often surprising parallels across problems of neurobehavioural integration and its development.

Issues

The gaps in our understanding between basic neuronal operations and even simple forms of behaviour are intimidating. To cite a single example, several decades of careful research on invertebrate 'pattern generators' has failed to provide a complete element by element explanation for rhythm production at the intact organism level (Selverston, 1980; Pearson, 1987). Given such circumstances, it is not surprising that a major emphasis in current neuroscience is toward progressive reductionism. We often understand machines best by taking them apart (Kandel & Schwartz, 1985). Yet, this can lead to an abandonment of behavioural relevance if contextual factors are ignored or controlled into oblivion, rather than being studied directly.

The 'simpler networks' approach (Fentress, 1976b; Selverston, 1985; Carew & Kelley, 1989) to the study of nervous systems and behaviour has led to a number of important model systems. Three points deserve emphasis, however. First, even these 'simpler' networks generate properties that still escape definitive analysis (Selverston, 1985). Secondly, many systems are studied in relative isolation, which precludes logical extrapolations to their operation in the intact organism (e.g. Harris-Warwick & Johnson, 1989). Thirdly, analogies to other neural networks can obscure the specialised properties of network diversity.

My argument in this essay is that unidirectional reductionism will never provide all the answers. Rather, investigators must adopt the three-pronged approach of (i) detailed evaluation of performance properties at the selected level of analysis, (ii) search for rules of connection with lower levels of analysis, *and* (iii) search for rules of connection with higher levels of organisation. Rules of reciprocity, complementarity, and transformation (to borrow from Robert Hinde's terminology) can be clarified only in this way. Equally important, generalisations must be derived from a prior appreciation for diversity in detail across levels, animals, behavioural forms, and functions. This is why the task is intimidating. Robert Hinde's frequent warning that investigators operate from a stance of humility in the face of diversity is critical.

Often, however, simplifying models are needed to help us keep our thoughts clear. To quote again from Robert Hinde:

Between the incredible complexity of patterns of neural firing and behaviour we need synthesizing variables such as motivation: prediction via all the physiological intermediaries would be hopelessly cumbersome   (Hinde, 1979, p. 34).

The challenge to future research is how to extrapolate important principles of operation that build upon diversity and the necessary simplifications that our model systems demand.

The burgeoning field of *neuroethology* (e.g. Fentress, 1976b; Guthrie, 1980; Ewert, 1980; Ewert, Capranica & Ingle, 1983; Camhi, 1984; Hoyle, 1984; Rauschecker & Marler, 1987; Guthrie, 1988) has provided an important counter to unilateral reductionism. Here I merely state a half dozen obvious contributions (see also, Fentress, 1983a, 1986).

1. Acceptance of the four cornerstones of ethological research: evolution, development, proximal causation, and function.
2. The employment of complex natural stimuli, rather than artificially restricted stimuli.
3. Evaluation of full patterns of behavioural performance in response to these stimuli plus central patterning mechanisms.
4. Examination of modulatory (e.g. 'motivational') as well as eliciting and pattern generating events.
5. Appreciation for species diversity and the importance of ecological sensitivity as well as developmental analyses in the study of diversity.

6. Examination of intra- and interspecific exchanges between animals as a complement to understanding the behaviour of individuals (e.g. social behaviour, predator–prey relations).

Most neuroethologists begin their investigations from a naturalist's fascination with the diversity of animal behaviour. They select species that offer not only special problems, but special insights into the search for more general principles of neurobehavioural organisation. They also combine the traditional ethological emphases upon description, classification, analysis and (tentative) synthesis of neurobehavioural properties and their rules of coherent expression. There are no grand theories, nor are any promised in the near future (Fentress, 1976a, 1986; Camhi, 1984). However, there are issues and themes relevant to future inquiries (for a list that nicely complements the above, see Bateson, 1988). It is these that I concentrate upon here. I do this in the sense of exploration, not final solution.

The bidirectional perspective

A common problem with strict unidirectional 'reductionistic' references to behaviour is that the richness and diversity of behavioural phenomena are not only controlled, but subsequently ignored. Mechanisms for non-existing phenomena are not interesting, however. The ethologist has much to offer here by dissecting natural streams of expression into component properties, and then evaluating how these properties cohere in the production of higher-order patterns. The point may seem obvious, but it is often ignored.

The derivative but less obvious position I shall advocate is that it can often be valuable to view the coherences across levels of inquiry as being mutually dependent (rather than unidirectional). I shall go further, and suggest that properties of 'pieces' in behaviour (and/or nervous systems) are in part *dictated* by the 'relations' that occur among these pieces in space and time (Figure 1). In brief, simple atomism in neuroscience will work no better than has simple atomism in chemistry and physics (Bohm, 1980).

This is the essence of what I seek to capture in the phrase, 'synthetic neuroscience'. The term synthetic here does not mean artificial at all, but quite the opposite. Synthetic neuroscience may be the only neuroscience that can address the questions of behavioural organisation that have fascinated ethologists for so many years (cf. the need for an 'integrative reduction' in cognitive neuroscience, as discussed in Sejnowski & Churchland, 1989).

Ethologists stress that many of the fundamental separations and interconnections relevant to an appreciation of nervous system operations can be ascertained only through behavioural analysis. The basic ethological strategy of looking at *components in context* provides an important guideline for neurobiological research as well. Behavioural coherences occur over time,

80

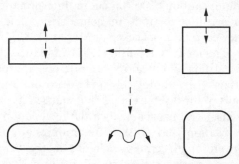

Figure 1. The analysis of neurobehavioural systems involves the abstraction of properties or 'units', which then must be evaluated for their connections to 'extrinsic' factors, including possible connections to other 'units' (top row). These abstracted 'units' may change their properties in time, partially through mutual interactions, which can in turn change subsequent rules of relation among the abstracted properties (bottom row). *Because of such interlocking dynamics in behavioural neuroscience, the very distinction between 'units' and their relations is often difficult to evaluate precisely.*

involve often changing relations among (and perhaps even properties within) parts, and by definition 'cross and re-cross' levels of organisation (to borrow a favourite phrase from Robert Hinde).

As emphasised by Mayr (1976), among others, evolution has some of its most direct consequences in animals upon behavioural phenotypes. It is often less important *how* animals achieve behavioural coherence in terms of particular machinery than *that* they achieve this coherence. This immediately alerts us to the likelihood that nervous system operations are constrained at complementary levels. There is no reason, other than tradition, to view one level of constraint as 'more fundamental' than another. Flexible means towards a common goal (Hinde & Stevenson, 1969) are commonplace in behaviour, and clearly offer important insights into nodes of flexibility and constraint of underlying nervous system operations. Further, divergent species may face similar problems of design that are reflected in analogous patterns of control (Lorenz, 1981). As illustration, the fine control of muscle tension in arthropods and mammals is achieved through convergent properties of feedback, although the details of underlying neural machinery are very different (Kennedy, 1976). It is possible, therefore, that behavioural *principles* can be found that represent common design problems and thus can tell us what underlying circuits must *do* (but not precisely how they do what they must do).

I think that careful argument by analogy can be helpful in many cases, as long as appropriate cautions are taken in interpretation. Comparative parallels between sensitive periods in neuroscience and behaviour have recently been reviewed by Rauschecker & Marler (1987), with considerable success. Similarly, Changeux & Konishi (1987) and Horn (1985) have shown how problems of learning and memory can often be approached with profit through a marriage of ethological and neurobiological perspectives. Although the details of the diverse studies summarised in these volumes vary widely, one can sense a rapproachment in the focus upon *themes* and even *principles* of organisation that cross more traditionally defined fields. Of course, many conventionally employed terms in the behavioural sciences (attention, learning, motivation, etc.) have long suggested a certain commonality in theme even though the details in specific cases may vary widely. The delicate task of comparative and multilevelled work is to highlight *both* similarities and differences as these are revealed through explicitly defined perspectives and measures (cf. Bohm, 1980).

One possibility that is currently generating much interest in many branches of natural science is that certain principles of order are reiterated (with transformations that can be defined) at complementary levels. The theory of fractals, literature on 'self-organising systems', synergetics, and bifurcation theory (e.g. reviews in Kugler & Turvey, 1987; Yates, 1987) are cases in point. It is premature to judge the likely success of such endeavours. However, they do provide some reason to seek possible conceptual parallels between Robert Hinde's recent 'higher-order' work on human social interactions/relationships and formally similar 'lower-order' problems that one encounters at the interface between ethology and neuroscience. In each case, for example, individual properties contribute to system profiles that may in turn constrain the performance of individuals. Let me emphasise that I view my task here as suggesting avenues for exploration, not final answers.

I have argued previously (Fentress, 1984; Fentress & McLeod, 1986) that the *conceptual* polarities of relative continuity–discontinuity (discreteness, specificity, etc.) and relative change–stability (process models versus structure models) recur across a wide range of time frames and levels of inquiry (see also chapters and editorial comments in Fentress, 1976a, e.g. Ch. 1). They can be usefully tackled, I believe, by focusing upon problems of *dynamic pattern formation*, where underlying organisational properties tread the delicate balance between tendencies toward self-organisation and contextual sensitivity. Robert Hinde's concerns with the dynamic, relational and multilayered properties of human social behaviour can in this abstract sense be reflected upon more simple patterns of animal action. This still ill-defined map leads toward the goals I explore here.

Diversity and the misuse of reified behavioural constructs

The insistence upon clear separation between working 'process' based constructs and too rigidly defined 'items' of behaviour has been a hallmark of Robert Hinde's own multiplexed approach to issues of behavioural organisation. I agree fully with him that it is all too easy, and common, for workers to mistake their words for things, and to mistake these abstracted 'things' at the behavioural level for circumscribed 'entities' (e.g. 'neural centres') at the biological level. Unfortunately, many otherwise promising forays into links between behavioural and neurobiological levels of organisation suffer from this *deficit of fallacious reification*. The problem becomes amplified when outdated approaches to behavioural organization are extrapolated in the guise of multidisciplinary research. 'Ethology has progressed' (Hinde, 1984, p. 391).

Robert Hinde responded, correctly I believe, to a previous review of 'neuroethology' (Hoyle, 1984) in these terms:

In attempting to understand the diverse phenomena of the living world, scientists must classify them into manageable groups, and they may use explanatory concepts whose utility subsequently turns out to be limited to a small range of phenomena or to a particular level of analysis. The progress of scientific understanding depends upon using these categories and concepts judiciously, valuing the advances they make possible, while at the same time recognizing their limitations

(Hinde, 1984, p. 391; emphasis in the original)

Our methods of description and classification, and our interpretation of these methods, largely dictate our subsequent approaches to mechanism, as well as to more broadly defined approaches to synthesis. A number of concrete examples can be cited, from which I select a small number here.

Behavioural units

Units of behaviour as commonly used (cf. Gallistel, 1980; Fentress, 1984) are in my view a sometimes convenient fiction (cf. Sherrington, 1906, on the concept of reflex). 'Units' of behaviour are like 'unitary drives' (Hinde, 1959) in at least three basic senses. First, almost all, if not all, behavioural units that we abstract contain heterogeneous properties that reveal themselves upon detailed analysis. Categories such as *fighting behaviour* and *grooming behaviour* are obviously useful when we desire to summarise broad functional end points in expression and the general routes through which these end points are expressed. However, finer dissections of the 'behavioural stream' almost inevitably reveal a heterogeneity of underlying processes. Robert Hinde's (Hinde & Steel, 1966; cf. Hinde & Stevenson, 1969) research on the components of nest-building behaviour in canaries is an obvious case

83

in point. Gathering, carrying and building in canaries are amongst those activities that indicate clearly the need to separate certain activity phases from others. Thus, any unitary neurobiological model of canary nest-building is doomed to failure.

There are two more subtle points in the quest for neurobehavioural units, to which I shall return later. The first of these is that our abstracted 'units' can change their internal properties as a function of the broader contexts within which they operate (cf. Figure 1). They can be *interdependent* rather than simply interactive. To the extent that this is true, the clear implication follows that abstracted 'pieces' in behaviour (or nervous system operations) are not necessarily more fundamental than are the coherences among these pieces. I think this abstraction echoes, in potentially important 'neuro-ethological' ways, Robert Hinde's recent research indicating that social interactions and relationships among people may not only emerge from activities defined at the individual level, but also reflect basic higher-order coherences that would otherwise be missed altogether.

The second point is that rules of relation can often be more 'simple' (regular) than are the operations of individually defined contributors to the overall relations examined. The idea is not a new one at all. For example, Lashley (1951) proposed his doctrine of 'motor equivalence' on the premise that animals and people often employ variable means toward the attainment of a singularly defined goal (such as when we make many mutually compensatory movements of the arms and head to ensure that the food on our fork is placed within our mouths and not our ears!). While the ideas of motor equivalence and its derivatives are obviously not new, we still do not have effective means for evaluating the multilevelled transformations that occur between constancy of end product and the often variable means by which this end product is produced (cf. Bernstein, 1987).

[*Here I come to the primary point of the present exercise. I believe strongly that common* conceptual problems *reiterate themselves across essentially* all *of the multiplexed and multilevelled inquiries Robert Hinde has pursued over his career. While I accept Robert Hinde's appreciation of diversity in nature as we observe it directly, I suspect he can also appreciate that individual human brains tend to carve up the world in similar ways that we can at present monitor only much more indirectly. I thus have no sense of embarrassment at all in suggesting that even Robert Hinde's recent insights into human social interactions and relationships might carry a more abstract message into the behavioural neurosciences.*]

Limitations to inference based upon classical ethological constructs

One of the strengths of early ethological work was the abstraction of manageable properties of behaviour and its control (Lorenz, 1950; Tinbergen, 1951). Perhaps foremost among these concepts was the 'fixed action pattern'. As Barlow (1977) noted in a detailed review, extrapolation of this concept took attention away from 'modal' properties around which potentially important variations in performance can be distributed. Precisely where one draws the line between 'modal action patterns' and actions with even greater variations is a moot point. It was also not always clear in many early studies whether concerns about variation were confined to an individual or distributed across individuals, dependent upon broader contexts of expression (such as in the co-articulation of human speech; Liberman, 1970; cf. Fentress, 1983a), or which properties of movement (such as amplitude, timing, or force) showed greater or lesser variation. Most importantly, there are often *relational invariants* among action properties that in themselves vary (cf. Bernstein, 1967; Golani, 1976). Many movement properties can be mutually compensatory, and even where the overt form of movement appears invariant, underlying neural and muscular events can be distributed and ordered differently between one expression and another.

Hoyle (1964), one of the innovative pioneers of 'neuroethology' (along with Bullock, Ewert, Griffin, Huber, Roeder, Wilson – and others), early demonstrated that in insect (locust) locomotion regular stepping movements often are *not* accompanied by 'fixed' patterns of electrical activity in the motor neurons. Huber (1983) has provided a masterly review of similar complexities (indeed, mysteries) in 'insect neuroethology'. Insects can often execute different 'programs simultaneously, for instance, grooming the antennae or feeding while singing … and even synchronize motor programs, such as stridulation and ventilation' (Huber, 1983, p. 93). Moreover, Huber emphasises that the same set of muscles and motor neurons can often be used for different movements (e.g. flight and wing stridulation in crickets), and that there are occasions where two 'motor programs' are incompletely separate (such as in transitions between hindleg stridulation and wing stridulation). Davis (1976) has argued from analogous examples in the sea slug *Pleurobranchia* that excessive compartmentalisation in our *thinking* about motor packages can prevent rather than enhance our appreciation of adjustments that are made by neuronal networks within broader expressive contexts.

Similar examples in diverse vertebrate species are commonplace (Fentress, 1984, 1990a, b; Fentress & McLeod, 1986; Grillner *et al.*, 1986; Davis, Jacobs & Schoenfeld, 1989). To cite an example related to the short-term patterning of behaviour, Stein, Mortin & Robertson (1986) have demonstrated that scratch reflexes in spinal turtles can undergo a variety of 'blends' which in turn reveal complex mixes of underlying neural circuit properties. With respect to ontogeny, Bekoff (1986) has provided evidence that the same neural networks may be involved in quite different patterns of movement in the egg and after hatching. Single networks can be both flexible and 'multifunctional'.

While many other examples could be cited, two central points emerge. First, the early ethological construct of fixed action patterns (FAP) was, and remains, a valuable heuristic. This is true *if*, to echo Robert Hinde's (1984) caution, the FAP construct is not used to imply an absolute distinction that is then extrapolated in its implications (e.g. to origins and control). Second, part of the problem has been the frequent tendency of earlier research workers to isolate properties of behavioural expression, and then fail to ask how the isolated properties might change when viewed in the broader context of the intact organism. A third point stressed by many current cognitive psychologists (e.g. Posner, 1978; Keele & Ivry, 1987) is that by focusing upon 'acts' as basic units, the possibility that there are operations that are shared amongst these 'acts' can be obscured (Figure 2). Thus, Keele & Ivry (1987) have shown that in human subjects cerebellar timing mechanisms are shared among motor performance properties and temporal perception. Similarly, Berridge, Fentress & Parr (1987) have reported evidence for timing mechanisms that can be shared by rodent grooming actions that differ greatly in their form.

Perhaps one should add the obvious caution that in a brief survey which touches upon insects, marine molluscs, and human performance, critical species differences may appear to be thrown under the proverbial academic rug. However, it is the *issue* of the importance of contextual factors in performance to the understanding of processes of control that I seek to emphasise here. That *issue* of 'acts' versus 'rules' or 'operations' is one that not only can, but must, be explored in greater depth, whatever the species.

Let us look at the complementary issue of excessive extrapolation in somewhat more detail. To many early ethologists, 'fixed action patterns' *necessarily* implied 'certainly programmed', which in turn *necessarily* implied 'genetically programmed'. One of the great achievements of ethology has been to move our investigations away from the sterile stance of reflexology in neuroscience and stimulus–response psychology. However, the enthusiasm with which many neurobiologists took up subsequent notions of necessary and sufficient 'command neurons/circuits' (Kupferman & Weiss, 1978), and 'central pattern generators' (reviewed by Selverston, 1980; plus papers in Barnes & Gladden, 1985; Selverston, 1985), has now proven to be a much too simple perspective. To cite but one example here, Pearson (1987) has

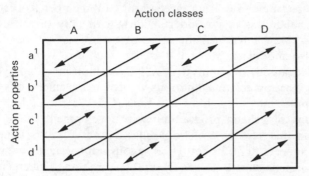

Figure 2. Categorisations by action classes (columns) and action properties (rows) can lead to orthogonal taxonomies. For any one set of observations, coherences among these criteria (represented by diagonal arrows) may be multiplicative and occur over variable numbers of taxonomic 'cells' (as indicated by arrow length). *The isolation of operations which both underlie a given act and also contribute to several acts can be important.*

reviewed data on both invertebrate and vertebrate species that indicate how the concept of isolated and invariant 'central motor programs' can reflect the isolated and invariant conditions under which neurophysiological investigations are conducted. When these circuits are evaluated at the intact organism level, and are thereby subjected to fluctuations in other circuit properties, their simplicity often disappears (for related review, see Harris-Warrick & Johnson, 1989).

Now this is a delicate point, and one that Robert Hinde (e.g. Hinde, 1970, 1984) has often cautioned us about, albeit in rather different contexts. It is akin to babies and bathwater (to take an analogy that fits more closely with Robert Hinde's current research interests). One does not want to revel in complexity for its own sake. Each of us needs to seek simplifications if we are not to get hopelessly bogged down. But we also need, from time to time, to remind ourselves that we have made these simplifications, and thus not reify or overgeneralise our initial concepts. There is a danger in being misunderstood by my neurobiological colleagues when I stress the contextual and variable properties of animal (not to mention, human) performance, and I hope to avoid that misunderstanding (cf. Berkinblitt, Feldman & Fukson, 1986, and Ewert, 1987, for recent related reviews). The late D. O. Hebb (an unabashed admirer of Robert Hinde's thinking) used to remind me often during his later years at Dalhousie that models and constructs are best designed when we can pick at them, and show their limitations.

Many other examples from the early ethological literature could be given.

One is that of the 'innate releasing mechanism'. I remember Robert Hinde telling me once that this is a wonderful idea, with only three flaws: the 'mechanism' is rarely innate (in the sense of 'preformed'), does not just release (can also modulate, etc.), and is not a unitary (not to mention neurologically localised) mechanism at all! Even molecular biologists are now beginning to appreciate limitations to isolated element by element analyses of complex integrative brain functions (Crick, 1979) and previously accepted notions of genetic programming in development (Stent, 1981). While I applaud this new sense of 'molecular humility' I also wonder if it would have been necessary if Robert Hinde's constant balancing between the analytic and synthetic aspects of behavioural research (cf. Tinbergen, 1963) had been appreciated earlier. There is great diversity in nature, as Robert Hinde has so often pointed out, but there is also the possibility of adopting critical scientific stances that can help us encompass this diversity. That is what a 'synthetic neuroscience' may help us accomplish.

To describe, and describe again

If one seeks a mechanism for a phenomenon, one must first define the phenomenon. Otherwise the very idea of mechanism becomes superfluous. In my view it has too often been the case in behavioural neurobiology that the very intricate issue of establishing appropriate, and alternative, behavioural taxonomies is ignored (Fentress, 1990a). Current ethology makes a tremendously important contribution in this regard. Not only is there a renewed insistence upon the explicit formulation about potentially alternate criteria for proper description and classification of behaviour, but in tandem one cannot help but appreciate the growing awareness that different perspectives yield different pictures. No one perspective is necessarily 'right' for all problems (cf. Bohm, 1980; Fentress, 1986, 1990a, b).

The important distinction between behavioural form and behavioural function (Hinde, 1970, 1984) is an obvious case in point. Actions that differ, often greatly, in their form may contribute to a common function, just as actions that are similar in their form may often contribute to different functions (Fentress, 1984, 1990a, b). The critical question for synthetic neuroscience is how one then takes the plethora of consistencies and variations to construct reasonable approaches to problems of behavioural control.

There clearly is no answer to this question at the present time. Therefore, it is useful to examine what different styles of description can reveal to us, and what they might obscure. The one stance to be avoided at all costs is that a single descriptive perspective can solve all problems. I am reminded here of the wonderfully civilised 'debate' between Richard Andrew and Robert

Hinde in a text on the analysis of communication in diverse species (Hinde, 1972). Richard Andrew, appropriately, focused upon the details of motor performance, while Robert Hinde, equally appropriately, focused upon the essential biological consequences of the often varied performance properties.

Categorisations of form 'versus' function of course represent an initial heuristic that can also obscure many subtleties as one crosses levels of inquiry. A simple movement profile, such as the swipe of a single paw, may be a statement of form at the initial behavioural level, but reveals the end product (consequence) of multiple neural and mechanical events as they operate within the constraints of an often variable environment (Bernstein, 1967).

Rodent grooming as illustration of issues

Much of my own research has been devoted to the organisation and control of rodent grooming as a mammalian behavioural assay for issues that I here lump under the heading of 'synthetic neuroscience'. As soon as one uses terms such as 'grooming' one is in danger of extrapolating from an often presumed function to more detailed suggestions of both form and control in motor performance. Clearly 'grooming' is a functional label, with diverse implications about control in different species, different individuals within a species, and even the same individual under different conditions (Fentress, 1972; Berridge & Fentress, 1986). Here the issue I wish to explore is how we can describe grooming from alternative, perspectives, including its expressive contexts. Later, I shall show how these alternative descriptive perspectives can yield different insights about mechanism (cf. recent multidisciplinary volume on grooming behaviour edited by Colbern & Gispen, 1988). No one of the descriptive perspectives can generate all of the insights we wish to achieve. The most fundamental conclusion from the descriptions is that grooming (as all actions in behaviour) represents a multilayered set of processes, each of which has a degree of separation from other processes but is also, to varying extents, responsive to the operation of these other processes.

Early explorations of 'interrupted ongoing behaviour'

I can trace many of the origins of this chapter to research I conducted as a student at Madingley, where Robert Hinde assisted Bill Thorpe through all phases of my DPhil studies. It was Robert Hinde who, in our very first Cambridge discussion, cautioned me about unitary behavioural labels that could obscure multiple meanings. (At that time I was tempted to link 'fear', 'timidity' and even 'domestication' as useful synonyms!). His advice was to take as complete records of ongoing behaviour in my voles (*Microtus agrestis* and *Clethrionomys britannicus*) as possible, to see how different classes of action fit together, and to evaluate changes in the animals' responses to experimental perturbations (e.g. a fake overhead moving predator) as a function of behavioural state. It became clear immediately that the voles were most likely to flee from rather than freeze in response to the overhead stimulus if they either were locomoting or *had been* locomoting shortly before the stimulus presentation. Never again did it seem reasonable to view behavioural 'causes' as producing their 'effects' outside the context of ongoing system states (cf. Wise, 1987, for state models in integrative neuroscience).

To this basic framework, Robert Hinde encouraged me to examine the separate and converging influences of multiple 'independent variables' (species, rearing conditions, ongoing behaviour, number of previous stimulus presentations, and so forth). It was in this way that I became fascinated by the observation that increases as well as decreases in apparently irrelevant grooming behaviour could occur as a systematic reflection of separate and combined qualitative, quantitative, and temporal factors. To account successfully for grooming and related actions it became necessary to untangle the 'nexus' of diverse causal relations (Fentress, 1968a, b). Component actions plus their individual control processes clearly lived in broader contexts.

Given ethological models at the time, some of my data were puzzling. It did not appear, for example, that all increases in grooming could be explained solely by means of *behavioural disinhibition*, although clearly at some level different classes of behaviour are mutually antagonistic. What the data did suggest as a supplementary consideration was that at moderate levels of activation, as well as during the early stages (warmup) of response to and subsequent recovery from events such as model predators, the probability, duration and even vigour of grooming movements could be enhanced. This suggested to me that both relatively non-specific (global) as well as specific (local) factors had to be taken into account. Further, the degree of specificity, as measured by the *integrated set of* incremental and decremental effects of stimulus presentations upon grooming, did not appear fixed but rather dynamically ordered along the broad dimension of 'effective stimulus intensity' (see Fentress, 1983b, for further discussion within the context of animal motivation). I thus began to wonder whether more dynamic and relational measures of behavioural control might be important to explore. I also became fascinated with lower-level descriptive patterns of movement coordination in actions such as rodent grooming. Perhaps similar organisational issues would repeat themselves at these lower levels.

Element chains and hierarchies

In our experience, all persons who observe rodent grooming sequences find it easy to dissect the 'behavioural stream' into component parts that are in turn related to one another over time by statistical rules of cohesion (Fentress, 1972; Fentress & Stilwell, 1973; Berridge *et al.*, 1987). Separations of face grooming from body grooming represent one obvious distinction based upon the orientation of individual grooming actions. Similarly, face grooming sequences can be subdivided into a number of subclasses, such as licking of the forepaws, low-amplitude movements around the mouth, higher-amplitude movements that cross the eyes or ears, and so forth (Fentress, 1972; Fentress & Stilwell, 1973; Berridge *et al.*, 1987).

These are multiplexed dissections, meaning that human observers often combine various attributes as forming natural categories (see discussions of categorical perception in Harnad, 1987). Once these perceptually defined action properties are dissected, the next question is how they relate to one another in time and across levels of expression, species, individual differences, etc.

One way to couch such questions formally is to ask how predictably a given abstracted action follows from its predecessors. Here an interesting and prevalent problem in ethology emerges, for often one's ability to predict subsequent actions is far greater than that revealed by formal quantitative rules expressed at a single level of inquiry (cf. Fentress, 1984). Clearly we, as behavioural investigators, often take into account factors that are not expressed in our formal models. This is especially true if we force our models into simple linear profiles.

One approach that we have found helpful (e.g. Fentress & Stilwell, 1973; Berridge *et al.*, 1987) is to arrange individually dissected items of behavioural performance into a descriptive hierarchical structure (cf. Dawkins, 1976; Cools, Spruijt & Ellenbroek, 1988; Sachs, 1988). This structure accompanies changing rules of transition among behavioural acts, rather as melodies are defined not so much by their individual notes but the changing rules of relation among these individual notes. The fact that the 'same' notes can contribute to several behavioural melodies is of fundamental importance (Fentress, 1981, 1990a, b).

Even this simple hierarchical perspective of rodent grooming (and other actions in other species) has a number of serious limitations, however (Fentress, 1983b, 1990a, b). Perhaps the most important of these is that the subtleties of contextual variables can easily become lost. At a purely descriptive level, the fine details of performance for individually abstracted actions can change with their broader expressive contexts (cf. co-articulation in human speech; Liberman, 1970). The 'units' in this sense are not 'units' at all, if the term 'unit' is meant to imply either total invariance or insensitivity to its broader realms of expression (cf. Figure 1). I see a commonality here with Robert Hinde's emphasis that human social interactions and development (Hinde, 1979; Hinde, Perret-Clermont & Stevenson-Hinde, 1985) must place equal status upon the 'intrinsic' properties of the individual and the sensitivities of the individual as a participant in social interactions and longer-term relationships. I think that nervous systems operate in the same way (cf. Minsky, 1985, on the 'society of mind').

A further limitation to classical hierarchical models is that they are typically couched in terms that suggest animals are performing only one action at a time. However, reasonably detailed analyses of rodent grooming indicate that animals are also faced with many problems of simultaneity in expression (such as maintaining balance, generating rhythms that may be restricted to or cross abstracted action classes, control of movement force, direction, and the like). This is one reason that careful ethological analyses can obligate neuroscientists to seek parallel as well as serial processing pathways in integrated action. As Robert Hinde has often stressed (e.g. 1982) the application of alternative descriptive frameworks can provide insights into mechanisms that would otherwise be ignored.

The critical issue is to recognise that singularly focused descriptions of behaviour may be anchored upon frameworks that are in themselves more or less arbitrary. This is why the application of alternative descriptive frameworks can often provide complementary perspectives. To give a single example, Berridge *et al.* (1987) found that grooming elements that differ in their form, such as paw-licking and forepaw sweeps just anterior to the mysticial vibrissae, may converge in their timing during transitions from licking to sweeping strokes. In this case timing properties, which are but one feature of individual movement classes based upon form, are shared amongst movements with different geometrical profiles. Such observations of *mutual embeddedness* often preclude simple decisions as to 'higher' or 'lower' movement properties.

Grooming in comparative perspective

In a recent study, Berridge (1990) has shown how careful descriptions of rodent grooming can provide comparative insights that also reflect upon models of neural control. 'Syntactic chains' (movements that fall within a defined global sequential structure; cf. Lashley, 1951), for example, showed broad commonalities among guinea-pigs, gerbils, hamsters, mice, rats and ground squirrels. Each species exhibited four basic sequential profiles previously described by Berridge *et al.* (1987) for laboratory rats (Figure 3), but with a number of both qualitative and quantitative differences. For example, both gerbils and ground squirrels often expressed chains that contained 'novel' action combinations not seen in rats. Compared to the other species the ground squirrels elongated elliptical strokes in the early sequence subphase, guinea-pigs inserted pauses between successive elliptical strokes, and mice showed strong alternating asymmetry in forepaw use rather than the bilateral symmetry seen in rats. The smaller rodents included more strokes per chain, and there was a strong positive correlation between ellipse cycle duration and body weight. The completion of movement chains ranged from 100 % for guinea pigs to 46 % for ground squirrels. Each species exhibited patterns of reciprocal movement transitions and perseveration of individual movement types (Berridge *et al.*, 1987) in spite of the differences in detail of sequential structure.

In these data we are faced with the common ethological dilemma of how to evaluate both commonalities and differences among underlying control processes. One of the interesting conclusions from Berridge's research is that global structural rules shared across species may be fundamental rather than merely emerging fortuitously from their lower-order elements. Higher-order invariances can be found between as well as within species, in spite of variations in movement form, symmetry, number and timing. Broad themes of serial reciprocity, perseveration and hierarchic clustering of movement types are also apparent in spite of differences in movement detail. To the neuroscientist such data suggest that different levels of descriptive order in behaviour are likely to have a certain independence in their control. *It remains a fundamental mystery, however, how nervous systems can achieve higher-order invariances through the adjustment of lower-order properties.*

Central–peripheral relations

A classic dichotomy in the ethological and neurobiological literature is that of central 'versus' peripheral control. This dichotomy, and others like it (e.g. higher 'versus' lower, specific 'versus' non-specific, and even nature 'versus' nurture) often reflect a confusion between heuristic separation and relational process. It is thus important to ask: (i) what is the *relative* contribution of X versus Y under specific conditions of measurement, and (ii) can this relative influence change with the overall dynamics of the behavioural systems in question?

Responsiveness to peripheral events. Here analytical ethology provides an important tool. By breaking down behaviour into its various properties of organisation it becomes possible to provide a precise evaluation. In our early studies of rodent grooming (e.g. Fentress, 1972; see also Fentress, 1988) we found that slow and complex movements were more easily disrupted by either

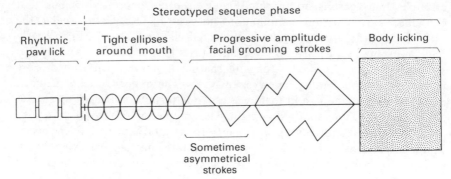

Figure 3. *Often it is useful to abstract major features of a behavioural sequence along a linear dimension, even though this represents many obvious simplifications.* In this figure four temporally distributed clusters of rat grooming motions are depicted as they occur during a 'stereotyped sequence phase' (Berridge *et al.*, 1987). This phase begins with rhythmic paw licking, followed by a series of tight ellipses of the forepaws around the mouth. The basic timing of these ellipses is then extrapolated to a series of grooming strokes around the face that increase in amplitude and duration, followed in turn by licking of the body. This linear sequencing co-occurs with other properties of movement perseveration and alternation, and hierarchical taxonomies can be used to account for transitional rules. The overall pattern is seen in a variety of rodent species, in spite of differences in movement detail. In rats, trigeminal deafferentation has little effect on the overall sequencing of movements in the stereotyped phase, even though actions may be distorted in their form (including the occasional intrusion of forelimb flails). Conversely, kainic acid lesions of the striatum typically preclude full sequence completion, even when individual actions are emitted in a normal form. The relevant salience of these peripheral and central manipulations also depends upon broader contexts of expression as well as sequence stereotypy.

phasic or tonic modifications of sensory input (tactile, proprioceptive) than were more rapid and stereotyped phases of the same sequence. Again, this appears to be a broad principle that is reflected in a number of species ranging from insects to man (Fentress, 1984). To cite but one invertebrate example, Wolf & von Helversen (1986) found that an auditory neuron in the acridid grasshopper 'switches off' during active stridulation (Figure 4). Removal of proprioceptive input led to incomplete switching off, and imposed leg movements reduced the sensitivity of the interneuron in a graded fashion. Two recent examples from mammals are: (i) Chapin (1987) who found that cutaneous sensory transmission in rats can be strongly modulated

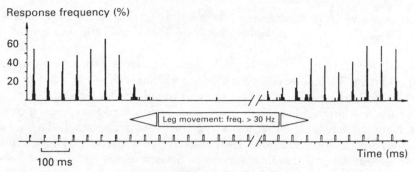

Figure 4. An invertebrate example where motor performance blocks the reception of sensory unit (Wolf & von Helversen, 1986). The 'G' auditory interneuron in acridid grasshoppers is suppressed in its response to auditory and vibratory stimuli during stridulation, and also declines in a graded fashion with imposed hindleg movements (shown here at greater than 30 Hz). *The resulting decreased sensitivity to extrinsic factors may have important analogues for attempts to understand the dynamics of self-organisation in neurobehavioural circuits more generally, although diversity in network properties must not be forgotten (see text).*

during movement, and (ii) Bushnell, Duncan & Lund (1987) who report variable gating of transmission of sensory information through the trigeminal system of cats during mastication. There are a number of related cases where strongly activated systems become tightly focused and block afferent signals that might otherwise influence the systems' properties (Fentress, 1976b, 1983b, 1984, 1990b). Schöner & Kelso (1988) have reviewed evidence that for diverse biological systems destabilisation often occurs during relaxation phases, marked by slowing of dynamic profiles and increased sensitivity to system perturbations.

A study by Berridge & Fentress (1986) demonstrated that the effects of trigeminal deafferentation in rats upon grooming movements varied with both the phase of grooming (rapid and stereotyped phases being less prone to disruption) and the broader contexts of grooming (e.g. grooming during ingestion tended to be less affected than did postprandial grooming). Interestingly, the laterality of tongue movements was affected more during ingestion than during postprandial grooming (a double dissociation). Berridge & Fentress (1987a) confirmed that 'syntactic' structure of grooming is relatively unaffected by trigeminal deafferentation procedures, even though the form of individual movements is often modified considerably. This supports the idea that central nervous system processes can be effective in generating integrated movement sequences rather independently of changes in sensory input. *The experiments as a group, however, argue strongly against any simple and invariant dichotomy between central and peripheral events.*

Central machinery. That central nervous system structures can be important in the sequential integrity of grooming behaviour was demonstrated by Berridge & Fentress (1987b) who found that kainic acid lesions of the corpus striatum often led to incomplete action sequences, even though the form of individual movements remained relatively intact. The same lesions could also produce response perseveration under special conditions, such as seen in paw-treading sequences of rats during infusion of taste substances (Berridge, Fentress & Treit, 1988). Together these data indicate the importance of careful fragmentation of behavioural profiles as well as explicit evaluation of the broader contexts within which any given property of behaviour is expressed. They also warn against simple models in that lesions of the corpus striatum can lead to either behavioural fragmentation or perseverant stereotypy as a function of action class and testing conditions.

It is not possible in this review to deal in detail with central circuitry, but several points deserve brief mention. First, when one speaks of a large and complex structure such as the corpus striatum it is important to realise that gross anatomical or physiological criteria can obscure internal heterogeneity. For example, the mammalian striatum has a rich mosaic structure with many anatomical and chemical specialisations (Gerfen, 1987), and different regions of the striatum can have quite specific effects upon different movement properties (Pisa & Schranz, 1988). Secondly, it is an error to think of all or part of the striatum as an 'island' of control, for there are many and typically recurrent connections to other brain regions (e.g. cortex and thalamus: Parent, 1986). Thirdly, although the mammalian striatum appears to play a broad role in the sequencing of behavioural events (Cools *et al.*, 1984), this must not draw our attention from the fact that it can do this at least in part through the gating of sensory information (Lidsky, Manetto & Schneider, 1985). Fourthly, the application of similar anatomical terms across vertebrate classes can lead to a confusion along a number of issues concerning origin, structural details and function (Parent, 1986).

One interesting model of striatal function in mammals is that it serves as a 'flexible glue' which contributes to the adaptive performance of various behavioural sequences (Fentress, 1990b). It may do this in part by shifting the effective *boundaries* of behavioural control systems, as reflected both in the balance of central and peripheral events and in modulating the specificity of underlying integrative processes (e.g. as measured by relations among classes of behavioural action: Fentress, 1976a). Brown (1988), for example, has recently reported evidence that the rat striatum can contribute importantly to the focusing of somatosensory events within multilevelled afferent networks. The mammalian striatum is especially well situated to play such a role, in that it links the cortex and subcortical structures through both highly specific and more widely distributed circuits (Gerfen, 1987).

Distributed circuit properties

The above illustrations make it clear that synthetic neuroscience must be concerned with multiplexed rules of relation among properties that we might otherwise wish to abstract, and study as isolated properties. *Both* separations and coherences among defined processes must be taken into account, as these operate together within the dynamic networks of intact organism function. While the point is not a new one, it deserves renewed emphasis in a period where progressive reductionism is often taken to provide ultimate (and complete) answers. It is precisely where and how nervous systems achieve their delicate balance between separation of activity properties, while at the same time linking these properties together into more global forms of expression, that many of our most critical future questions lie (cf. Wise, 1987). Progress in our thinking here has been slow.

Many years ago von Holst & von St Paul (1963) cautioned ethologists and neuroscientists against seeking simple brain 'centres' for the organisation of complex activities. Rather, they sought to isolate level dependent *operations* that together formed the nexus of brain–behaviour relations. While their techniques of electrical stimulation (chickens) were in many ways crude by modern standards, their thinking has been supported by many recent advances in neuroethology and elsewhere. We can indeed admire the modern ring of their proposition that: 'One may think that it might be economical to distribute the neurons serving a given function over a wide area, and to intersperse them with those serving other functions – namely, when cross-relationships among these functions are called for' (p. 1).

Today many neuroscientists are stressing the distributed and degenerate (non-isomorphic equivalents) of nervous system processing (e.g. Edelman, 1987; Sejnowski & Churchland, 1989). These developments reflect the dual recognition that complex neurobehavioural functions involve the cooperative participation of many brain regions, and that even individual elements within a region can serve multiple functions. A given function defined at the behavioural level can also be mediated by a wide range of individual element activities, with relative weightings that may change in time. Importantly, these properties are not confined to vertebrate nervous systems, but appear in the invertebrate world as well (e.g. Selverston, 1985; Carew & Kelley, 1989).

I close this section with the metaphorical suggestion that there is an intriguing conceptual parallel between the 'society of behaviour' at the individual organism level and emergent properties that one sees in social interactions and longer-term relationships (Hinde, 1979; cf. Minsky, 1985). In each case, before mechanisms can be understood properly, we must obtain descriptive frameworks that clarify degrees of coherence and stability amongst 'individual' properties of performance, with the added awareness that these relational descriptions reveal properties that cannot be extrapolated from studies confined to their isolated (individual) components. This is not an argument for complexity for its own sake; indeed, the relational properties of behaviour, even at the individual organism level, can yield simplifying organisational principles that would be missed by data confined to a lower order of description.

The integrative nexus

Such considerations lead naturally to what Robert Hinde has often called the 'nexus' of causal relations in behaviour. Nervous systems are partially compartmentalised, to be sure (Posner & Petersen, 1990), but they also operate along converging and diverging pathways, often with distributed re-entrant loops, that can make the localisation of global function an exceptionally difficult task (Edelman, 1987; Edelman, Gall & Cowan, 1990). I have tried to suggest above that part of the difficulty in this task is that varying forms of behavioural taxonomy clarify certain properties of expression while potentially obscuring others. Unitary 'boxes connected by arrows' taxonomies often do not work, in part because they too easily draw our attention away from the properties of the arrows that in turn may affect the properties of the boxes. Are more flexible approaches needed when we think about nervous system properties, and (more importantly) are they workable? Obviously I would not have asked this question if I did not think its answer was in the affirmative direction. I say affirmative direction only because the answer is at present very incomplete.

Dynamic network analyses (towards a behaviourally relevant 'DNA')

Let us presume that neural subsystems are both separable *and* interconnected. I do not see any alternative to that presumption. Let us also presume that these subsystems have intrinsically distinctive properties (operations), that their degrees of separation and interconnection are dynamically ordered, that these dynamic rules of interconnection reflect the properties of the subsystems, and that the interconnections in turn affect (to a greater or lesser degree) the properties of the abstracted subsystems. Finally, let us presume that control systems, as behavioural actions, can be cross-classified by different taxonomic criteria, and that no one classification will serve all purposes. If those presumptions are correct, which I believe they are at least for what we commonly call 'higher brain functions', the question is how one proceeds to perform any analysis at all!

The key ingredients are to (i) accept that our definitions of systems are always abstractions (and that other abstractions are possible), (ii) anchor these abstractions to precisely defined behavioural criteria (not necessarily 'acts', but other abstracted properties such as timing events, etc.), (iii) analyse the 'intrinsic' properties of these abstracted systems in as much detail as is feasible, and (iv) see if and how these properties change as the broader contexts within which these abstracted systems exist are changed. In brief, the approach is to evaluate *relative* system isolation within a dynamic and multilevelled framework.

Such considerations emphasise two important points. First, the richness of intact organism behaviour (and neural control) can only be revealed when 'intrinsic' system properties are combined with manipulations of their 'extrinsic' surround. Secondly, the changes in expression that one often sees by adopting this simple framework are also rule given. By establishing these rules of transformation in expression, one can often come closer to the study of mechanism in a deterministic sense than if one merely subverts variation to an issue of statistical noise. In other words, there may be multideterministic regularities in performance that 'single mechanism' models miss altogether.

In higher organisms, such as primates, the search for polymorphic networks represents a major challenge to future research (cf. Edelman, 1987). It is clear that even at the level of movement, models will have to take into account principles of population coding. To cite a striking recent example, Georgopoulos and his colleagues (e.g. Georgopoulos, 1988) have recorded from a large sample of neurons in the motor cortex of rhesus monkeys that were trained to move their arms in a precise manner. They found that individual neurons were broadly turned with respect to the direction of arm movements. That is, these cells have a preferred direction of movement but are not narrowly restricted to movements in one particular direction. However, if the *vector sum* of a population of such neurons is calculated, *then* the direction of arm movements can be accounted for with remarkable accuracy. The inescapable conclusion is that individual neurons each contribute broad-band and even variable activity patterns that are synthesised together in behavioural performance. Most striking is the recent observation (Georgopoulos *et al.*, 1989) that when a monkey was confronted with a mental rotation task, the vector sum of these neuronal populations could actually be visualised to rotate in time. Careful behavioural dissections employed with explicit considerations of synthesised sums of neuronal activity provide a clarity of picture that would otherwise be unavailable.

Recent theoretical models in neuroscience have attempted to place greater

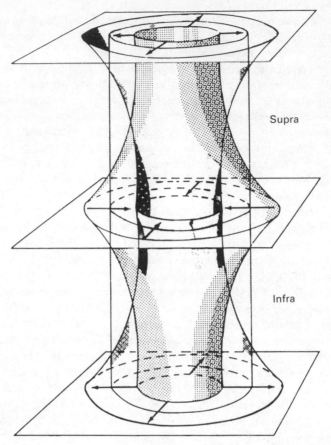

Figure 5. A schematic of 'group confinement' from Edelman (1987) where there is a complementary focusing of activity between somatosensory cortical layer IV and supra plus infra cortical layers. Core excitation accompanied by lateral inhibitory circuits can increase and decrease the focus, or specificity, of processing boundaries within and across layers. Thus, as larger regions of layer IV receive excitation from thalamic sources along with increased excitation in other layers, a restriction of the excitatory core is produced in layer IV through increased inhibition. Conversely, expansion of layer IV restricts the excitatory focus in supra and infra layers. *This schematic highlights how organisational boundaries can be dynamically ordered in complex and distributed patterns of neuronal activity. As such it places doubt on models that treat control pathways in unitary fixed terms.*

emphasis upon the dynamic relations among participating neural processes (cf. Schöner & Kelso, 1988). One of the important features of many of these models is the incorporation of core activation fields with inhibitory surrounds. A second feature is the reciprocal linkage among different functional pathways and neural regions. For example (Figure 5), Edelman (1987) has employed such a reciprocal centre–surround model to depict how cortical layers can expand and restrict their focus of operation in time (cf. Fentress, 1976a, 1984 for a similar, behaviourally based, model).

Network modulations and polymorphic codes

I return at this point to my general proposition that neurobehavioural systems, at multiple levels, represent a still poorly understood balance between tendencies toward intrinsic control and sensitivities to more broadly defined contextual variables. Indeed, I believe that it is this necessity for systems to be *both* interactive and self-organising (ISO) that is the major conceptual stumbling block for many issues in ethology and neuroscience alike (cf. earlier treatments in Fentress, 1976a, 1983a, 1984). Developmental studies in both neuroscience and behaviour represent similar challenges, albeit along a protracted time scale (e.g. Purves, 1988; Constantine-Paton, Cline & Debski, 1989).

Even in moment to moment performance, individual neurons can operate over many different time-scales, and with varying degrees of specificity. For example, Burrows (1985) has shown that for locusts non-spiking interneurons may have a relatively tonic and widespread effect on motor output neurons. Burrows goes on to argue that when both spiking and non-spiking interneurons are considered as integrated populations even superficially clear separations into motor control and sensory integration 'are oversimplifications' (p. 122). 'The separation of action becomes blurred when other aspects of both types of local interneuron are considered' (ibid.), and behavioural context is important to a full evaluation of neural circuit properties. In vertebrate brains there may be well over 50 neuronal types that also vary greatly in the specificity and time course of their operations (Sejnowski & Churchland, 1989). As illustration, cells utilising noradrenaline, serotonin, dopamine, acetylcholine and γ-aminobutyric acid (GABA) often have effects that contribute more obviously to global and tonic modulations of neural operations than in the detailed patterning of these operations. Full appreciation of how these local variations in specificity and time course map onto more integrated behavioural functions represents a major challenge for future research.

There is now clear neurobiological evidence that modulatory substances can restructure circuit properties, in both vertebrate and invertebrate species

(Marder, 1984; Davis *et al.*, 1989). One of the interesting concepts to derive from this work is that neural networks are often 'polymorphic' in their properties. Thus, Getting & Dekin (1985) have shown that in the marine mollusc, *Tritonia*, swimming networks are reconfigured into different functional circuits depending upon the behavioural state of the animal (Figure 6). The analysis by Getting & Dekin (1985) has also demonstrated that clear separations between motor neurons, central pattern generators, and command neurons are often difficult to maintain. Many neurons are multifunctional in ways that cross these early neuroethological boundaries. Finally, this study and related research (e.g. chapters in Barnes & Gladden, 1985; Selverston, 1985; Carew & Kelley, 1989; Davis *et al.*, 1989) have indicated that dynamic circuit attributes, such as pattern generation, are commonly 'emergent properties' that involve the participation of variable ensembles of individual elements.

Operations, networks and the localization of complex functions

The distinction between unitary behavioural acts and multiplexed underlying operations has led to remarkable recent advances in our thinking about complex functions, including those involved in human cognitive processing. Human as well as animal brains operate with an often remarkable degree of modularity (separation) of selective operations, but these specialised operations are also richly interconnected through distributed networks in the production of intact performance (Posner & Petersen, 1990). It is precisely this balance between separation and interconnection that represents perhaps the most enduring conceptual challenge in all of neuroscience (cf. Edelman, 1987). As illustration, Posner & Petersen (1990) review data (e.g. performance plus positron emission tomography [PET scan]) showing that performance of a language task may be both separable from and influence visual orienting. In their words: 'This result is compatible with the view that visual orienting involves systems separate but interconnected with those used for language processing' (p. 35). It remains difficult to conceptualise the subtleties of such dual statements about separation *and* interconnection, although in broad outline they often match available observations.

Figure 7 presents representative data from such analyses (Petersen *et al.*, 1988). As in neuroethology, this diagram represents an attempt to link behavioural operations with a formal (flow diagram) representation of anatomical regions by which these operations are mediated. There is a constraining assumption that the 'box' operations remain sufficiently independent to ensure their basic properties are unaltered by the patterns of connectivity observed (and more broadly possible). A more fully dynamic

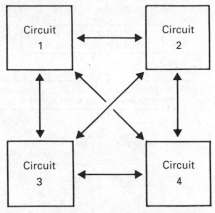

Figure 6. A summary diagram from Getting & Dekin (1985) to depict how a neural network in *Tritonia* can become reconfigured into different functional circuits. Such 'polymorphic' network properties often preclude the isolation of single neural elements to a single function, and may also blur distinctions between earlier heuristics of command, pattern generation and even motor output. The authors conclude that: 'The pattern of activity displayed by a neuronal circuit depends on a complex interaction between the nature of the inputs to the system, the nature of the synaptic interactions among the neurons, and the intrinsic membrane properties of the neurons themselves' (p. 17). *In most animal nervous systems a number of diverse interactive and self-organising* [ISO] *properties are likely to be distributed widely in the production of integrated action patterns.*

and relational approach to higher brain control processes deserves further clarification.

[*A number of years ago, Brookhart* (1979) *stated one of the fundamental issues well:* '. . . *we must devise ways to determine whether or not parts of the system function with the whole in the same way they do in isolation . . . learning how a system subcomponent behaves in a carefully defined and constrained set of circumstances gives us no guarantee that our subcomponent will behave according to the same rules if the circumstances were changed'* (p. 299).]

Ongoing states, hidden influences and boundary definitions

There are several final points that deserve emphasis for any attempts to construct unifying perspectives in neuroscience and behaviour. First, as emphasised in the ethological literature under the heading of 'motivation', ongoing system states can strongly modulate both the effectiveness and direction of influence of impinging processes. This commonly observed fact

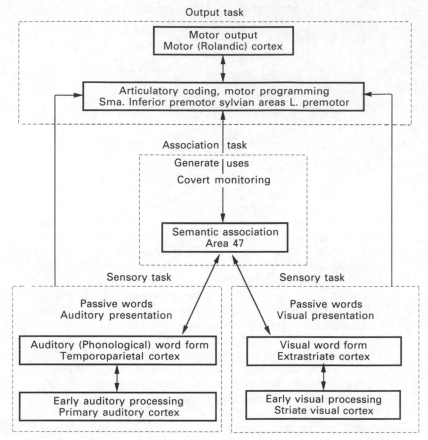

Figure 7. A schematic network (redrawn from Petersen *et al.*, 1988) for positron emission tomographic [PET; cerebral blood flow imaging] studies of lexical processing in human subjects. Basic features of this representation are that (a) individual operations can be isolated, (b) these operations are broadly localised anatomically, and (c) complete performance is mediated through a distributed neural network. Subtraction methods (dashed boxes) were used to distinguish between PET records of chronometrically and spatially distributed sensory, semantic association and motor output task properties. The solid boxes indicate possible levels of coding along with their associated anatomical loci. From these data the authors emphasise multiple-route (network) processing, rather than serial single-route (linear) control. They note: 'There are many alternative networks consistent with the conditions under which the areas are activated, but this arrangement represents a simple design consistent with our results, and some convergent experiments from other types

provides further impetus to the construction of models that are not only dynamic but also sensitive to changing relations of defined 'intrinsic' and 'extrinsic' variables (cf. Wise, 1987). Secondly, variables can often have a 'covert' influence. There is increasing neurobiological evidence that events defined as being 'outside' a sensory receptive field may influence responses to events that occur 'within' a receptive field (see review in Allman, Miezin, & McGuinnes, 1985). As illustration, Moran & Desimone (1985) have shown that cells in the cat prestriate cortex are often modulated in their response to events 'within' their receptive fields, even though the same cells show no response to these 'outside' events presented alone. In a recent study, Clemo & Stein (1988) found that in the cat superior colliculus nearly half the neurons recorded exhibited modification of 'within-field response' to one or more sites outside the traditionally defined receptive field boundaries. In each case the very definition of organisational boundaries may thus be dependent upon particular *combinations* of even 'hidden' events that the investigator takes into account.

Thirdly, higher-order 'behavioural fields' are commonly synthesised into complex configurations from *sets* of interacting events that may themselves be much more simply organised (e.g. topographically arranged; see Konishi, 1986, on the coding of sensory space in barn owls). One can expect 'hidden' as well as obvious influences within and across modalities will be revealed in the future. With rare exceptions these more complex network events have not been subjected to systematic investigation. A striking exception in the human literature concerns 'blindsight', where events that escape conscious verbal report can nonetheless influence subsequent verbal evaluations of controlled stimuli (Marshall & Halligan, 1988).

Our knowledge of higher-order networks through which behaviourally reflected events segregate and recombine remains very incomplete. It is here that ethologists, joined with their neurobiological colleagues, may make particularly important contributions. There is reason to suspect that future progress will depend upon systematic evaluations of the separate and combined manipulation of events along quantitative, qualitative and temporal domains (Fentress, 1976 a, b). These domains are not entirely independent, and in concert they may influence our views about such fundamental issues as specificity and localisation of neurobehavioural operations (cf. Fentress, 1984, 1990a).

One point I have attempted to emphasise in this chapter is that future

of studies' (p. 588). *The extent to which these abstracted network properties, both within and between 'boxes', might be modulated or even reconfigured in detail by associated manipulations remains incompletely explored.*

Table 1. *This table summarises 12 abstracted features in integrated performance networks addressed in the text. In addition to the importance of evaluating events as they occur within a broader 'nexus' of operations, future investigators will do well to address dynamic organizational processes at complementary levels*

Organisational dynamics: a dozen summary principles

1. Overlap plus population codes can lead to precision.

2. Boundary (field) size can vary, and thus can overlap – precision (specificity).

3. Boundary (field) size is measurement dependent, and can reflect covert influences.

4. Coding is multiply represented (with specialised subjunctions but also some redundancy), and same elements can be part of multiple actions (polymorphic networks).

5. Nervous system appears to cross-categorise behaviour into actions, dimensions and operations (polymorphous representation).

6. Processing occurs, often simultaneously, at a number of levels, which in turn have complex rules of *bidirectional* cross-talk.

7. Relational constancies are commonplace, and may imply a degree of *mutual moulding* of event properties.

8. Functional systems are dynamically ordered as well as relational, with patterns that emerge, dissolve, and reform.

9. 'Extrinsic' events are relatively defined, and necessarily operate against ongoing state of system.

10. Rules of extrinsic influence (e.g. facilitate versus respecify) are complex and may be threshold dependent.

11. Generalisation networks within and across defined systems remain poorly understood.

12. The combination of ethological analyses of patterned expression and neural analyses of dynamic networks are important for the clarification of both system boundaries and mechanism operations, in both the integration and development of behaviour.

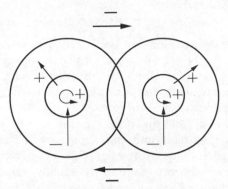

Figure 8. One way to conceptualise a number of observations on neurobehavioural system *boundaries* is through a combination of central autocatalytic cores and surrounding inhibition. Two partially overlapping system representations are shown. The proposition for further experimentation is that core excitation is accompanied by lateral inhibition, which in turn both focuses the excitatory core and blocks penetration by 'extrinsic' system events. While for the purposes of illustration the figure is drawn for localised fields, in practice these interactive and self-organising [*ISO*] system properties may be widely distributed. Empirical predictions encompassed by this conceptualisation include (a) broad band excitation and receptivity at low levels of activation, (b) increased specificity and insulation at high levels of activation, and (c) a common tendency for low levels of 'extrinsic' input to facilitate ongoing system dispositions while higher levels of input are more likely to respecify the system's intrinsic properties. *This simple model has been applied with considerable success to problems of behavioural integration, and it may have useful analogues in the study of development (see Fentress, 1976b, 1983b, 1984, 1989 and 1990b for more detailed discussions).*

progress will depend upon conceptual as well as analytic refinement in our treatment of neural network and behavioural boundaries. In a brief review that became available as I was completing this chapter, Altman & Kien (1990) have argued that even for *Aplysia* networks, 'substantial new insights into the functioning of the networks that produce biologically meaningful behaviour will need more than technical prowess' (p. 82). They go on to add, 'the new observations from molluscs, leeches and cats reinforce the urgent need to think about the neural organisation of behaviour in new ways rather than simply continuing to analyse connections between neurones' (ibid). One approach that appears promising is the application of dynamic theory models (Abraham & Shaw, 1982; Schöner & Kelso, 1988) to neural networks as they operate in different functional configurations.

John C. Fentress

Towards unifying perspectives: centres and surrounds

My goal in the preceding sections has been to show how in both ethology and neuroscience there has been an important trend to move away from models that emphasise unitary and totally isolable events. This necessitates a delicate stance. Clearly behavioural and neural events must have a degree of modularity (separation) if they are to exist at all. Further, I have tried to indicate that the goal of localising neural operations relevant to behavioural functions is both important and promising. At the same time I have endeavoured to suggest that seeking rules of dynamic interconnection across complementary levels of organisation is equally important. From the beginning of this chapter I have also attempted to pay more than superficial homage to the ethologists' appreciation for diversity in nature.

It is from this combination of efforts that one must seek possible common themes of organisation. The most important theme is that of organisational dynamics. Twelve, somewhat arbitrary, subthemes are summarised in Table 1.

One broad conceptualisation that appears useful at both the behavioural and neurobiological level is a view of integrative systems that operate within a dynamic balance of autocatalysis and surround inhibition (Figure 8). Such systems exhibit the combined properties of interaction with a more broadly defined surround and self-organisation. Extrinsic events can either facilitate or respecify the sytems' properties in part as a function of their relative levels of activation. With greater 'extrinsic' activation ongoing system states are more likely to be respecified, whereas with stronger 'intrinsic' activation external events are likely to have a reduced impact (see also Fentress, 1976a, 1983a, b, 1984, 1990b).

I believe that this basic 'centre–surround' conceptualisation can be applied to a variety of neurobehavioural control systems, and that it also offers a way to link our thoughts about central–peripheral dynamics and integrative specificity. The reason for this latter statement is that in both central–peripheral relations and relations among different classes of behaviour (and/or operations) one senses that strong activation is often accompanied by (i) increased resistance to surrounding activities, and (ii) a narrowing of focus into more restricted domains (cf. Fentress, 1976b, 1984). One metaphor for such actions is that of a searchlight that not only moves between possible domains of activation, but also one that narrows its beam with increasing activation (cf. Crick, 1984). Now it is important not to take such metaphors too simply or literally. For example, 'focused' operations need not be localised within any given anatomical structure, but are often likely to be distributed across a wide population of spatially separable elements.

108

However, the metaphor does appear to open useful areas of investigation. Wise & Desimone (1988) note that temporal lobe receptive fields for objects in primates can be very large, but once one object is selected the response to other objects diminishes 'almost as if the receptive field "shrinks" around the attended stimulus'. They thus argue for an analogy between receptive field dynamics and higher-order 'attentional fields'. Konishi (1986) has demonstrated that for the processing of spatial information in barn owls, fields in a distributed network can exhibit contrast enhancement through lateral inhibition. The previously cited reference to 'switching-off' of an auditory interneuron in the acridid grasshopper (Wolf & von Helversen, 1986; see Figure 4) involves similar considerations, as does the more general model by Edelman (1987) on neural dynamics (see Figure 5).

Many formal ('neural network') models are now being proposed that have autocatalysis and lateral inhibition as primary ingredients, and these are being extended into problems of pattern formation during ontogeny. As illustration, von der Malsburg & Singer (1988) have demonstrated how the amplification of small fluctuations combined with inhibition of surrounding states might account for ocularity domains in the mammalian visual cortex. Most models of this type emphasise excitatory processes with a lower threshold and more limited domain of influence than surrounding inhibition (cf. Gierer, 1988). An exciting, but still imperfectly tested, possibility is that through such models one may find a common framework through which integrative and developmental dynamics might be linked in the future.

Today, many developmental neurobiologists are re-emphasising conceptual frameworks not dissimilar to current thinking in the ethological literature. Particularly significant is the realisation that cellular events in development can only be understood through a perspective that encompasses the dynamic balance among tendencies toward interaction with a more broadly defined surround and self-organisation. As Constantine-Paton *et al.* (1989) stated: 'Those of us interested in the developmental effects of activity have come a long way to rediscover that the developing brain is an interactive self-organizing system with dynamic properties that can change qualitatively when broken down into individual cellular elements' (p. 280). Both *degrees of interaction* and the often diverse consequences of interaction when *combined with self-ordering dispositions* provide major foci for current neurobiological as well as ethological research.

What is the 'bottom-line' of these considerations? I think it is that we, as investigators, have tremendous difficulty in formulating integrative processes within a framework that is truly dynamic, relational and multilayered. When one pursues such a position the data become more complex than simple static, unitary and linear models can possibly encompass. Perhaps the single most difficult task for the investigator in behavioural neuroscience is to see

Table 2. *This table provides a partial elaboration on integrative parameters in ethology and neuroscience that can focus future investigations. (1) A major argument in this chapter is that events must be extracted but also viewed with broader expressive contexts. (2) Action patterns have a number of formal properties (such as timing, relations to body referents, sequencing, relations to external referents, force and parallel expression), each of which may be isolable in its control. (3) Activities can terminate through both intrinsic and extrinsic sources. (4) There are multiple perspectives relevant to issues of system modularity (independence–interdependence). (5) A valuable approach is to evaluate how events are 'co-ordered' as well as organised in isolation (a small set of possibilities is indicated). (6) The evaluation of dynamic boundary problems will involve a set of considerations that include (a) invariance among individual properties, (b) events that may be degenerate (substitutable) and distributed, (c) interactive/self-organising parameters within and across levels, (d) extrinsic influences that may range from simple transfer of information through various transformations to cases where events serve to trigger intrinsic system properties, (e) separation of instructional influences from those that have modulatory functions or that respecify system properties through selective processes, and (f) clarification of the routes and limits by which these extrinsic influences are generalised.*

Some integrative parameters

---

1. When activity occurs (e.g. expressive context)

2. Form activity takes
   - (a) Temporal (duration/rhythm/acceleration/velocity/phase relations)
   - (b) Spatial (body referents)
   - (c) Sequential (melodies)
   - (d) Directional (environmental referents)
   - (e) Force (intensity)
   - (f) Simultaneity (chords)

3. When activity terminates
   - (a) Self-termination
   - (b) Extrinsic termination
     - (i) new sensory events
     - (ii) antagonistic actions

4. Independence–interdependence
   - (a) Modularity/modality (isolation)
   - (b) Interaction
   - (c) Mutual moulding/interpenetration
   - (d) Hierarchical cohesions

5. Co-order
   (a) Animal and environment
   (b) Acts/operations
   (c) Within/between limb segments – limbs
   (d) Rotational/planar/conical movements (EW)
   (e) Muscle/neural populations

6. Dynamic boundaries/networks
   (a) Relational invariants
   (b) Degenerate/distributed networks
   (c) *ISO* processes within/across levels (hierarchy)
   (d) Transfer/transform/trigger
   (e) Instruct/modulate/select
   (f) Generalisation networks
       (i) within modules/modalities
       (ii) synergistic
       (iii) antagonistic
       (iv) cross-level

how properties can be both isolable *and* interconnected, and to pursue the deeper implications of this dynamic polarity at multiple levels as well as across complementary time frames. In Table 2 I have outlined some of the major parameters of integrative networks that deserve further study.

The ontogeny of integrative networks: challenges for the future

Space limitations preclude a full exploration of possible parallels between integrative and developmental events in this chapter, and even if more space were available the arguments would remain incomplete (see Fentress, 1989). However, there are a few broad thematic commonalities that can be addressed. The first is that in studies of both integration and development, analytical ethology and synthetic neuroscience are likely to converge on the study of dynamic pattern formation. As I am confident will be reflected in other chapters of this volume, it is the combined separation and synthesis of events that offer challenges for the study of both development and integration in behaviour.

Classic dichotomies as 'nature versus nurture' are conceptual kin to issues of 'central versus peripheral' or, at a slightly more abstract level, even 'specific versus non-specific'. In each case we make heuristic divisions to order our initial thoughts, but soon come faced with the limitations of these divisions. The pathways of connection involve complex networks rather than simple linear chains, with ongoing system states being equally important to

111

Table 3. *Some possible parallels in the organisation of integrative and developmental events are suggested. (1) The degree of specificity of extrinsic influences as well as system properties may be dynamically ordered, as in facilitation versus respecification of ongoing system trajectories. (2) With increased system specification (e.g. through lateral inhibition) systems may reduce their sensitivity to a given set of extrinsic events. (3) One possibility, in need of much further study, is that many extrinsic events operate with a dual threshold, where global facilitation of system properties becomes replaced by respecification of these properties. (4) In both integrative and developmental nexus operations events may generalise along a number of imperfectly explored alternative pathways, such as on the basis of movement form versus functional behavioural class. [A point that could not be covered fully in this chapter is that degraded or incomplete influences may often be amplified or 'filled in' by ongoing system states, thus reinforcing the difficulty of any simple dichotomies between intrinsic and extrinsic influences.]*

Possible parallels between integration and development

---

1. Early and low levels of activation – relative non-specificity
   (a) Broad range of patterns facilitated
   (b) Frequent mutual facilitation (induction) among incompletely differentiated systems
   (c) Initiated trajectories often dependent upon, and easily disrupted by, changes in periphery

2. Later and higher levels of activation – more narrowly focused trajectories
   (a) Autocatalytic central core with expanding inhibitory surrounds
   (b) Mutual inhibition among systems assists specification (differentiation)
   (c) Focused trajectories become less dependent upon and less easily disrupted by surround

3. Dual-threshold hypothesis – incorporation of peripheral events
   (a) Low level/near target perturbations – *Enhance ongoing predispositions* (low level, minimal distortion)
   (b) High level/far from target perturbations – *Respecify ongoing trajectories* (high level, greater distortion)

4. Generalisation networks – options and hypotheses
   (a) Based upon physical form/physiological proximity
   (b) Based upon functional networks that are physically dispersed
   (c) Fill in gaps when activation incomplete or degraded
   (d) Both cooperative and competitive depending upon mix of qualitative, quantitative, and temporal parameters

---

extrinsic perturbations. Even rules of specificity within these networks are likely to be dynamically ordered, with a broad tendency of systems to become self-organised through interactions with their surround (for example, see Meinhardt, 1982, on the generation of structural patterns in ontogeny). Accompanying this self-organisation one can expect modulated sensitivities to surrounding events. Interactions within networks can be either antagonistic or synergistic, and these patterns at present remain poorly understood. More speculatively, I suspect that in both integrative and developmental systems the degree of specification from extrinsic events is likely to be threshold dependent in an interesting way. Low levels of activation, even when slightly 'off target' are expected to facilitate ongoing states whereas at a higher threshold respecification of these events will be more common (Fentress, 1981, 1989, 1990b). Finally, the generalisation networks for a given 'experience' are likely to operate across multilayered functional criteria rather than in terms of any simple physical dimension.

Table 3 provides a slightly expanded version of these possible thematic parallels between integration and development. As such the table is less a summary of known facts than it is a map for the possible acquisition of new facts.

Conclusion

In this chapter I have attempted to demonstrate possible rules of contact between ethology and neuroscience, while at the same time pointing towards limitations in our existing databases. I have tried, in as explicit terms as possible, to illustrate that a broad approach that stresses the dynamic, relational and multilayered nature of neurobehavioural events is critical. The primary conceptual problem remains how we can think of neurobehavioural systems both in terms of their constituent parts and in terms of their higher-order rules of connectivity. I have concluded with some speculations as to where future research might take us.

I hope it is clear how frequently I have borrowed from the research and the thinking of Robert Hinde. I do believe that he is correct in his insistence that ethology is not so much an island unto itself as it is an attitude towards inquiry that can have many exciting implications. In some sense it may not matter, therefore, whether we are speaking of interactions and relationships among individual persons or individual neurons. In each case we must try to isolate the properties of the participants and also ask the often more difficult question of how these participants work together to perform within emergent patterns of orders.

Acknowledgements

I had the privilege to attend a series of presentations given by Robert Hinde at the University of Waterloo in Canada as I was preparing this manuscript.

His insightful dissections and syntheses of human social behaviour at this conference on child development indeed provided the basic framework from which I have prepared the present chapter. This may seem odd given that my chapter has as its assigned focus a much more narrow ('simple') viewpoint about animal behaviour than Robert Hinde presented. However, Robert Hinde's concerns with the diversity of behaviour, and the need to construct explanations that are dynamic, relational, and multilevelled brought to the forefront are things I have been struggling with over the years. To the limits of my ability I have sought to prepare this paper in the spirit of critical inquiry and lively exploration that Robert Hinde's own contributions have so often engendered among his students, his colleagues and his many friends. I owe him warm thanks for his unwavering support along many scientific and personal fronts over the years that I have had the privilege to know him.

I thank Pat Bateson for his invitation to contribute to this special volume. Pat Bateson also provided constructive comments on an earlier draft of this paper, while reminding me in patient terms that clocks tick. My contribution was supported in part by grants from the Medical Research Council of Canada and the Natural Sciences and Engineering Research Council of Canada. Kathleen Bloom made it possible for me to attend the Waterloo Conference. Wanda Danilchuk helped with the manuscript preparation. I thank them both.

References

Abraham, R. H. & Shaw, C. D. (1982). *Dynamics – The Geometry of Behavior*. Santa Cru: Aerial Press, Inc.

Allman, J., Miezin, F. & McGuinnes, E. (1985). Stimulus specific response from beyond the classical receptive field: Neurophysiological mechanisms for local–global comparisons in visual neurons. *Annual Review of Neuroscience*, 407–30.

Altman, J. S. & Kien, J. (1990). Highlighting *Aplysia*'s networks. *Trends in Neurosciences*, **13** (3), 81–2.

Barlow, G. W. (1977). Modal action patterns. In *How Animals Communicate*, ed. T. A. Sebeok, pp. 98–134. Bloomington, Indiana: Indiana University Press.

Barnes, W. J. P. & Gladden, M. H. (ed.) (1985). *Feedback and Motor Control in Invertebrates and Vertebrates*. London: Croom Helm.

Bateson, P. (1988). Epilogue: An ethological overview. In *Aims and Methods in Neuroethology*, ed. D. M. Guthrie, pp. 301–5. Manchester: Manchester University Press.

Bekoff, A. (1986). Ontogeny of chicken motor behaviours: Evidence for multi-use limb pattern generating circuitry. In *Neurobiology of Vertebrate Locomotion*, ed. S. Grillner, P. S. G. Stein, D. G. Stuart, H. Forssberg and R. M. Herman, pp. 433–53. Hampshire, England: Macmillan.

Berkinblitt, M. B., Feldman, A. G. & Fukson, O. I. (1986). Adaptability of innate motor patterns and motor control mechanisms. *Behavioural and Brain Sciences*, **9** (4), 585–99.

Bernstein, N. (1967). *The Co-ordination and Regulation of Movements*. New York: Pergamon Press.

Berridge, K. C. (1990). Comparative fine structure of action: Rules of form and sequence in the grooming patterns of six rodent species. *Behaviour* (in press).

Berridge, K. C. & Fentress, J. C. (1986). Contextual control of trigeminal sensorimotor function. *Journal of Neuroscience*, **6**, 325–30.

Berridge, K. C. & Fentress, J. C. (1987a). Deafferentation does not disrupt natural rules of action syntax. *Behavioural Brain Research*, **23**, 69–76.

Berridge, K. C. & Fentress, J. C. (1987b). Disruption of natural grooming chains after striatopallidal lesions. *Psychobiology*, **15** (4), 336–42.

Berridge, K. C., Fentress, J. C. & Parr, H. (1987). Natural syntax rules control action sequence of rats. *Behavioural Brain Research*, **23**, 59–68.

Berridge, K. C., Fentress, J. C. & Treit, D. (1988). A triggered hyperkinesia induced in rats by lesions of the corpus striatum. *Journal of Experimental Neurology*, **99**, 259–68.

Bohm, D. (1980). *Wholeness and the Implicate Order*. London: Routledge & Kegan Paul.

Brookhart, J. M. (1979). Convergence on an understanding of motor control. In *Posture and Movement*, ed. R. E. Talbott and D. R. Humphrey, pp. 295–303. New York: Raven Press.

Brown, L. L. (1988). The function of dopamine in the striatum: A sharpener of sensory information? *Society for Neuroscience Abstracts*, 287.4.

Burrows, M. (1985). Nonspiking and spiking local interneurons in the locust. In *Model Neural Networks and Behavior*, ed. A. I. Selverston, pp. 109–25. New York: Plenum Press.

Bushnell, M. C., Duncan, G. H. & Lund, J. P. (1987). Gating of sensory transmission in the trigeminal system. In *Higher Brain Functions: Recent Explorations of the Brain's Emergent Properties*, ed. S. P. Weiss, pp. 211–37. New York: John Wiley.

Camhi, J. M. (1984). *Neuroethology*. Sunderland, Mass.: Sinauer.

Carew, T. J. & Kelley, D. B. (ed.) (1989). *Perspectives in Neural Systems and Behavior*. New York: Alan R. Liss.

Changeux, J.-P. & Konishi, M. (ed.) (1987). *The Neural and Molecular Bases of Learning*. Chichester/New York: John Wiley.

Chapin, J. K. (1987). Modulation of cutaneous sensory transmission during movement: Possible mechanism and biological significance. In *Higher Brain Functions: Recent Explorations of the Brain's Emergent Properties*, ed. S. P. Weiss, pp. 181–209. New York: John Wiley.

Clemo, H. R. & Stein, B. E. (1988). Examination of receptive field surrounds in somatosensory neurons in cat superior colliculus. *Society for Neuroscience Abstracts*, **50**, 17.

Colbern, D. L. & Gispen, W. H. (ed.) (1988). *Neural Mechanisms and Biological Significance of Grooming Behaviour. Annals of the New York Academy of Sciences, Vol. 525. Grooming Behavior.* New York: New York Academy of Sciences.

Constantine-Paton, M., Cline, H. T. & Debski, E. A. (1989). Neural activity, synaptic convergence, and synapse stabilization in the developing central nervous system. In *The Assembly of the Nervous System*, ed. L. T. Landmesser, pp. 279–300. New York: Alan R. Liss.

Cools, A. R., Jaspers, R., Schwarz, M., Sontag, K. H., Vrijmoed-de Vries, M. & van den Bercken, J. (1984). Basal ganglia and switching motor programs. In *The Basal Ganglia: Structure and Function,* ed. J. S. McKenzie, R. E. Kemm, and L. N. Wilcock, pp. 513–44. New York: Plenum Press.

Cools, A. R., Spruijt, B. M. & Ellenbroek, B. A. (1988). Role of central dopamine in

ACTH-induced grooming behavior in rats. In *Neural Mechanisms and Biological Significance of Grooming Behaviour*, ed. D. L. Colbern & W. H. Gispen. *Annals of the New York Academy of Sciences, Vol. 525*, pp. 338–49. New York: New York Academy of Sciences.

Crick, F. H. C. (1979). Thinking about the brain. In *The Brain: A Scientific American book*. New York: W. H. Freeman (original article in September 1979 issue of *Scientific American*).

Crick, F. H. C. (1984). The function of the thalamic reticular complex: The searchlight hypothesis. *Proceedings of the National Academy of Sciences (USA)*, **81**, 4586–90.

Davis, M., Jacobs, B. L. & Schoenfeld, R. I. (1989) (ed.). *Modulation of Defined Vertebrate Neural Circuits. Annals of the New York Academy of Sciences, Vol. 563*. New York: New York Academy of Sciences.

Davis, W. J. (1976). Behavioral and neuronal plasticity in mollusks. In *Simpler Networks and Behavior*, ed. J. C. Fentress, pp. 224–238. Sunderland, Mass.: Sinauer.

Dawkins, R. (1976). Hierarchical organization: A candidate principle for ethology. In *Growing Points in Ethology*, ed. P. P. G. Bateson and R. A. Hinde, pp. 7–54. Cambridge: Cambridge University Press.

Edelman, G. M. (1987). *Neural Darwinism: The Theory of Neuronal Group Selection*. New York: Basic Books.

Edelman, G. M., Gall, W. E. & Cowan, W. M. (ed.) (1990). *Signal and Sense: Local and Global Order in Perceptual Maps* (in press).

Ewert, J.-P. (1980). *Neuroethology: An Introduction to the Neurophysiological Fundamentals of Behavior* (translation of the German edition of 1976). Berlin: Springer-Verlag.

Ewert, J.-P. (1987). Neuroethology of releasing mechanisms: Prey-catching in toads. *The Behavioral and Brain Sciences*, **10** (3), 337–68.

Ewert, J.-P., Capranica, R. R. & Ingle, D. J. (ed) (1983). *Advances in Vertebrate Neuroethology (NATO ASI Series)*. New York: Plenum Press.

Fentress, J. C. (1968a). Interrupted ongoing behaviour in voles (*Microtus agrestis* and *Clethrionomys britannicus*): I. response as a function of preceding activity and the context of an apparently 'irrelevant' motor pattern. *Animal Behaviour*, **16**, 135–53.

Fentress, J. C. (1968b). Interrupted ongoing behaviour in voles (*Microtus agrestis* and *Clethrionomys britannicus*). II. extended analysis of intervening motivational variables underlying fleeing and grooming activities. *Animal Behaviour*, **16**, 154–67.

Fentress, F. C. (1972). Development and patterning of movement sequences in inbred mice. In *The Biology of Behavior*, ed. J. Kiger, pp. 83–132. Corvallis: Oregon State University Press.

Fentress, J. C. (1976a). Dynamic boundaries of patterned behavior: Interaction and self-organization. In *Growing Points in Ethology*, ed. P. P. G. Bateson and R. A. Hinde, pp. 135–69. Cambridge: Cambridge University Press.

Fentress, J. C. (ed.) (1976b). *Simpler Networks and Behavior*. Sunderland, Mass.: Sinauer.

Fentress, J. C. (1981). Sensorimotor development. In *The Development of Perception: Psychobiological Perspectives*, ed. R. N. Aslin, J. R. Alberts and M. R. Petersen, pp. 293–318. New York: Academic Press.

Fentress, J. C. (1983a). The analysis of behavioral networks. In *Advances in*

Vertebrate Neuroethology, ed. J. P. Ewert, R. R. Capranica and D. J. Ingle, pp. 939–68. New York: Plenum Press.

Fentress, J. C. (1983b). Ethological models of hierarchy and patterning of species-specific behavior. In *Handbook of Neurobiology: Motivation*, ed. E. Satinoff and P. Teitelbaum, pp. 185–234. New York: Plenum Press.

Fentress, J. C. (1984). The development of coordination. *Journal of Motor Behavior*, **16**, 99–134.

Fentress, J. C. (1986). Ethology and the neural sciences. In *Relevance of Models and Theories in Ethology*, ed. R. Campan and R. Zayan, pp. 77–107. Toulouse: Privat, I.E.C.

Fentress, J. C. (1988). Expressive contexts, fine structure, and central mediation of rodent grooming. In *Neural Mechanisms and Biological Significance of Grooming Behaviour*, ed. D. L. Colbern & W. H. Gispen. *Annals of the New York Academy of Sciences, Vol. 525*, pp. 18–26. New York: New York Academy of Sciences.

Fentress, J. C. (1989). Developmental roots of behavioral order: Systemic approaches to the examination of core developmental issues. In *Systems and Development*, ed. M. R. Gunnar & E. Thelen. *The Minnesota Symposia on Child Psychology: Vol. 22*, pp. 35–76. Hillsdale, NJ: Erlbaum.

Fentress, J. C. (1990a). The categorization of behavior. In *Explanation and Interpretation in the Study of Animal Behavior: Comparative Perspectives*, ed. M. Bekoff and D. Jamieson. Boulder, CO: Westview Press (in press).

Fentress, J. C. (1990b). Organizational patterns in action: Local and global issues in action pattern formation. In *Signal and Sense: Local and Global Order in Perceptual Maps*, ed. G. M. Edelman, W. E. Gall and W. M. Cowan.

Fentress, J. C. & McLeod, P. (1986). Motor patterns in development. In *Handbook of Behavioral Neurobiology, Vol. 8. Developmental Processes in Psychobiology and Neurobiology*, ed. E. M. Blass, pp. 35–97. New York: Plenum Press.

Fentress, J. C. & Stilwell, F. P. (1973). Grammar of a movement sequence in inbred mice. *Nature*, **244**, 52–53.

Gallistel, C. R. (1980). *The Organization of Action: A New Synthesis*. Hillsdale, NJ: Erlbaum.

Georgopoulos, A. P. (1988). Neural integration of movement: Role of motor cortex in reaching. *FASEB Journal*, **2**, 2849–57.

Georgopoulos, A. P., Lurito, J. T., Petrides, M., Schwartz, A. B. & Massey, J. T. (1989). *Science*, **243**, 234–6.

Gerfen, C. R. (1987). The neostriatal mosaic: The reiterated processing unit. In *Neurotransmitter Interactions in the Basal Ganglia*, ed. M. Sandler, C. Feuertein and B. Scatton, pp. 19–29. New York: Raven Press.

Getting, P. A. & Dekin, M. S. (1985). *Tritonia* swimming: A model system for integration within rhythmic motor systems. In *Model Neural Networks and Behavior*, ed. A. I. Selverston, pp. 3–20. New York: Plenum Press.

Gierer, A. (1988). Generation of spatial order in the developing nervous system. In *Organization of Neural Networks: Structures and Models*, ed. W. von Seelen, G. Shaw and U. M. Leinhos, pp. 127–39. Weinheim: VCH Verlagsgesellschaft.

Golani, I. (1976). Homeostatic motor processes in mammalian interactions: A choreography of display. In *Perspectives in Ethology*, ed. P. P. G. Bateson and P. H. Klopfer, pp. 69–134. New York: Plenum Press.

Grillner, S., Stein, P. S. G., Stuart, D. G., Forssberg, H. & Herman, R. M. (ed.) (1986). *Neurobiology of Vertebrate Locomotion*. Hampshire, England: Macmillan Press.

Guthrie, D. M. (1980). *Neuroethology*. London: Blackwell.
Guthrie, D. M. (ed.) (1988). *Aims and Methods in Neuroethology*. Manchester: Manchester University Press.
Harnad, S. (ed.) (1987). *Categorical Perception: The Groundwork of Cognition*. New York: Cambridge University Press.
Harris-Warwick, R. M. & Johnson, B. R. (1989). Motor pattern networks: Flexible foundations for rhythmic pattern production. In *Perspectives in Neural Systems and Behavior*, ed. T. J. Carew and D. B. Kelley, pp. 51–72. New York: Alan R. Liss.
Hinde, R. A. (1959). Unitary drives. *Animal Behaviour*, 7, 130–41.
Hinde, R. A. (1970). *Animal Behavior: A Synthesis of Ethology and Comparative Psychology* (2nd edn). New York: McGraw-Hill.
Hinde, R. A. (ed.) (1972). *Non-verbal Communication*. Cambridge: Cambridge University Press.
Hinde, R. A. (1979). *Towards Understanding Relationships*. London: Academic Press.
Hinde, R. A. (1982). *Ethology: Its Nature and Relations with other Sciences*. Oxford/New York: Oxford University Press.
Hinde, R. A. (1984). Ethology has progressed. *Behavioral and Brain Sciences*, 7, 391.
Hinde, R. A. & Steel, E. A. (1966). Integration of the reproductive behaviour of female canaries. *Symposia of the Society for Experimental Biology*, 20, 401–26.
Hinde, R. A. & Stevenson, J. G. (1969). Goals and response control. In *Development and Evolution of Behaviour*, ed. L. R. Aronson, E. Tobach, J. S. Rosenblatt and D. S. Lehrman, pp. 216–37. New York: Freeman.
Hinde, R. A., Perret-Clermont, A.-N. & Stevenson-Hinde, J. (ed.) (1985). *Social Relationships and Cognitive Development: A Fyssen Foundation Symposium*. Oxford: Clarendon Press.
Horn, G. (1985). *Memory, Imprinting, and the Brain: An Inquiry into Mechanisms*. Oxford: Clarendon Press.
Hoyle, G. (1964). Exploration of neuronal mechanisms underlying behavior in insects. In *Neural Theory and Modeling*, ed. R. F. Reiss, pp. 346–76. Palo Alto, Calif.: Stanford University Press.
Hoyle, G. (1984). The scope of neuroethology. *Behavioural and Brain Sciences*, 7, 367–412.
Huber, F. (1983). Implications of insect neuroethology for studies on vertebrates. In *Advances in Vertebrate Neuroethology*, ed. J.-P. Ewert, R. R. Capranica and D. J. Ingle. New York: Plenum Press.
Kandel, E. R. & Schwartz, J. H. (1985). *Principles of Neural Science* (2nd edition). New York/Amsterdam/Oxford: Elsevier.
Keele, S. W. & Ivry, R. I. (1987). Modular analysis of timing in motor skill. In *The Psychology of Learning and Motivation, Vol. 21*, ed. G. H. Bower, pp. 183–228. New York: Academic Press.
Kennedy, D. (1976). Neural elements in relation to network function. In *Simpler Networks and Behavior*, ed. J. C. Fentress, pp. 65–81. Sunderland, Mass.: Sinauer.
Konishi, M. (1986). Centrally synthesized maps of sensory space. *Trends in Neurosciences*, 9 (4), 163–8.
Kugler, P. N. & Turvey, M. T. (1987). *Information, Natural Law, and the Self-Assembly of Rhythmic Movement*. Hillsdale, NJ: Erlbaum.
Kupfermann, I. & Weiss, K. (1978). The command neuron concept. *Behavioural and Brain Sciences*, 1, 3–39.

Lashley, K. S. (1951). The problem of serial order in behavior. In *Cerebral Mechanisms in Behavior*, ed. L. A. Jeffries, pp. 112–36. New York: John Wiley.

Liberman, A. M. (1970). The grammars of speech and language. *Cognitive Psychology*, **1**, 301–23.

Lidsky, T. I., Manetto, C. & Schneider, J. S. (1985). Considerations of sensory factors involved in motor functions of the basal ganglia. *Brain Research Reviews*, **9**, 133–46.

Lorenz, K. (1950). The comparative method in studying innate behaviour patterns. *Symposia of the Society for Experimental Biology*, **4**, 221–68.

Lorenz, K. Z. (1981). *The Foundations of Ethology*. New York: Springer-Verlag.

Marder, E. (1984). Mechanisms underlying neurotransmitter modulation of a neuronal circuit. *Trends in Neurosciences*, **7**, 48–53.

Marshall, J. C. & Halligan, P. W. (1988). Blindsight and insight in visuo-spatial neglect. *Nature*, **336**, 766–7.

Mayr, E. (1976). *Evolution and the Diversity of Life: Selected Essays*. Cambridge, Mass.: The Belknap Press of Harvard University Press.

Meinhardt, H. (1982). Generation of structures in a developing organism. In *Developmental Order: Its Origin and Regulation*, pp. 439–61. New York: Alan R. Liss.

Minsky, M. (1985). *The Society of Mind*. New York: Simon & Schuster.

Moran, J. & Desimone, R. (1985). Selective attention gates visual processing in extrastriate cortex. *Science*, **229**, 782–4.

Parent, A. (1986). *Comparative Neurobiology of the Basal Ganglia*. New York: John Wiley.

Pearson, K. G. (1987). Central pattern generation: A concept under scrutiny. In *Advances in Physiological Research*, ed. H. McLennan, J. R. Ledsom, C. H. S. McIntosh and D. R. Jones, pp. 167–85. New York: Plenum Press.

Petersen, S. E., Fox, P. T., Posner, M. I., Mintun, M. & Raichle, M. E. (1988). Positron emission tomographnic studies of the cortical anatomy of single-word processing. *Nature*, **331**, 585–9.

Pisa, M. & Schranz, J. A. (1988). Dissociable motor roles of the rat's striatum conform to a somatopic model. *Behavioral Neuroscience*, **102**, 429–40.

Posner, M. I. (1978). *Chronometric Explorations of Mind*. Hillsdale, NJ: Erlbaum.

Posner, M. I. & Petersen, S. E. (1990). The attention system of the human brain. *Annual Review of Neuroscience*, **13**, 24–42.

Purves, D. (1988). *Body and Brain. A Trophic Theory of Neural Connections*. Cambridge, Mass.: Harvard University Press.

Rauschecker, J. P. & Marler, P. (ed.) (1987). *Imprinting and Cortical Plasticity: Comparative Aspects of Sensitive Periods*. New York: John Wiley.

Sachs, B. D. (1988). The development of grooming and its expression in adult animals. In *Neural Mechanisms and the Biological Significance of Grooming Behaviour*, ed. D. L. Colbern and W. H. Gispen, *Annals of the New York Academy of Sciences*, *Vol. 525*, pp. 1–17. New York: New York Academy of Sciences.

Schöner, G. & Kelso, J. A. S. (1988). Dynamic pattern generation in behavioral and neural systems. *Science*, **239**, 1513–20.

Sejnowski, T. J. & Churchland, P. S. (1989). Brain and cognition. In *Foundations of Cognitive Science*, ed. M. I. Posner, pp. 301–56. Cambridge, Mass.: MIT Press.

Selverston, A. I. (1980). Are central pattern generators understandable? *The Behavioural and Brain Sciences*, **3**, 535–71.

Selverston, A. I. (ed.) (1985). *Model Neural Networks and Behavior*. New York: Plenum Press.

Sherrington, C. S. (1906). *The Integrative Action of the Nervous System*. New Haven: Yale University Press.

Stein, P. S. G., Mortin, L. I. & Robertson, G. A. (1986). The forms of a task and their blends. In *Neurobiology of Vertebrate Locomotion*, ed. S. Grillner, P. S. G. Stein, D. G. Stuart, H. Forssberg and R. M. Herman, pp. 201–16. Hampshire, England: Macmillan Press.

Stent, G. S. (1981). Strength and weakness of the genetic approach to the development of the nervous system. *Annual Review of Neuroscience*, **4**, 163–94.

Tinbergen, N. (1951). *The Study of Instinct*. Oxford: Clarendon Press.

Tinbergen, N. (1963). On aims and methods of ethology. *Zeitschrift für Tierpsychologie*, **20**, 410–33.

von der Malsburg, C. & Singer, W. (1988). Principles of cortical network organization. In *Organization of Neural Networks: Structures and Models*, ed. W. von Seelen, G. Shaw and U. M. Leinhos, pp. 109–26. Weinheim: VCH Verlagsgesellschaft.

von Holst, E. & von St. Paul, U. (1963). On the functional organization of drives. *Animal Behaviour*, **11**, 1–20. (First published in German, *Naturwissenschaften*, **47**, 409–22.

Wise, S. P. (ed.) (1987). *Higher Brain Functions: Recent Explorations of the Brain's Emergent Properties*. New York: John Wiley & Sons.

Wise, S. P. & Desimone, R. (1988). Behavioural neurophysiology: Insights into seeing and grasping. *Science*, **242**, 736–41.

Wolf, H. & von Helversen, D. (1986). 'Switching-off' of an auditory interneuron during stridulation in the acridid grasshopper *Chorthippus biguttulus* L. *Journal of Comparative Physiology*, **158** (A), 861–71.

Yates, F. E. (ed.) (1987). *Self-organizing Systems: The Emergence of Order*. New York: Plenum Press.

—5—

Cerebral function and behaviour investigated through a study of filial imprinting

Gabriel Horn

One of Robert Hinde's many major contributions to knowledge is his book *Animal Behaviour* (1966). The book is subtitled *A Synthesis of Ethology and Comparative Psychology*. In the sense that he demonstrates continuities between seemingly diverse ideas, and unites them into a complex, majestic whole, the book is indeed a synthesis. But it is more than that: in exploring mediating physiological processes Hinde also provides us with an analysis of animal behaviour. A quick glance through the book reveals the extraordinary range of mediating processes that he considers. These include the neural mechanisms involved in the control of locomotion; in the encoding and representation of sensory stimuli and the feedback control of sensory input (corollary discharge); in stimulus selection, including attentive behaviour; in arousal; in the response to novelty; and also the neuroendocrine mechanisms controlling sexual behaviour, hunger and thirst. In the two decades or so that have elapsed since the first edition of *Animal Behaviour* appeared, advances in some of these fields have been little short of spectacular. Much as I would wish to give an account of these developments as a tribute to Hinde's immense contributions, I am not competent to do so; and even if I were, the space required would be at least equal to that of several volumes of *Animal Behaviour*. Instead, I will concentrate on developments in areas in which I have direct experimental experience.

Both Hinde and I have an interest in learning. For Hinde, this interest took him to study (i) aspects of song-learning in chaffinches (Hinde, 1958), (ii) habituation, through his enquiries into the waning of the 'mobbing' response of chaffinches to predators (Hinde, 1954a, b, 1960) and (iii) imprinting (Hinde, 1955, 1962; Hinde, Thorpe & Vince, 1956). It is perhaps not without significance that a number of individuals who have taken the analysis of these forms of learning from the behavioural to the neural level, have at one time

121

or another worked at Madingley, and so would have come under Hinde's influence.

The analysis of birdsong was pursued through a beautiful series of experiments by Nottebohm and by Konishi and their collaborators (see Nottebohm, 1980; Konishi, 1985). My own experimental work on the neuronal mechanisms of habituation was carried out in the 1960s (see Horn, 1970). During that decade several laboratories were intensively studying this form of learning, and the convergence of ideas from the behavioural and the neural levels of analysis was so encouraging that Hinde and I organised a conference in 1969 bringing together workers who had been following the different approaches (Horn & Hinde, 1970). The evidence at that time suggested that: (i) the habituation of at least some behavioural responses could be accounted for in terms of a progressive reduction of impulse discharges in the neural circuit mediating the response, (ii) this depression was brought about by activity in the circuit, and in that sense was 'self-generated', (iii) the depression was a consequence of a reduction in the release of neurotransmitter at certain synapses in the circuit, (iv) the change in transmitter release was probably brought about through a change in the movement of calcium ions at the depressed synapses, (v) dishabituation could be brought about by changing the membrane potential of the depressed presynaptic terminals, and (vi) many of the more subtle aspects of behavioural habituation could be accounted for by relatively simple arrangements of neural circuits possessing synapses with the above properties (see various contributions in Horn & Hinde, 1970). In the years that followed further support for many of these findings and suggestions appeared, and the analysis of habituation was extended especially at the cellular level (for review see Castelucci, Carew & Kandel, 1978; Carew, 1989).

Hinde's work on imprinting was conducted in the mid-1950s; and as his involvement in this form of learning began to wane my interest began to wax. This interest did not become translated into experimental work until I met Hinde's former research student Pat Bateson. Our approach to the analysis of imprinting was to start at the behavioural level and work 'downward' towards the neural level. But some surprises were to come and the direction of analysis was to be a two-way affair. I have attempted to give a flavour of this interaction in what follows.

From behaviour to brain

Soon after hatching, young domestic chicks (*Gallus gallus domesticus*) follow their mothers. This following response is not only elicited by the natural mother: a chick will approach a wide range of visually conspicuous objects, especially if they are moving. After a period of exposure to such an object the chick develops a social attachment to it. When this 'training' or 'imprinting' object is near, the chick emits contentment calls, and approaches it; if the object is moving away, the chick follows it. In addition, instead of approaching other conspicuous objects as it would have done in the naïve state, the chick now avoids them (see Spalding, 1873). As a result, when given a choice between a novel and a familiar object the chick approaches the familiar one. In this sense the chick recognises the object it had previously seen; so we may infer that the chick learned the characteristics of the object during the period of exposure. The learning process is known as filial imprinting (Lorenz, 1935/37; Hinde, 1955; Bateson, 1966; Sluckin, 1972).

Because filial imprinting is usually measured by a locomotor approach response, this form of learning has most extensively been studied in precocial species – those whose young show well-coordinated locomotor activity within a few hours of birth or hatching. However, there is no *requirement* that the underlying learning process must be tied to a locomotor response. Klopfer & Hailman (1964), for example, exposed domestic Vantress–Cross chicks to models of life-sized mallard duck decoys. Those chicks which did not follow the decoy during training, but sat watching it, showed the same subsequent preference as the initial 'followers', although not as strongly (see also Baer & Gray, 1960).

Imprinting is a particularly attractive form of learning for analysing mechanisms at the neural level. One important attraction is that some of the consequences of exposing a chick to a training object are often dramatic and may easily be measured: a chick may run the equivalent of 1 km in an hour in attempting to reach the training object (Horn, Rose & Bateson, 1973a). An additional attraction is that, by incubating eggs in darkness and by maintaining the chicks in darkness until they see the training object, a few hours after hatching, the experimenter may be confident that no other information derived from visual experience has been stored in the brain; and the chances of successfully detecting neural changes which are associated with the first visual experience are accordingly increased.

In the studies of imprinting described below, chicks were trained by exposing them to a visually conspicuous object. Most experiments employed the following procedures (see McCabe *et al.*, 1982). After hatching, chicks were reared in individual compartments in a dark incubator until they were between 15 and 30 hours old. The chicks were then placed individually in running wheels (Figure 1*d*), the centre of which stands some 50 cm from an imprinting stimulus (see Figure 1*a, b, c*). The chicks were exposed to the stimulus for between 1 and 4 hours, depending on the experiment, and the number of revolutions made by the wheel as the chick attempted to approach the training object was recorded ('approach activity'). A chick's preference was subsequently determined by exposing the chick to the familiar object and

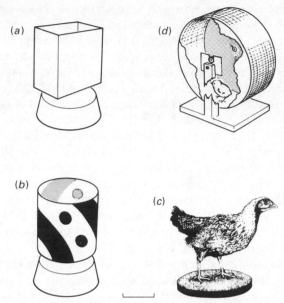

Figure 1. Training procedures and some training objects. In many of the experiments described in this chapter chicks were placed individually in a running wheel (*d*) facing the training object which was placed some 50 cm away (*a*). For the purposes of illustration one of the opaque sides of the running wheel is shown partly removed. The chick ran on the wire mesh. The training object illustrated in (*a*) is a box which, when activated, rotated about the base and was illuminated from within. The two larger surfaces were often coloured red, the narrower sides being black. The cylinder in object (*b*) was also illuminated from within and rotated about the base. (*c*) is the stuffed skin of a jungle fowl. Scale bar = 10 cm. (After Horn, 1985.)

to a novel object in succession. A measure of preference is given by the relative strength of the chick's approach to these objects.

If the storage process underlying imprinting involves changes in the connections between neurones then changes in protein and RNA metabolism may be expected to occur in those brain regions in which storage takes place. To examine this possibility one group of chicks was exposed to a conspicuous object, one group was exposed to diffuse light from an overhead lamp and one group was maintained in darkness. Training was found to be associated with an increase in the incorporation of radioactive lysine into protein and of radioactive uracil into RNA in the dorsal part (forebrain roof) of the cerebral hemispheres (Bateson, Horn & Rose, 1972). Although these results were clear-cut their interpretation is not since there are many ways in which the trained chicks differed from their controls and the biochemical changes may have been related to some or all of these differences. A number of control procedures was therefore devised to determine whether the biochemical changes were specifically related to the learning process, or whether they reflected some side-effects of training. The evidence provided by these procedures suggested that the biochemical changes were closely related to the learning process because (i) when visual input was restricted to one cerebral hemisphere by dividing the supra-optic commissure and occluding one eye with a black patch, incorporation was higher in the forebrain roof of the 'trained' hemisphere than the 'untrained' hemisphere (Horn, Rose & Bateson, 1973b), (ii) the magnitude of incorporation was positively correlated with a measure of how much the chicks had learned, but was not correlated with a variety of other measures of the chick's performance (Bateson, Horn & Rose, 1975), and (iii) the increase associated with training is not a result of some short-lasting effect of sensory stimulation (Bateson, Rose & Horn, 1973).

Since the biochemical changes were closely tied to the learning process of imprinting it was necessary, for a more detailed analysis of these changes, to enquire whether they were localised to restricted regions within the forebrain roof. Using an autoradiographic technique (Horn & McCabe, 1978), an increased incorporation of radioactive uracil into RNA was found in the intermediate and medial part of the hyperstriatum ventrale (Horn, McCabe & Bateson, 1979), a region referred to as IMHV (see Figure 2). Subsequently, the same region, and an adjacent part of the medial hyperstriatum ventrale, have been reported by other research groups to be involved in visual (Kohsaka *et al.*, 1979) and auditory imprinting (Maier & Scheich, 1983), as well as in passive avoidance learning (Rose & Csillag, 1985; Davies, Taylor & Johnson, 1988).

If IMHV plays a crucial role in the storage of information, then destruction of the region should prevent the acquisition of a preference through imprinting, and impair the retention of an acquired preference. Both of these predictions were confirmed in a number of lesion studies which involved the bilateral destruction of IMHV (McCabe, Horn & Bateson, 1981; McCabe *et al.*, 1982; Takamatsu & Tsukada, 1985). Similar lesions to other brain regions (i) a visual projection area known as the Wulst, and (ii) the lateral cerebral area, had no such effects (Johnson & Horn, 1987; McCabe *et al.*, 1982; Takamatsu & Tsukada, 1985).

The poor performance of the IMHV-lesioned chicks in the preference test could be accounted for if, for example, some sensory or motor functions were impaired by the lesion, or if the chicks lacked the motivation to approach the training object. However, the fact that chicks with these lesions peck at objects as accurately as sham-operated controls and that lesioned and

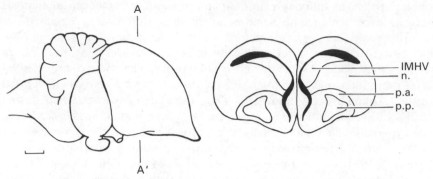

Figure 2. Outline drawing of the chick brain. The vertical lines AA′ above and below the drawing of the lateral aspect (left diagram) indicate the plane of the coronal section outline (right diagram) of the brain. Abbreviations: IMHV, the intermediate and medial part of the hyperstriatum ventrale; n., neostriatum; p.a., paleostriatum augmentatum; p.p., paleostriatum primativum. Scale bar = 2 mm. (After Horn & Johnson, 1989.)

control chicks, allowed to move about freely, could not be distinguished from each other even by experienced observers (McCabe *et al.*, 1981, 1982), all imply that there were no gross motor or motivational deficits in the lesioned birds. This implication is supported by the finding that these birds are able to perform certain other learning tasks (see below). It is also worth emphasising that the biochemical studies, which first implicated IMHV in imprinting, were correlative and did not involve any intervention that might impair the chicks' behaviour; the lesion studies served to test predictions based on the correlative studies, and the predictions were met. When all the experimental results are taken together, the most likely explanation of the behaviour of the IMHV-lesioned chicks is that they are unable to recognise the training object.

Many theories of the neural basis of memory suppose that a particular experience or event leads to the formation or strengthening of pathways in the brain (James, 1890) through changes in the size or number of synaptic junctions (Tanzi, 1893; Cajal, 1911; Hebb, 1949). Such changes occur widely in the central and peripheral nervous systems during normal growth and development, and frequently occur after injury. Thus the occurrence of these changes is not alone evidence that they play a role in memory. To be confident that a neural change plays such a role, it is necessary to demonstrate that the change is exclusive to learning and occurs in a brain region in which information is known to be stored (see Horn *et al.*, 1973a). The evidence presented above suggests that IMHV is such a region. A series

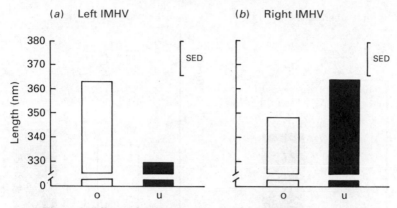

Figure 3. Effects of training on the length of the postsynaptic densities of synapses in IMHV. Mean values are shown according to hemisphere and treatment. Data for axospinous and axodendritic synapses are combined. Chicks were either exposed to the imprinting stimulus for 20 min (u, undertrained chicks, black bars) or for 140 min (o, overtrained chicks, open bars). Data for the left IMHV are shown in diagram (*a*) and for the right IMHV in diagram (*b*). For each side the standard error of the difference (SED) between mean values from undertrained and overtrained chicks are shown. Further training led to a significant increase in the lengths of the postsynaptic densities in the left IMHV only. (After Bradley *et al.*, 1981.)

of experiments was therefore conducted to enquire whether imprinting leads to changes in the structure of synapses in the left and right IMHV (Bradley, Horn & Bateson, 1979, 1981; Horn, Bradley & McCabe 1985).

In the first experiments two groups of chicks were used. Both groups were dark-reared until they were approximately 21 hours old. One group was then exposed to an artificial imprinting stimulus for 20 minutes (undertrained), the other group exposed to the stimulus for 140 minutes (overtrained). After training the right and left IMHV regions were removed and studied using the electron microscope. Quantitative sampling techniques were used to measure various aspects of synapse morphology, including the number of synapses per unit volume of brain tissue, and the mean size of axonal terminal swellings, the synaptic boutons. At chemical synapses, in which transmission is mediated by a neurotransmitter, pre- and postsynaptic elements are separated by a narrow cleft. At vertebrate synapses part of the postsynaptic membrane is thickened and is known as the postsynaptic density (PSD); the mean lengths of the PSD in right and left IMHV respectively were determined. Overtrained chicks differed from the undertrained chicks in only one measure of synapse structure: the mean length of the PSD was increased.

127

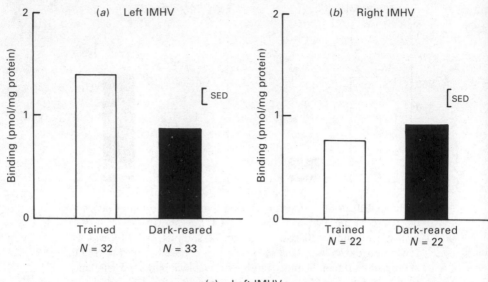

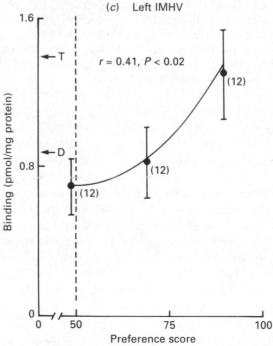

Figure 4. The effects of training on NMDA-sensitive binding of L-[³H]glutamate to membranes from the IMHV. Data for the left and right IMHV are shown in (a) and (b) respectively. In these figures

This change occurred only in left IMHV synapses (Figure 3). Synapses on dendrites occur in two forms, axodendritic and axospinous. Axodendritic synapses are found on the shafts of dendrites; axospinous synapses are found on small, balloon-shaped structures, the dendritic spines. The data shown in Figure 3 are based on measurements from the two types of synapses without distinction. The study of Bradley *et al.* (1981) was subsequently extended by increasing the number of chicks and adding a group of dark-reared chicks (Horn *et al.*, 1985). With this larger sample enough data were available to analyse separately the measurements from each type of synapse. When this was done the effects of training were found to be restricted to axospinous synapses: the mean length of the PSDs in the left IMHV of overtrained chicks was approximately 17% greater than the corresponding mean values for the two other groups of birds.

When neurotransmitter molecules are liberated from the presynaptic bouton they diffuse into the synaptic cleft and bind to receptors which are present in the postsynaptic density (Fagg & Matus, 1984). A consequence of this interaction between neurotransmitter and receptor protein is that ion channels may open. If the synapse is excitatory, the net ion flux will

---

mean values are shown together with the standard error of the differences (SED) between the means from trained and dark-reared chicks. N = number of samples, each sample comprising material from three chicks. (*a*) Left IMHV. Binding in the trained group was significantly higher than in the dark-reared group (matched-pairs t = 3·46; df = 30; $P < 0.005$). (*b*) Right IMHV. These samples were taken from the chicks which also contributed to the samples summarised in (*a*). There were no significant effects of training on binding in the right IMHV samples (t = 0·91). (*c*) Relationship between NMDA-sensitive binding in the left IMHV and preference score, both corrected by linear regression to constant approach during training as a result of a partial correlation analysis. The higher the preference score, the greater the chick's preference for the training stimulus and the greater the strength of imprinting. Preference scores of 100 and 0 indicate that in the preference test all activity was directed to the imprinting and novel objects respectively. The 'no preference' score of 50 is indicated by the vertical broken line. Arrow D indicates the mean binding in the left IMHV of dark-reared chicks and arrow T the mean binding in trained chicks in the experiments on which (*a*) is based. Each point represents a mean of 12 values. The standard error bars for binding (vertical) and for preference score (horizontal) are given. The curve is a polynomial fitted to all 36 points by least-squares regression. Note that T is close to the mean of the group with the highest mean preference score. (For further details see McCabe & Horn, 1988.)

depolarise the postsynaptic cell membrane and may lead to the discharge of an impulse along the axon. At least some axospinous synapses in the mammalian central nervous system are excitatory and possess receptors for the excitatory amino acid L-glutamate (Nafstad, 1967; Storm-Mathisen, 1977; Nadler *et al.*, 1978; Errington, Lynch & Bliss, 1987). Membranes with these receptors bind the radioactive isotope L-[^{3}H]glutamate. If imprinting leads to an increased number of receptors for this amino acid, then membranes prepared from the left IMHV of trained chicks should bind more L-[^{3}H]glutamate than corresponding membranes from dark-reared chicks. McCabe & Horn (1988) found that this was indeed the case. However, there are several sub-types of receptor for L-glutamate. One of these subtypes is defined by the action of the selective agonist *N*-methyl-D-aspartate (NMDA). McCabe & Horn (1988) found a significant increase in NMDA-sensitive binding in the left IMHV of trained chicks compared with that in dark-reared controls; there were no such differences in right IMHV binding (Figure 4*a*, *b*).

Whilst these results were consistent with the results of the electron microscope studies of IMHV described above (compare the pattern of mean values in Figures 3*a*, *b* and 4*a*, *b*), many ambiguities remained in the interpretation of the data. The trained birds were visually experienced, the dark-reared birds were not, so that the differences in NMDA-sensitive binding could be a result of these and other, consequential differences. To clarify these ambiguities, a group of chicks was exposed to the training stimulus and given a preference test immediately before being killed. The strength of the chick's preference for the familiar object relative to a novel object was measured and expressed as a preference score (McCabe *et al.*, 1982). The preference score was positively correlated with NMDA-sensitive binding in the left IMHV. The corresponding correlation coefficient for NMDA-sensitive binding in the right IMHV was not significant. Bateson & Jaeckel (1976) found that approach activity during training is correlated with preference score. It is therefore possible that the observed correlation between NMDA-sensitive binding and preference score reflects a relation between binding and locomotor activity during training. Binding and preference scores were therefore corrected for training approach activity, using the method of partial correlation. There was a significant positive partial correlation between NMDA-sensitive binding in the left IMHV and preference score (see Figure 4*c*). The chicks with the lowest mean corrected preference score performed at chance; the corresponding mean binding for this group is not significantly different from that in the left IMHV of the dark-reared chicks of the previous experiments (see Figure 4*a*). The partial correlation between NMDA-sensitive binding in the right IMHV and preference score was not significant.

The increase in binding in the left IMHV is very likely due to an increase in the number of receptors (McCabe & Horn, 1988). This increase cannot simply be attributed to side effects of the training procedure for several reasons. (i) The studies that led to the localisation of IMHV and to the demonstration of the crucial role of this region, especially of the left IMHV (Cipolla-Neto, Horn & McCabe, 1982), in information storage had controlled for these and other side-effects of training. (ii) An effect of arousal would be expected to be expressed in behaviour, e.g. the more aroused the chicks, the more vigorously would they be expected to approach the red box during training. However, the partial correlation coefficient between NMDA-sensitive binding and preference score was significant when the effect of approach activity during training was held constant. This latter finding also demonstrates that differences in locomotor activity during training cannot account for the correlation between binding and corrected preference score. (iii) Light exposure *per se* does not account for the findings, since the corrected mean left IMHV binding in chicks that had been exposed to the red box for 140 minutes, but had not developed a preference for it, was closely similar to the mean left IMHV binding of dark-reared chicks. These considerations suggest that the change in receptor binding is not a side-effect of training, but that learning leads to an increase in the number of NMDA-type receptors in the left IMHV.

The selective preference of the imprinted chicks for the familiar object is evidence that these chicks recognise this object. It is possible, therefore (Horn, 1962), that the increased number of excitatory receptors leads to an increased efficacy of synaptic transmission in the left IMHV and hence forms a basis for this recognition memory (see also Horn & McCabe, 1990). Although the molecular mechanisms which bring about the changes in the postsynaptic density are not known, the consequences of the changes, and of the increased number of NMDA receptors, are likely to be subtle in several ways. (i) The ion channels associated with the NMDA receptors will pass current only under certain conditions: the receptors must be activated by their neurotransmitter *and* the postsynaptic cell must be excited through ion channels associated with other receptors (Nowak *et al.*, 1984). At the behavioural level, such conditions could have interesting consequences. For example, the presentation of a familiar object may activate the afferent fibres to the synapses which, through training, have an increased number of NMDA receptors. The activated afferent fibres may release L-glutamate which binds to these receptors. The postsynaptic cell may not respond to the presynaptic signal unless the cell is depolarised by some other input. This input may be generated by, for example, neurones whose activity is controlled by the attentional state of the animal; that is, attentional mechanisms may exercise some control of the flow of signals through the memory systems of the brain (Horn, 1970). Other controlling inputs may be from neural systems underlying affective states of the animal or from neuronal assemblies representing other memories. (ii) Calcium ions flow inwards through NMDA-channels (MacDermot *et al.*, 1986). This influx may lead to and maintain changes in the structure of the postsynaptic density and influence its interactions with proteins in the cytoskeleton of the dendritic spine. If this view proves to be correct, it may be that prolonged inactivity of a previously modified synapse may lead to a regression of the modification and so to a corresponding loss of the specific memory with which these synapses are involved.

It is clear that many questions remain to be answered in addition to those which are implicit in the considerations outlined in the above paragraph. For example, do the structural changes in axospinous synapses, and the changes in NMDA receptors, occur at the same synapses; are all axospinous synapses in the left IMHV affected by training or are the changes restricted to a sub-population of them; and are the changed synapses interconnected as in a Hebbian cell-assembly (Hebb, 1949)? While a change in number of NMDA receptors might, as suggested, increase synaptic efficiency, other possibilities exist and need to be explored. For example, the increase in NMDA receptors may play only a 'permissive' role in the cellular mechanisms of memory: the increase might permit a relatively large influx of calcium into the cell to initiate other changes, for example in synapse structure, after which NMDA receptor numbers may return to lower levels.

NMDA receptors have been implicated in the processes that control certain forms of plasticity in the developing nervous system (Cline, Debski & Constantine-Paton, 1987; Rauschecker & Hahn, 1987; Kleinschmidt, Bear & Singer, 1987). The implied link between developmental processes and learning is not wholly unexpected (see also Brown & Horn, 1990). Changes occur in the morphological and functional properties of neurones during the course of ontogeny; in some systems the direction of these changes is such that neurones largely lose their capacity for plastic change as their synaptic connections become stabilised in the course of development and maturation (Hubel & Wiesel, 1970; Olson & Freeman, 1980; Knusden & Knusden, 1986). A similar direction of change may occur as a result of learning in neural circuits specialised for storage. Thus Horn *et al.* (1973a) suggested that neurones within the memory systems of the brain may remain plastic until they become engaged in the storage process associated with a specific learning experience. Thereafter the synaptic connections may become stabilised although, as suggested above, this stabilisation may require active maintenance.

From brain to behaviour

In the study in which autoradiography was used to determine whether or not training led to localised biochemical changes in the forebrain, the training object was an artificial one (Horn *et al.*, 1979). Indeed, artificial visual objects had been used as training stimuli in all our earlier experiments as well. However, in a series of four experiments in which the effects of brain lesions on imprinting were studied, one of the training objects was artificial (Figure 1*a*) and the other was the stuffed skin of a jungle fowl (Figure 1*c*). Both of these stimuli were illuminated and moved. After a given period of training (see p. 123) the chicks were given a sequential preference test and a preference score adjusted (see legend to Figure 4). In a preliminary experiment the 'attractiveness' of the box and fowl were adjusted by varying the intensity of illumination and the speed of movement, so that for a given period of training, the mean preference score of box-trained chicks did not differ significantly from that of the fowl-trained chicks.

The type of training stimulus (box or fowl) used in the four lesion experiments referred to above did not seem to influence the outcome of the results. Therefore, the preference scores of the box-trained chicks had been combined with those of the fowl-trained chicks in each experiment. However, when the data for all four experiments were analysed together, a different picture emerged (Horn & McCabe, 1984). IMHV-lesioned chicks which had been trained on the box performed at chance, achieving an overall mean preference score which was not significantly different from 50 % (Figure 5*a*); IMHV-lesioned chicks which had been trained on the fowl had a clear preference for that object (Figure 5*b*), a preference which was slightly, though significantly, smaller than that of their sham-operated controls. The mean preference scores of the two sham-operated control groups were not significantly different from each other. In contrast, the mean preference scores of the two lesioned groups differed significantly from each other. Thus, lesions to IMHV had a profound effect on the mean preference score of box-trained birds, but only a small effect on the mean preference score of the fowl-trained birds.

Two other procedures also teased apart an effect of the training object. In the first experiment one group of chicks received a drug (DSP-4) which reduces the concentration of catecholamines in the brain. Chicks which had received an injection of this drug and had been exposed to a rotating red box performed at chance in the sequential preference test. In contrast, drug-treated chicks which had been exposed to the fowl had a strong preference for the fowl in the test, though the strength of the preference was significantly less than that of the fowl-trained controls which had received an injection of distilled water instead of the drug (Davies, Horn & McCabe, 1985). This

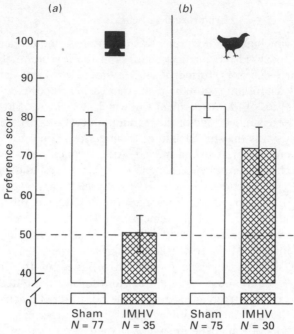

Figure 5. Summary of data from experiments in which preference scores were impaired by lesions of IMHV. The scores (see legend to Figure 4) for chicks with lesions of IMHV and sham-operated controls are set out according to the stimulus to which the chicks were exposed during the training period. Means ± SEM for chicks trained with the box (*a*) and with the jungle fowl (*b*). The standard errors may be used to compare the means against the chance, no preference scores of 50. Sham = sham operated control chicks; IMHV refers to chicks with lesions of this brain region. N = number of chicks. (Based on data from Horn & McCabe, 1984.)

pattern of results – a strong preference for the training object by the controls, performance at chance by the box-trained experimental birds, and a clear, though slightly impaired, preference for the training object by the fowl-trained experimentals – is very similar to that found in the lesion studies (Figure 5). The second procedure which provided further evidence of stimulus-dependent effects involved an analysis of plasma testosterone concentrations. The mean preference score of fowl-trained chicks which had received an injection of testosterone was higher than for those chicks which had not received the hormone. Furthermore, there was a significant positive correlation between plasma testosterone concentration and preference score in the fowl-trained birds. This correlation was significant even amongst fowl-trained birds which had not received testosterone; that is, the correlation between preference score and testosterone concentration held over the physiological range of concentrations of the hormone. In contrast to these findings in fowl-trained birds, exogenous testosterone was without effect on the preference scores of box-trained chicks; nor was there a significant correlation between preference score and plasma testosterone concentration in these birds (Bolhuis, McCabe & Horn, 1986).

Although we had no clear evidence that the behavioural responses elicited by the naturalistic stuffed fowl differed from those elicited by the artificial red box the results of the neural and endocrine studies compelled us to be alert to the possibility that such differences might exist. We had been forced, so to speak, to move 'upwards' from studying brain function to studying behaviour.

Evidence for such differences came from a different experimental approach (Bolhuis, Johnson & Horn, 1985; Johnson, Bolhuis & Horn, 1985). In these studies chicks were subjected to various procedures and the chicks' preferences for the box and fowl were then tested. These experiments differed from earlier ones in that the chicks had not seen either the box or the stuffed fowl before the test. Furthermore, unlike most of the previous studies in which a chick's preference was measured in a test which involved presenting novel and familiar stimuli separately (the sequential test), in this study the two objects were presented together using the simultaneous choice test of Bateson & Wainwright (1972). Apart from the obvious differences between the two tests, the simultaneous test provides a more sensitive measure of the chick's preference by providing a more sensitive measure of the chick's approach activity (see Horn, 1985, pp. 156–7).

The central finding of the experiments of Bolhuis *et al.* (1985) and Johnson *et al.* (1985) can be summarised quite briefly. Chicks were raised in individual compartments of an incubator and when they were approximately 24 hours old were placed in a running wheel for a total of 2 hours. They were then returned to the incubator. The chicks were given a simultaneous choice test (test 2) *either* 2 hours (test 1) *or* 24 hours (test 2) after having been removed from the wheel. *Until the chicks were given the preference test they had been kept in darkness.* At test 1, the chicks performed at chance, expressing no preference. At test 2, the chicks preferred the jungle fowl. Control chicks which had remained in the incubator all the time, until the test, performed at chance in the test.

These experiments suggest that some aspects of the chicks' experiences of the wheel (e.g. handling, opportunity to move about in the wheel) were necessary for the expression of the preference for the fowl. The experiments also suggest that, over the period studied, this preference does not appear simply with the passage of time. Because the preference appeared in the

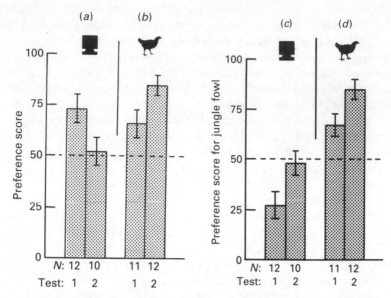

Figure 6. Mean preference scores ($\pm$ SEM) in test 1 and test 2 for box-exposed (*a*), (*c*) and fowl-exposed (*b*), (*d*) chicks. In (*a*) and (*b*), preference scores were calculated from the expression:

$$\frac{100 \times \text{distance travelled by trolley as chick attempted to approach the familiar conspicuous object}}{\text{total distance travelled by the trolley}}$$

Thus the score of 100 indicates that the chicks directed all their approach activity towards the training object, 0 that all the approach activity was directed toward the novel object; a score of 50 indicates that activity was directed equally to the two objects. In (*c*) and (*d*) the preference scores in (*a*) and (*b*) were expressed as preferences for the stuffed jungle fowl (thus 100 signifies that all approach was directed toward the fowl, 0 that approach was directed towards the box). $N =$ number of chicks in each group. (Results based on data from Johnson *et al.*, 1985.)

absence of prior visual experience, it was referred to as an *emerging predisposition*.

The emerging predisposition can be detected in previously trained as well as in visually naïve chicks. Thus, in the experiments of Johnson *et al.* (1985) the preferences of young chicks were measured either approximately 2 hours (test 1) or 24 hours (test 2) after exposure to a red box or a stuffed fowl. Preferences were measured using the simultaneous choice test. At test 1 the chicks preferred the object to which they had previously been exposed, whether it had been the stuffed fowl or the red box (Figure 6*a*, *b*). However, at test 2 the pattern of results was different. The mean preference of the fowl-trained chicks in this test was significantly stronger than that of the fowl-trained chicks in test 1; in contrast, the mean preference scores of the box-trained chicks in test 2 was significantly less than that of the box-trained chicks in test 1 (Figure 6*a*, *b*). In other words, it appeared as if the preferences of the fowl-trained chicks had strengthened with the passage of time, whereas those of the box-trained chicks had weakened. Johnson *et al.* (1985) found that chicks (light-exposed) which had been placed in a running wheel and exposed to diffuse white light, but not to the box or to the fowl, showed a similarly increasing preference for the fowl over time when tested in the same way.

Since the box and fowl were both present in the simultaneous choice test, the preferences may be expressed in terms of approach to the stuffed fowl irrespective of a chick's prior experience. The mean preference scores shown in Figure 6*a*, *b* are used in Figure 6*c*, *d*, but expressed now as mean preferences for the stuffed fowl. Chicks which had been exposed to the box and which preferred this object in test 1 necessarily had a low preference for the stuffed fowl. All chicks tested approximately 24 hours after training (test 2), however, showed a significantly greater preference for the stuffed fowl than those tested at approximately 2 hours (test 1), regardless of the training stimulus. The mean values shown in Figure 6*c*, *d* are again plotted in Figure 7. This figure also includes the mean preference scores of the light-exposed chicks referred to above. These scores may be used as a baseline for measuring the effects of training on mean preference scores at the appropriate testing times. The mean preference scores of the light-exposed chicks changed over time. Accordingly, the baseline level from which the acquired preferences were measured also changes with time (Figure 7, Δy), and so is different at test 2 from that at test 1. The difference between the mean preference score of an experimental group and that of the light-exposed group is k_i. This difference provides a measure of the preferences acquired by the chick for one of the conspicuous objects as a result of being exposed to it during training. In test 1 the mean preference score of the chicks exposed to the box was less than that of the light-exposed controls by 19·2% (Figure 7, k_1). The corresponding difference for the chicks exposed to the fowl is almost identical, 20·7% (Figure 7, k_2), but in the opposite direction of the scale used in this figure. The preferences of all three groups of chicks shift towards the jungle fowl from test 1 to test 2. Is this shift associated with the loss of the preference acquired through training? If the acquired preference is lost we should expect (Figure 7) k_3 to be less than k_1 and k_4 to be less than k_2. In order to test this hypothesis the mean preference scores of the light-exposed birds in each test were subtracted from the preference score of each

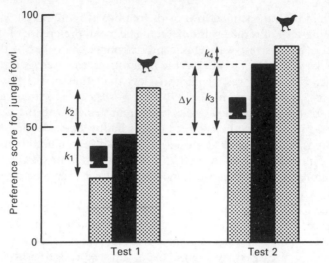

Figure 7. A model for the interaction between acquired preferences and a developing predisposition. All mean preference scores are expressed as preferences for the stuffed fowl. Broken lines represent the base lines in test 1 and test 2 set by the respective groups of light-exposed chicks (black bars). Δy represents the difference in mean preference score between the light-exposed chicks in test 1 and in test 2. k_i represents the effects of prior exposure, to the red box (k_1 and k_3) or to the jungle fowl (k_2 and k_4). See text for further discussion. (After Johnson *et al.*, 1985.)

trained bird at the same test. The resulting adjusted scores were subjected to an analysis of variance. The adjusted scores of the experimental birds were not significantly affected by the time of testing (test 1 or test 2), implying that the acquired preferences are not lost; they are stable over the period studied, notwithstanding the emergence of the predisposition for the fowl.

This result, together with the finding that the relative preference for the jungle fowl increases from test 1 to test 2 suggests that the preferences of the experimental chicks are affected by two underlying processes: (i) a developing predisposition which becomes apparent as an increase in preference for the jungle fowl by the light-exposed chicks and (ii) a learning process through which chicks come to recognise particular objects to which they have been exposed. Whether or not these two processes may be related in some way to the activity of the different neural systems revealed by the physiological studies (pp. 133–5) is an issue which is taken up below (p. 141).

In all the experiments in which the emerging preference had been studied, the chicks were placed in the running wheels when they were approximately a day old. The results of further experiments suggested that there is a sensitive period for the emergence of the preference: if chicks are placed in the wheel before or after this period the preference for the fowl is not present in the 24-hour test (Johnson, Davies & Horn, 1989).

Once developed, the predisposition might serve as a filter for incoming signals, allowing only information about stimuli that resemble conspecifics to be processed for learning. If this were so, not only might the bird preferentially approach such stimuli, but it might be unable to learn about other objects through being exposed to them. However, Bolhuis, Johnson & Horn (1989a) have shown that chicks are able to learn the characteristics of, and come to prefer, an artificial object even though there is strong presumptive evidence that the chicks' predisposition to approach the fowl has appeared. Nevertheless, if chicks are exposed to an imprinting object during the sensitive period for the predisposition, they form a stronger attachment to an object resembling a conspecific than to an artificial object (Boakes & Panter, 1985; Bolhuis & Trooster, 1988). This effect is not revealed by a preference test (see Figure 7: $/k_1/ = /k_2/$) but has been shown in experiments designed to change an acquired preference (Bolhuis & Trooster, 1988). These authors showed that it is more difficult to modify the preference of a fowl-trained chick than that of a box-trained chick. These findings are consistent with the interaction model of preference formation described above (see Horn & McCabe, 1984; Johnson et al., 1985). If exposed to a conspecific at the appropriate time chicks are predisposed to approach it; subsequently they learn the characteristics of that individual. At the neural level at least two systems are engaged, IMHV in the learning process and the system outside IMHV in the process controlling the predisposition (see p. 140). If an artificial stimulus, such as the box, is first presented the chick learns about it and is subsequently able to recognise it (Bolhuis et al., 1989a). But if given a choice between the box and the fowl, the predisposition and the learning process seem, at both the behavioural and neural levels of analysis, to 'pull' in opposite directions. In the case, then, of attachment to the natural mother the interactions between predisposition and learning appear to be synergistic; whereas for the box, an artificial mother surrogate, the interaction does not appear to be synergistic and may even be antagonistic. It should follow from these considerations that when the sensitive period for the predisposition has passed the strength of attachment to the fowl should no longer be greater than to an artificial object. Recent work by M. Johnson, J. Bolhuis and G. Horn (unpublished) suggests that this is indeed the case.

What aspects of the stuffed fowl are critical, and serve as 'targets' for the emerging preference? This question was addressed in a series of experiments which involved giving chicks a simultaneous choice test. In this test one object was always the intact stuffed fowl (see Figure 1c), but the second test object was varied (Johnson & Horn, 1988). These experiments suggested that the target of the emerging preference was the head and neck region of the fowl. However, experiments using as test objects a stuffed Gadwall duck or a stuffed polecat demonstrated that *the configuration of features essential for the predisposition is neither species-specific nor even class-specific*. It remains unclear whether or not certain features of the region are more important than others. That the eyes may play a role (see for example Coss, 1972; Scaife, 1976a, b) is consistent with a lack of species-specificity in this change of behaviour.

In considering the possible implications of their findings Horn & McCabe (1984) suggested *inter alia* that two neural systems may be involved in controlling the response of a chick to the fowl. One of these systems, they suggested, is within IMHV and the other outside this brain region. The two systems were considered to play different roles in the recognition of conspecifics: the system outside IMHV is concerned with the recognition of the general features of conspecifics whereas IMHV is involved in recognising the features of particular individuals. These features must be learned; and IMHV, it was proposed, is involved in the learning process whether the chick learns the markings of its own mother or the characteristics of an artificial object such as the red box.

Three predictions arise from these proposals concerning conspecifics. First, that intact young chicks are capable of learning the characteristics of individual adult fowl, and, secondly, that ablation of IMHV precludes such learning. These two predictions have been confirmed (Johnson & Horn, 1987). Moreover, the impaired ability of IMHV-lesioned birds to recognise individual conspecifics extends into adult life (Bolhuis *et al.*, 1989b). A third prediction is that ablation of IMHV will not impair the emerging predisposition. This prediction has also been confirmed (Johnson & Horn, 1986).

The evidence that the emerging predisposition is to the face and neck region, or to features contained within it, raises the possibility that the putative recognition system involved, lying outside IMHV, is responsive to the features of the face and neck, and may have some of the properties of 'face neurones' which have been described in the temporal cortex of monkeys (Bruce, Desimone & Gross, 1981; Perret, Rolls & Caan, 1982) and sheep (Kendrick & Baldwin, 1987). Whether or not this is so will only be known if it proves possible to localise a region of the brain which is crucially involved in the predisposition.

We do not yet know what it is about the period in the running wheel that gives rise to the emergence of the predisposition. Handling the chick is an obvious possibility, but other non-specific experiences have not been excluded. The finding of an emerging predisposition for some features possessed by conspecifics is reminiscent of the findings of Klopfer (1967) in his studies of the preferences of young Peking ducklings. From these studies he concluded: 'It looked as if some kind of innate preference existed that had to be activated by the experience of following...' Whether movement was the important factor in Klopfer's studies, or some other non-specific factor associated with following, is not known. One way of thinking about the action of non-specific factors, such as arousal, is to suppose that they have physiological consequences which lead to a modification of chicks' preferences. What these physiological consequences may be is not known, though the possibility that they involve hormones may be worth exploring. Thus arousal, and even minor degrees of stress, may lead to a change in the hormonal state of an animal (cf. Kruhlich, Hefco & Read, 1974). Furthermore, Bolhuis *et al.* (1986) have shown that the strength of preference of fowl-trained chicks for the fowl is correlated with the concentration of testosterone in the plasma. In addition, the relatively long time taken by some hormones to exert certain of their effects is consistent with the relatively long time taken for the predisposition to be expressed. Whilst these views are speculative they at least have the merit of being experimentally testable. Testable speculation may be pushed still further by supposing (see above) that neurones in the putative system outside IMHV which support the emerging preference for the jungle fowl, have properties similar to face-detecting neurones. In the chick such a system would not be expected to be functional prior to the emergence of the predisposition, perhaps because transmission between neurones in the system is ineffective. Transmission across these synapses may become effective, and the system 'functionally validated', soon after the chick has been in the running wheel – or, in more natural circumstances, soon after it begins to move about. Such functional validation could be achieved through hormonal action, the hormone initiating intraneuronal events which lead to efficient synaptic transmission. Once operational, neurones in the face-detecting system may be excited by impulses evoked by the sight of the natural mother who may possess a combination of features which optimally trigger these neurones. If such neurones control orientation and approach behaviour, the chick is likely to direct its activity selectively to the parent and, as suggested above, gradually learn its characteristics in a process which engages neurones in IMHV.

The term 'imprinting' was originally used by Lorenz (1935/37) in the context of the following response of birds. Hence it is easy enough to suppose that the rules governing the following response also apply to the learning process. Whilst there is good evidence of a sensitive period for the following response, as there is for the predisposition, it does not follow that there is a sensitive period for the learning process, or that there is anything 'peculiar' about this process (cf. Lorenz 1935/37). Sluckin & Salzen (1961) have emphasised the perceptual side of the learning process, as have Hinde (1962), Bateson (1966, 1971), and Kovach, Fabricius & Fält (1966). Sluckin used the term 'exposure learning', since it 'refers unambiguously to the perceptual registration by the organism of the environment to which it is exposed' (Sluckin, 1972, p. 109; see also Thorpe, 1944). Such learning is not restricted to birds, but occurs widely even amongst mammals (see for example Hinde, 1962; Sluckin, 1972).

The general situation, or context in which learning takes place, influences the outcome of a training procedure (see Mackintosh, 1982). So also, of course, does the motivational state, previous experience and age of the animal. Furthermore, it has become apparent that animals have predispositions to learn some things and not others even though the tasks seem of similar difficulty. In other words, learning is constrained and predisposed in many ways (see, for example, Hinde & Stevenson-Hinde, 1973). The influence of such predispositions is, perhaps, nowhere more powerful than in very young animals. The central nervous system of the newborn, or newly hatched animal cannot be thought of as a *tabula rasa* on which is inscribed the characteristics of viewed objects. Thus Goren, Sarty & Wu (1975) found that human newborns, whose median age was 9 minutes postpartum, turned their eyes and heads further to follow a schematic face than to follow a variety of 'scrambled' faces. Goren *et al.* wrote that all the persons with whom the infant could have had visual contact were capped, gowned and masked so that the infant had not been exposed to a face before testing. Nevertheless, the infants may have 'seen' their attendants' eyes, become familiar with them and later followed the eye stimuli of the schematic face. This is not a plausible explanation of the infants' responses since two of the scrambled faces also contained eye stimuli, but were not followed as far as the schematic face. In the light of their findings Goren *et al.* considered that an infant 'enters the world predisposed to respond to any face' (see also Johnson, 1987). Chicks also have predispositions, responding differently to objects of certain colours, size and contrast (see Fabricius & Boyd, 1953; Schaefer & Hess, 1959; Kovach, 1971). Indeed Hinde (1961) suggested that for some species, objects resembling the natural mother may be optimal for eliciting following behaviour, a prescient suggestion given the evidence set out above concerning the emerging predisposition. This predisposition interacts with information acquired through learning. In the natural situation, where the chick is exposed to patterned light and is able to move around freely, the predisposition may emerge very rapidly (Bolhuis *et al.*, 1985). The young chick may then attend to the face and neck of its own mother, rather than to inanimate objects, learn specifically about the features of this region and so come to recognise her on the basis of these features.

Conclusion

Robert Hinde has made massive contributions to the behavioural sciences. I hope that the work outlined in this chapter will give him some pleasure, for he formulated many of the questions which this work has attempted to address. His own contributions have extended far beyond the paths that I have explored. Extensive and diverse as his contributions have been, a single theme unites them – the nature of relationships. He has explored this in several contexts: in filial imprinting in birds, in the relationship between parents and their young in non-human and human primates, in the relationship between pairs of individuals, between individuals and society, and between societies. In all of these enterprises he has brought not only penetrating new insights but an ability to sift the trivial from the major issues; not only to formulate the right questions, but to act to resolve them and, where it has not been possible to resolve them, then to draw attention to them. Nowhere is this more apparent than in his commitment to understanding the nature of aggression and war, and the dangers to life on earth of allowing, uncontrolled, those human activities which degrade the environment. Behavioural scientists have not always acted in the most humane of ways (see for example Müller-Hill, 1988); but Robert Hinde has done, and continues to do so.

References

Baer, D. M. & Gray, P. H. (1960). Imprinting to different species without overt following. *Perceptual Motor Skills*, **10**, 171–4.

Bateson, P. P. G. (1966). The characteristics and context of imprinting. *Biological Reviews*, **41**, 177–220.

Bateson, P. P. G. (1971). Imprinting. In *Ontogeny of Vertebrate Behavior*, ed. H. Moltz, pp. 369–87. New York: Academic Press.

Bateson, P. P. G., Horn, G. & Rose, S. P. R. (1972). Effects of early experience on regional incorporation of precursors into RNA and protein in the chick brain. *Brain Research*, **39**, 449–65.

Bateson, P. P. G., Horn, G. & Rose, S. P. R. (1975). Imprinting: Correlations between behaviour and incorporation of (^{14}C) Uracil into chick brain. *Brain Research*, **84**, 207–220.

Bateson, P. P. G. & Jaeckel, J. B. (1976). Chick's preferences for familiar and novel conspicuous objects after different periods of exposure. *Animal Behaviour*, **24**, 386–90.

Bateson, P. P. G., Rose, S. P. R. & Horn, G. (1973). Imprinting: lasting effects on uracil incorporation into chick brain. *Science*, **181**, 576–8.

Bateson, P. P. G. & Wainwright, A. A. P. (1972). The effects of prior exposure to light on the imprinting process in domestic chicks. *Behaviour*, **42**, 279–90.

Boakes, R. & Panter, D. (1985). Secondary imprinting in the domestic chick blocked by previous exposure to a live hen. *Animal Behaviour*, **33**, 353–65.

Bolhuis, J. J., Johnson, M. H. & Horn, G. (1985). Effects of early experience on the development of filial preferences in the domestic chick. *Developmental Psychobiology*, **18**, 299–308.

Bolhuis, J. J., Johnson, M. H. & Horn, G. (1989a). Interacting mechanisms during the formation of filial preferences: the development of a predisposition does not constrain learning. *Journal of Experimental Psychology: Animal Behavior Processes* (in press).

Bolhuis, J. J., Johnson, M., Horn, G. & Bateson, P. (1989b). Long-lasting effects of IMHV lesions on social preferences in domestic fowl. *Behavioral Neuroscience*, **103**, 438–41.

Bolhuis, J. J., McCabe, B. J. & Horn, G. (1985b). Androgens and imprinting. Differential effects of testosterone on filial preferences in the domestic chick. *Behavioral Neuroscience*, **100**, 51–6.

Bolhuis, J. J. & Trooster, W. J. (1988). Reversibility revisited: Stimulus-dependent stability of filial preference in the chick. *Animal Behaviour*, **36**, 668–74.

Bradley, P., Horn, G. & Bateson, P. P. G. (1979). Morphological correlates of imprinting in the chick brain. *Neurosciences Letters Supplement*, **3**, S84.

Bradley, P., Horn, G. & Bateson, P. (1981). Imprinting: an electron microscopic study of chick hyperstriatum ventrale. *Experimental Brain Research*, **41**, 115–20.

Brown, M. W. & Horn, G. (1990). Are specific proteins implicated in the learning process of imprinting? *Developmental Brain Research*, **52**, 294–7.

Bruce, C., Desimone, R. & Gross, C. G. (1981). Visual properties of neurons in a polysensory area in superior temporal sulcus of the macaque. *Journal of Neurophysiology*, **46**, 369–84.

Cajál, S. R. (1911). *Histologie du Système Nerveux de l'Homme et des Vertébrés, Vol. 2*. Paris: Maloine.

Carew, T. J. (1989). Developmental assembly of learning in *Aplysia*. *Trends in Neurosciences*, **12**, 389–94.

Castelluci, V. F., Carew, T. J. & Kandel, E. R. (1978). Cellular analysis of long-term habitation of the gill-withdrawal reflex of *Aplysia californica*. *Science*, **202**, 1306–8.

Cipolla-Neto, J., Horn, G. & McCabe, B. J. (1982). Hemispheric asymmetry and imprinting: the effect of sequential lesions to the hyperstriatum ventrale. *Experimental Brain Research*, **48**, 22–7.

Cline, H. T., Debski, E. A. & Constantine-Paton, M. (1987). *N*-methyl-D-aspartate receptor antagonist desegregates eye-specific stripes. *Proceedings of the National Academy of Sciences (USA)*, **84**, 4342–5.

Coss, R. G. (1972). Eye-like schemata: their effect on behaviour. PhD dissertation, University of Reading.

Davies, D. C., Horn, G. & McCabe, B. J. (1985). Noradrenaline and learning: the effects of the noradrenergic neurotoxin DSP4 on imprinting in the domestic chick. *Behavioral Neuroscience*, **100**, 51–56.

Davies, D. C., Taylor, D. A. & Johnson, M. H. (1988). The effects of hyperstriatal lesions on one-trial passive-avoidance learning in the chick. *Journal of Neuroscience*, **8**, 4662–6.

Errington, M. L., Lynch, M. A. & Bliss, T. V. P. (1987). Long-term potentiation in the dentate gyrus: induction and increased glutamate release are blocked by D(-)aminophonovalerate. *Neuroscience*, **20**, 279–94.

Fabricius, E. & Boyd, H. (1952/53). Experiments on the following reactions of ducklings. *Wildfowl Trust Annual Report*, **6**, 84–9.

Fagg, G. E. & Matus, A. (1984). Selective association of *N*-methyl aspartate and quisqualate types of L-glutamate receptor with postsynaptic densities. *Proceedings of the National Academy of Sciences (USA)*, **81**, 6876–80.

Goren, C. C., Sarty, M. & Wu, P. Y. K. (1975). Visual following and pattern discrimination of face-like stimuli by newborn infants. *Pediatrics*, **56**, 544–9.

Hebb, D. O. (1949). *The Organization of Behavior*. New York: Wiley.

Hinde, R. A. (1954a). Factors governing the changes in strength of a partially inborn response, as shown by the mobbing behaviour of the chaffinch (*Fringilla coelebs*). I. The nature of the response, and an examination of its course. *Proceedings of the Royal Society of London B*, **142**, 306–31.

Hinde, R. A. (1954b). Factors governing the changes in strength of a partially inborn response, as shown by the mobbing behaviour of the chaffinch (*Fringilla coelebs*). II. The waning of the response. *Proceedings of the Royal Society of London B*, **142**, 331–58.

Hinde, R. A. (1955). The modifiability of instinctive behaviour. *Adv. Sci.*, **12**, 19–24.

Hinde, R. A. (1958). Alternative motor patterns in chaffinch song. *Animal Behaviour*, **6**, 211–18.

Hinde, R. A. (1960). Factors governing the changes in strength of a partially inborn response, as shown by the mobbing behaviour of the chaffinch (*Fringilla coelebs*). III. The interaction of short-term and long-term incremental and decremental effects. *Proceedings of the Royal Society of London B*, **153**, 398–420.

Hinde, R. A. (1961). The establishment of the parent–offspring relation in birds, with some mammalian analogies. In *Current Problems in Animal Behaviour*, ed. W. H. Thorpe and O. L. Zangwill, pp. 175–93. Cambridge: Cambridge University Press.

Hinde, R. A. (1962). Some aspects of the imprinting problem. In *Evolutionary Aspects of Animal Communications: Imprinting and Early Learning*, pp. 129–38. London: Symposium of the Zoological Society of London.

Hinde, R. A. (1966). *Animal Behaviour* (2nd edition, 1970). McGraw-Hill, New York.

Hinde, R. A. & Stevenson-Hinde, J. (ed.) (1973). *Constraints on Learning*. London: Academic Press.

Hinde, R. A., Thorpe, W. H. & Vince, M. A. (1956). The following response of young coots and moorhens. *Behaviour*, **9**, 214–42.

Horn, G. (1962). Some neural correlates of perception. In *Viewpoints in Biology*, ed. J. D. Carthy and C. L. Duddington, pp. 242–85.

Horn, G. (1970). Changes in neuronal activity and their relationship to behaviour. In *Short-term Changes in Neural Activity and Behaviour*, ed. G. Horn and R. A. Hinde, pp. 567–606. Cambridge: Cambridge University Press.

Horn, G. (1985). *Memory, Imprinting, and the Brain*. Oxford: Clarendon Press.

Horn, G., Bradley, P. & McCabe, B. J. (1985). Changes in the structure of synapses associated with learning. *Journal of Neuroscience*, **5**, 3161–8.

Horn, G. & Hinde, R. A. (ed.) (1970). *Short-term Changes in Neural Activity and Behaviour*. Cambridge: Cambridge University Press.

Horn, G. & Johnson, M. H. (1989). Memory systems in the chick: dissociations and neuronal analysis. *Neuropsychologia*, **27**, 1–22.

Horn, G. & McCabe, B. J. (1978). An autoradiographic method for studying the incorporation of uracil into acid-insoluble compounds in the brain. *Journal of Physiology*, **275**, 2–3 P.

Horn, G. & McCabe, B. J. (1984). Predispositions and preferences. Effects on imprinting of lesions to the chick brain. *Animal Behaviour*, **32**, 288–92.

Horn, G. & McCabe, B. J. (1990). The time course of *N*-methyl-D-aspartate (NMDA) receptor binding in chick brain after imprinting. *Journal of Physiology* (in press).

Horn, G., McCabe, B. J. & Bateson, P. P. G. (1979). An autoradiographic study of the chick brain after imprinting. *Brain Research*, **168**, 361–73.

Horn, G., Rose, S. P. R. & Bateson, P. P. G. (1973a). Experience and plasticity in the central nervous system. *Science*, **181**, 506–14.

Horn, G., Rose, S. P. R. & Bateson, P. P. G. (1973b). Monocular imprinting and regional incorporation of tritiated uracil into the brains of intact and 'split-brain' chicks. *Brain Research*, **56**, 227–37.

Hubel, D. H. & Wiesel, T. N. (1970). The period of susceptibility to the physiological effects of unilateral eye closure in kittens. *Journal of Physiology*, **206**, 419–36.

James, W. J. (1890). *The Principles of Psychology*. New York: Henry Holt.

Johnson, M. H. (1987). Brain maturation and the development of face recognition in early infancy. *Behavior and Brain Research*, **26**, 224.

Johnson, M. H., Bolhuis, J. J. & Horn, G. (1985). Interaction between acquired preferences and developing predispositions during imprinting. *Animal Behaviour*, **33**, 1000–6.

Johnson, M. H., Davies, D. C. & Horn, G. (1989). A sensitive period for the development of a predisposition in dark-reared chicks. *Animal Behaviour*, **37**, 1044–5.

Johnson, M. H. & Horn, G. (1986). Dissociation of recognition memory and associative learning by a restricted lesion of the chick forebrain. *Neuropsychologia*, **24**, 329–40.

Johnson, M. H. & Horn, G. (1987). The role of a restricted region of the chick forebrain in the recognition of individual conspecifics. *Behavior and Brain Research*, **23**, 269–75.

Johnson, M. H. & Horn, G. (1988). Development of filial preferences in dark-reared chicks. *Animal Behaviour*, **36**, 675–83.

Kendrick, K. M. & Baldwin, B. A. (1987). Cells in temporal cortex of conscious sheep can respond preferentially to the sight of faces. *Science*, **236**, 448–50.

Kleinschmidt, A., Bear, M. F. & Singer, W. (1987). Blockade of "NMDA" receptors disrupts experience-dependent plasticity of kitten striate cortex. *Science*, **238**, 355–8.

Klopfer, P. H. (1967). Is imprinting a Cheshire cat? *Behavioral Science*, **12**, 122–9.

Klopfer, P. & Hailman, J. P. (1964). Perceptual preferences and imprinting in chicks. *Science*, **145**, 1333–4.

Knusden, E. I. & Knusden, P. F. (1986). The sensitive period for auditory localisation in barn owls is limited by age, not by experience. *Journal of Neuroscience*, **6**, 1918–24.

Kohsaka, S.-I., Takamatsu, K., Aoki, E. & Tsukada, Y. (1979). Metabolic mapping of chick brain after imprinting using [^{14}C]2-deoxyglucose. *Brain Research*, **172**, 539–44.

Konishi, M. (1985). Birdsong: from behavior to neuron. *Annual Review of Neuroscience*, **8**, 125–70.

Kovach, J. K. (1971). Effectiveness of different colors in the elicitation and development of approach behaviour in chicks. *Behaviour*, **38**, 154–68.

Kovach, J. K., Fabricius, E. & Fält, L. (1966). Relationship between imprinting and perceptual learning. *Journal of Comparative and Physiological Psychology*, **61**, 449–54.

Kruhlich, L., Hefco, E. & Read, C. B. (1974). The effects of acute stress on the secretion of LH, FSH, prolactin and GH in the normal rat, with comments on their statistical evaluation. *Neuroendocrinology*, **16**, 293–331.

Lorenz, K. (1935). Der Kumpan in der Umwelt des Vogels. *Journal für Ornithologie*, **83**, 137–213; 289–413.

Lorenz, K. (1937). The companion in the bird's world. *Auk*, 245–73.

McCabe, B. J., Cipolla-Neto, J., Horn, G. & Bateson, P. (1982). Amnesic effects of bilateral lesions in the hyperstriatum ventrale of the chick after imprinting. *Experimental Brain Research*, **48**, 13–21.

McCabe, B. J. & Horn, G. (1988). Learning and memory: regional changes in N-methyl-D-aspartate receptors in the chick brain after imprinting. *Proceedings of the National Academy of Sciences (USA)*, **85**, 2849–53.

McCabe, B. J., Horn, G. & Bateson, P. P. G. (1981). Effects of restricted lesions of the chick forebrain on the acquisition of filial preferences during imprinting. *Brain Research*, **205**, 29–37.

MacDermot, A. B., Mayer, M. L., Westbrook, G. L., Smith, F. J. & Barker, J. L. (1986). NMDA-receptor adrenalin increased cytoplasmic calcium concentration in cultured spine neurones. *Nature*, **321**, 519–22.

Mackintosh, N. J. (1983). *Conditioning and Associative Learning*. Oxford: Clarendon Press.

Maier, V. & Scheich, H. (1983). Acoustic imprinting leads to differential 2-deoxy-D-glucose uptake in the chick forebrain. *Proceedings of the National Academy of Sciences (USA)*, **80**, 3860–4.

Müller-Hill, B. (1988). *Murderous Science: Elimination by the Scientific Selection of Jews, Gypsies and others*. Oxford: Oxford University Press.

Nadler, J. V., White, W. F., Vaca, K. W., Perry, B. W. & Cotman, C. W. (1978). Biochemical correlates of transmission mediated by glutamate and aspartate. *Journal of Neurochemistry*, **31**, 147–55.

Nafstad, P. H. J. (1967). An electron microscope study of the termination of the perforant path fibers in the hippocampus and the fascia dentata *Z. Zellforsch. Mikrosk. Anat.*, **76**, 532–42.

Nottebohm, F. (1980). Brain pathways, for vocal learning in birds: a review of the first 10 years. *Prog. Psychobiol. physiol. Psychol.*, **9**, 86–124.

Nowak, L., Bregestovski, P., Ascher, P., Herbert, A. & Prochiantz, A. (1984). Magnesium gates glutamate-activated channels in mouse central neurones. *Nature*, **307**, 462–5.

Olson, C. R. & Freeman, R. D. (1980). Profile of the sensitive period for monocular deprivation in kittens. *Experimental Brain Research*, **39**, 17–21.

Perret, D. I., Rolls, E. T. & Caan, W. (1982). Visual neurones responsive to faces in the monkey temporal cortex. *Experimental Brain Research*, **47**, 329–42.

Rauschecker, J. P. & Hahn, S. (1987). Ketamine–xylazine anaesthesia blocks consolidation of ocular dominance. *Nature*, **326**, 183–5.

Rose, S. P. R. & Csillag, A. (1985). Passive avoidance training results in lasting changes in deoxyglucose metabolism in left hemisphere regions of chick brain. *Behavioral and Neural Biology*, **44**, 315–24.

Salzen, E. A. (1966). The interaction of experience, stimulus characteristics and exogenous androgen in the behaviour of domestic chicks. *Behaviour*, **26**, 286–322.

Scaife, M. (1976a). The response to eye-like shapes by birds. I. The effect of context: a predator and a strange bird. *Animal Behaviour*, **24**, 195–9.

Scaife, M. (1976b). The response to eye-like shapes by birds. II. The importance of staring, pairedness and shape. Effect of context: a predator and a strange bird. *Animal Behaviour*, **24**, 200–6.

Schaefer, H. H. & Hess, E. H. (1959). Color preferences in imprinting objects. *Zeitschrift für Tierpsychologie*, **16**, 161–72.

Sluckin, W. (1972). *Imprinting and Early Learning*. London: Methuen.

Sluckin, W. & Salzen, E. A. (1961). Imprinting and perceptual learning. *Quarterly Journal of Experimental Psychology*, **13**, 65–77.

Spalding, D. A. (1873). Instinct, with original observations on young animals. *Macmillan's Magazine*, **27**, 282–93 (reprinted in 1954 in *Br. J. anim. Behav.*, **2**, 2–11).

Storm-Mathisen, J. (1977). Glutamic acid and excitatory nerve endings: reduction of glutamic acid uptake after acotomy. *Brain Research*, **120**, 379–86.

Takamatsu, K. & Tsukada, Y. (1985). Neurobiological basis of imprinting in chick and duckling. In *Perspectives on Neuroscience from Molecule to Mind*, ed. Y. Tsukada, pp. 187–206. Berlin: Springer-Verlag.

Tanzi, E. (1893). I fatti e le induzioni nell' odierna istologia del sistema nervoso. *Riv. sper. Freniat. Med. leg Alien. ment*, **19**, 419–72.

Thorpe, W. H. (1944). Some problems of animal learning. *Proceedings of the Linnean Society of London*, **156**, 70–83.

—6—

How does the environment influence the behavioural action of hormones?

J. B. Hutchison

Some years ago at a conference, I heard an endocrinologist remark that detailed behavioural analysis has never added anything of substance to our understanding of how hormones affect behaviour. Somewhat stunned, my immediate reaction was to reach for the 'Blue Book' (Hinde, 1970) which has always provided the telling reference or clinching argument to refute this view. No other volume at that time provided such a wealth of critical argument and factual material to correct the impression that relationships between hormones and behaviour are 'simple'. As Robert Hinde has pointed out many times, a distinction can be drawn between the physiological level of analysis with successive sub-levels, which increasingly depend on molecular methodologies, and the psychological level which searches for laws governing observed regularities in behaviour (see Hinde, 1990 for further discussion). Interpretation of the results of physiological manipulation may require the reduction of sexual behaviour to its simplest elements and exclusion of individual differences. On the other hand, the behavioural scientist interested in the way in which discrete items of individual behaviour are integrated into functional sequences has to take a more global view. In the context of rapidly changing, individually different behavioural interactions, the reductionist approach of the physiologist may not be relevant. The problem is to bring the two approaches together.

In the early 1960s, Hinde's work was one of the first attempts to accommodate the methods of the ethologist to those of the physiologist. In my opinion, one of the reasons that he was able to do this so successfully was a background which made it possible to find the right species for the problem. He also knew a great deal about the life cycle of many avian species including the canary, on which many of these classical studies were performed (Hinde, 1955, 1958). A second important point is that this work

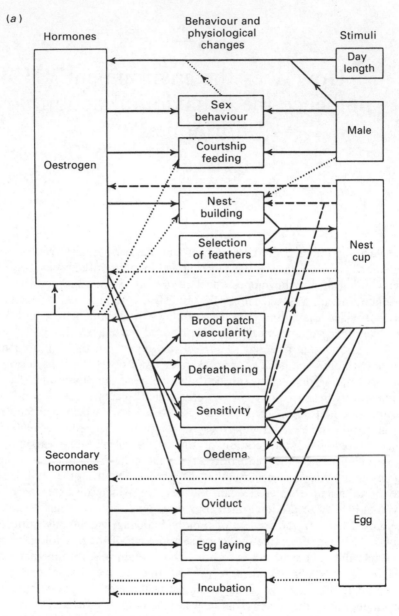

Figure 1. (*a*) For legend see facing page.

(*b*)

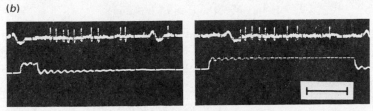

Figure 1. (*a*) The relationships between hormones, behaviour, somatic development and environmental stimuli in the canary (modified from Hinde, 1970). (*b*) Unit responses (upper trace) of a slowly adapting 'mini-dome' (approximately 20 μm in diameter) located superficially on the partly defeathered brood patch skin of a female canary. Units were recorded from a micro-electrode positioned in the dorsal root ganglion of a skin sensory nerve. Displacements of the stimulus probe (lower trace) were close to threshold (2 μm movement) and maintained for different durations (time scale 20 ms). From Hutchison and Konishi (unpublished data).

was concerned very much with the way in which the animal interacts with its environment during the reproductive cycle. The precisely synchronised endocrine changes required for the integration of nesting behaviour in the female canary formed the bulk of Hinde's research on hormonal mechanisms. These studies demonstrated the importance of temporal changes in the action of ovarian hormones not only on the female's behaviour, but also on hormone-sensitive somatic features which were shown to be correlated with changes in nesting behaviour (Figure 1*a*).

The complexity of the relationship between environment, behaviour and the reproductive physiology, or the 'causal nexus' as Hinde (1987) termed it, appears to defy analysis. Is there any hope of pinning down causal mechanisms that might satisfy both the ethologist and the behavioural physiologist? Future advances in this field must surely depend on continuing to combine this type of approach with advances in physiology. This chapter is not meant to be an exhaustive review of how earlier principles derived from ethologically based research can be applied to future work. It develops the theme that the approach pioneered by Hinde (and contemporaneously by Lehrman and his colleagues, 1965) can lead to new ways of studying how environmental stimuli influence hormone-sensitive brain mechanisms of behaviour. Specifically, the paper describes how the formation of behaviourally effective hormones within the male brain may be influenced by internal factors (e.g. reproductive condition of the male), and by environmental events (e.g. socio-sexual stimuli and photoperiod) both in the adult and during development.

Behavioural action of hormones

How do environmental stimuli and steroid hormones interact to bring about changes in behaviour? A great deal of evidence from studies of avian species shows that circulating concentrations of androgen are influenced by seasonal environmental factors such as light and food resources or social stimuli (see Wingfield, 1983; Wingfield & Moore, 1986 for further discussion). These act over a relatively long time period via the neuroendocrine system to regulate the release of neurohormones and ultimately the gonadotrophins that regulate interstitial cell production of androgen from the testes. In view of the action of environmental factors, testicular output of androgens is likely to differ between males with different individual histories.

Rapid changes in the environment, especially those arising from vocal stimuli, have also long been recognised to influence the organisation of sexual behaviour. Is there any evidence that elevation in circulating androgen, resulting for example from sexual interaction, leads to changes in male behaviour? In many cases, short-term changes in androgen level are probably a consequence of sexual interaction rather than a cause of behavioural change (Hutchison, 1990). The view that hormones cause changes in behaviour can also be criticised on theoretical grounds derived from ethological work. For example, apparently 'simple' sexual activities of the male can be shown to be part of a complex network of behavioural events. These have to be seen in the context of the changing relationship between male and female during the reproductive cycle. To give one example, Hinde (1970) has shown that copulatory attempts of chaffinches, observed in the field, result in conflicting tendencies in the female to flee from the male, attack the male, or solicit copulation. Each may involve different motivational states. The behaviour of the male during sexual interaction is unlikely to depend, therefore, on the unitary effect of a male hormone on a single brain mechanism underlying male sexual behaviour (see Hinde, 1960 for discussion of unitary drives).

Despite the difficulties of behavioural interpretation, there are some interesting interspecies differences in the response of the male neuroendocrine system to social cues which have been observed from field studies (Wingfield *et al.*, 1990). In males of monogamous species, the temporal patterning of androgen secretion is determined by behavioural cues. Polygynous species are, on the other hand, less responsive to such cues, and there appears to have been evolutionary selection for males with maximised testosterone levels irrespective of social environment. It is worthwhile considering, therefore, how androgen affects male behaviour in a monogamous species in which environmental stimuli clearly affect the neuroendocrine system. The ring dove (*Streptopelia risoria*) is one such monogamous species. Moreover, the

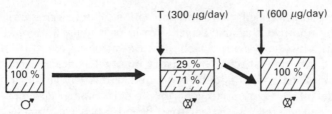

Figure 2. Individual differences in behavioural responsiveness of male ring doves to androgen. A large sample of sexually active, experienced male ring doves were castrated and injected with testosterone (T) 30 days later. A proportion showed no courtship when tested for behaviour with a female, but did so if the dosage was doubled (see Hutchison, 1974).

work of Lehrman and his colleagues showed many years ago that temporal changes in behaviour of this species depend upon a reciprocal relationship between the endocrine systems of the male and the female (Lehrman, 1965).

Before discussing this specific example, it is worthwhile considering some constraints on the behavioural actions of sex hormones. The first and most important principle for the purposes of this chapter is that while androgens influence behaviour mainly by direct action on the brain, the effectiveness of these hormones depends on factors governing the sensitivity of target tissues. This means that there is not necessarily a direct relationship between the amount of hormone in the blood and the degree of behavioural response to the hormone (Hutchison, 1978). Theoretically, androgen action on the brain is influenced in two ways which are not mutually exclusive: the hormone itself can change in amount and availability, or the sensitivity to the hormone of brain mechanisms mediating behaviour can change. Hormonal sensitivity depends not only on the genetic constitution of the individual (McGill, 1978) and previous behavioural experience, but also on environmental stimuli involved in social interaction. Evidence for individual differences in behavioural sensitivity to testosterone, which can be related directly to neural factors, is difficult to find. However, there have been a few studies. For example, differences in the behavioural responsiveness to androgen of adult, sexually experienced male doves can be demonstrated easily using the classical castration and testosterone therapy procedures (Figure 2). The behavioural effectiveness of androgen (testosterone) implants in the preoptic area of male doves also declines with time after the male is castrated, suggesting that local sensitivity of the behavioural 'substrate' in the brain to androgen changes according to the hormonal status of the animal. Social stimuli (e.g. vocalisations) reduce the decline in brain sensitivity to testosterone (Hutchison, 1978), indicating that environmental effects may interact with hormone action.

The second principle is that while the action of androgen is largely on the brain itself and hypothalamic target sites in particular, hormones influence peripheral sensory systems which in turn mediate input to the brain. Evidence for hormonal action on sensory input which leads to change in the behaviour of male birds is difficult to find. However, Hinde showed that under the influence of oestrogen, the female canary develops a highly vascular, defeathered and oedematous brood patch which is synchronised with ovarian and oviduct development (Hinde & Steel, 1964; R. E. Hutchison, Hinde & Bendon, 1968). The brood patch facilitates the transfer of heat to the eggs during incubation and also receives sensory input which affects behaviour. Shortly before laying the first egg, the female selects feathers instead of grass to line the nest. Tactile input associated with the texture and shape of the nest is involved. During this phase of nesting behaviour, the sensitivity of the brood patch skin, measured by a leg flexion response to tactile stimulation, rapidly increases. The change in brood patch skin sensitivity appears to be related to oestrogen (Hinde & Steel, 1964; Hinde, 1965). The question of interest is whether oestrogens affect somatosensory input and how this is achieved. Is the increase in tactile sensitivity due to hormone-dependent changes in responsiveness to mechano-receptive input within the somatosensory areas of the brain or to a change in skin sensitivity itself? As Mark Konishi and I found, there are minute, highly sensitive mechanoreceptors ('mini-domes') on the brood patch skin which are quite similar to mammalian touch spots. Using a single unit electrophysiological procedure to find the absolute threshold of sensitivity in mechanoreceptive units, we found that the mini-domes of the canary have the slowly adapting mechanoreceptive properties that appear to be suitable for textural analysis of the lining of the nest (Figure 1*b*). But the absolute sensitivity of these mechanoreceptors does not change during the repro-ductive cycle. It seems possible, therefore, that there is a hormone-dependent change in distribution of these mechanoreceptors in the skin during development of the brood patch. However, the perception of afferent input within somatosensory areas of the brain may also change under the influence of oestrogen. These alternatives and the major question of how sex hormones influence somatosensory input related to behaviour has yet to be resolved for any species.

To summarise the main points: (i) individuals differ in behavioural responsiveness to hormones; (ii) sex hormones affect behaviour by action on both the brain and sensory system; (iii) environmental factors such as socio-sexual stimuli influence the effectiveness of hormones on behaviour. Bearing these points in mind, I shall discuss our studies, largely carried out on the male ring dove, which explore one type of brain mechanism linking environmental changes and the action of androgen on behaviour.

Brain enzymes and adult behaviour

Recently, there has been an explosive increase in knowledge of the physiology of sex hormones and their cellular effects. A generally accepted model of hormonal steroid action suggests that the hormone after binding to intracellular receptors regulates gene expression in target tissues and the biological activity of the cell. However, additional steps have to be considered in the male, because androgens are extensively metabolised. Formation of active metabolites precedes binding by intracellular receptors. Oestrogens are known to be formed from androgens by a metabolic pathway consisting of an enzyme system, aromatase, which occurs in many tissues including ovary, skin and fat cells. The enzyme is also found in the brain cells of all vertebrates examined so far (see Callard, 1984; Hutchison & Steimer, 1984 for reviews). Whether the same aromatase occurs in all of these tissues is not yet known. Moreover, the brain metabolism of androgens is far more complex than analysis of this single enzyme system might suggest. We have shown that in the male ring dove at least two concepts can be applied to the problem. The first is that steroid metabolising enzyme systems both 'activate' (form active metabolites for behaviour) and 'inactivate' androgens (form behaviourally inactive metabolites). Both processes influence effective levels of testosterone in the brain. The second concept is that the delicate balance between inactivation and activation of the active hormone in brain cells is influenced both by circulating hormone levels and environmental stimuli (Figure 3).

The literature on the behavioural role of androgens is largely derived from studies of copulatory behaviour in male rodents (Baum, 1979; Holman & Hutchison, 1982; Steel & Hutchison, 1987 for reviews). A significant part of this work has concentrated on establishing whether oestrogenic metabolites can substitute for testosterone circulating as a pro-hormone. In our work on the ring dove, we have adopted a different approach by analysing behavioural interactions, occurring during pre-copulatory courtship, which change rapidly over time. This has been possible because the male ring dove shows a rapid alternation between two types of courtship behaviour, aggressive patterns (chasing and bowing) and nest-orientated patterns (Hutchison, 1978). Male courtship consists of the expression of two motivational systems and provides an excellent model for studying the effects of hormones on linked control mechanisms, operating under changing stimulus conditions in the laboratory. The threshold model shown in Figure 3 is based on the idea that brain mechanisms underlying courtship depend on a single hormone, testosterone. Circulating testosterone is known to increase rapidly following interaction with the female and then fall (see Hutchison, 1990 for review). Aggressive courtship appears to require higher levels of testosterone than nest-orientated behaviour. Therefore, aggressive behaviour with the higher

155

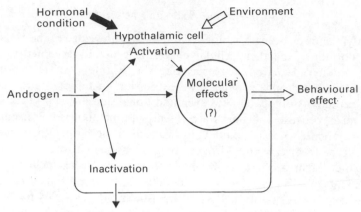

Figure 3. Cellular events in the action of androgen on the brain mechanisms of behaviour. Androgens are 'activated' to behaviourally effective hormones or inactivated to behaviourally ineffective metabolites by enzymes. Active hormones influence gene expression.

threshold of sensitivity to testosterone would fall out of the male repertoire in conditions of low circulating androgen level later in the cycle. This model, while parsimonious, does not account for the fact that the mechanisms controlling courtship are separable experimentally (Hutchison, 1978; Hutchison & Steimer, 1984). A dual hormone model is probably more appropriate. The reasons are two-fold. First, oestradiol is effective for nest-orientated behaviour, but is virtually ineffective for aggressive courtship. The synthetic oestrogen, diethylstilboestrol, which binds specifically to oestrogen receptors, has similar effects. Second, androgens which are not converted to oestrogen (5α-dihydrotestosterone, and the synthetic androgen, methyltrienolone R1181, which binds specifically to androgen receptors) are effective for aggressive courtship, but have little effect on nest-orientated behaviour (Hutchison *et al.*, 1989). Oestrogen-sensitive mechanisms in the brain appear, therefore, to be important in determining when and to what degree the male shows nest-orientated behaviour.

In view of the low concentrations of circulating oestradiol in male blood and the fact that aromatase occurs in brain cells, it seemed likely that oestrogen is formed centrally from testosterone. Sexual interaction between the male and female is known to increase the secretion of both luteinising hormone (LH) and testosterone in this species. Therefore, a working hypothesis is that the transition to nest-orientated behaviour early in the reproductive cycle depends on increasing concentrations of oestrogen building up in the brain during the initial part of the reproductive cycle. The functional importance of this transition seems clear in that females paired with males that show prolonged bouts of aggressive behaviour do not show normal reproductive development and do not lay eggs (Lovari & Hutchison, 1975; Hutchison & Lovari, 1976).

Detailed knowledge of the brain metabolism of androgen is required to develop this idea further. While working at Madingley, I was fortunate in being joined at this stage of the project by Thierry Steimer, a Swiss biochemist fresh from post-doctoral military training, who combined an active interest in behaviour with a capacity for doing innovative biochemistry on a shoe-string. His combat training was especially useful, because he had to take all the radio-isotopically labelled brain samples three miles by bicycle across an embryonic motorway that formed a mud barrier between Madingley and the many scintillation counters in the Department of Zoology in Cambridge. Even Robert Hinde, who was suspicious of what he called 'biochemical gobbledygook' came to terms with this attempt at pioneering biochemistry which had a behavioural end point.

We developed an *in vitro* micro-assay which enabled us to examine the metabolism of testosterone in small brain-tissue samples. The details, drawbacks and advantages of these techniques are considered elsewhere (Hutchison & Steimer, 1984). This radiometric assay had to be sensitive enough to measure metabolites in individual males if experimental groups of animals in different behavioural or endocrine conditions were to be compared statistically. Our procedure differed from the standard biochemical methods of the time which normally involved pooling tissue from different individuals. The latter procedure is as undesirable as summing different components of behaviour from different animals if statistical analysis is to be used. Aromatisation of testosterone was found to be limited to localised areas of the ring dove brain, notably the preoptic area, anterior hypothalamus and posterior hypothalamus. The former two areas are known to be associated with male courtship behaviour. Formation of oestrogen from testosterone also occurred in the living animal, since oestradiol could be chemically identified *in vivo* in preoptic cell nuclei of males injected with isotopically labelled [^{3}H]-testosterone.

One of our initial findings was that a prediction of the 'single hormone threshold model' (Figure 4) was incorrect. Due to the activities of competing metabolic pathways in the brain, the relationship between circulating testosterone and testosterone level in the preoptic area cannot be linear. However, as predicted by the model, at lower testosterone concentrations, metabolism is biased towards oestrogen levels optimal for nest-orientated behaviour. At higher concentrations the aromatase enzyme, which has a high substrate affinity (low K_m, $< 10^{-8}$ M), becomes saturated. More testosterone remains unmetabolised and available for effects on aggressive components of behaviour or metabolism by inactivating enzymes (Figure 4). The threshold

157

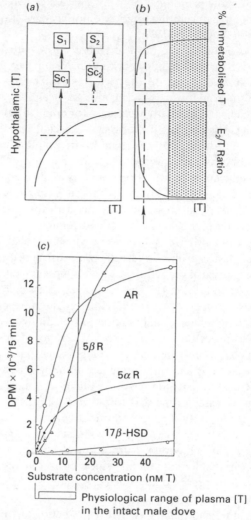

Figure 4. (*a*) Single-hormone threshold model for units of sexual behaviour with different levels of responsiveness to androgen. Hypothalamic testosterone (T) level, which is assumed to increase in the brain with elevation in plasma concentration, activates androgen-sensitive cell populations SC1, SC2 with differing thresholds of sensitivity (dotted line) to T concentration specifically associated with brain systems S1, S2 integrating units of sexual behaviour. In the example taken from dove courtship behaviour, hypothalamic T is assumed to rise to concentrations below threshold for SC2 (further details from Hutchison, 1978, and Hutchison & Steimer, 1984). (*b*)

model can be explained physiologically in terms of the kinetic properties of the aromatase and other androgen-metabolising enzyme systems.

Environmental effects

What evidence is there that environmental stimuli affect the metabolic formation of behaviourally effective hormones? Our evidence for a link between environment and the preoptic aromatase systems was derived in a circuitous way which depended mainly on a behavioural experiment. Males that had been castrated for 2–3 months appeared to be unresponsive to the behavioural effects of testosterone (Figure 5). In other words, the sensitivity to testosterone of mechanisms underlying male courtship behaviour appeared to decline with time after elimination of gonadal steroids. However, long-term castrates were responsive to much smaller doses of oestradiol than testosterone. This suggested to us that the activity of the aromatase system in the preoptic area could change in relation to internal physiological conditions, in this case the prolonged lack of circulating steroids. We tested, therefore, whether injected steroids (testosterone in the first instance) in long-term castrates could change preoptic aromatase activity. Our prediction was that the injected testosterone would have a 'priming effect' on the brain aromatase system. The results were unexpectedly dramatic. Androgen treatment over several days resulted in a massive increase (at least 5-fold) in preoptic aromatase activity after a period as short as 12 hours. Since these experiments were carried out *in vitro*, and involved tracking a radiolabelled product of the catalytic reaction, [³H]-oestradiol, there is no question of

---

The curve plotted for percentage of unmetabolised testosterone shows that as a result of metabolic activity, [T] in preoptic cells is not lineally related to substrate concentration *in vitro*. Therefore, preoptic [T] is unlikely to be related directly to plasma concentration (compare to single hormone threshold model). The oestradiol/testosterone ratio (lower centre diagram) is shown as a function of substrate [T] *in vitro*. At high [T] in the upper physiological range, the ratio is very low. But at lower concentrations, the ratio increases. Where substrate availability is limited in intact cells, the ratio is likely to be much higher. (*c*) *In vitro* study of enzymes involved in androgen metabolism. Changes in active and inactive metabolites when testosterone concentration is increased in the male dove preoptic area (kinetic data obtained using [T] varying from 1 to 40 nM: Steimer and Hutchison, unpublished data). AR, aromatase activity; 5β R, 5β-reductase activity; 5α R, 5α-reduced; 17β-HSD, 17β-hydroxysteroid dehydrogenase. At low physiological concentrations of T, aromatase activity is higher than the activity of other enzymes of steroid metabolism.

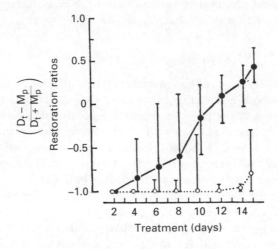

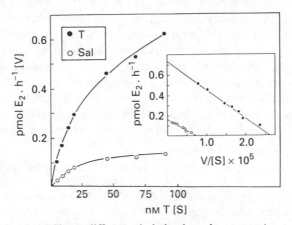

Figure 5. (*a*) Shows difference in behavioural response (nest soliciting) of long-term castrated doves to injected testosterone (solid line, 300 μg/day) or oestradiol (dotted line, 30 μg/day) plotted relative to precastration behaviour. Testosterone begins to affect nest soliciting by day 14. (*b*) Compares aromatase activity in the preoptic area of castrated male doves treated with testosterone (solid circles) or saline (open circles). Kinetic data obtained using varying testosterone (T) concentrations (panel insert, Eadie-Hofstee Plot) shows that the Michaelis constant (K_m) is unaffected by androgen treatment, and suggests that the enzyme is induced (modified from Steimer & Hutchison, 1981).

injected unlabelled testosterone contaminating the experiment. Kinetic studies of the enzyme showed that the increase in activity is due to 'induction' of the enzyme which probably involves synthesis of new enzyme rather than activation of existing aromatase (Steimer & Hutchison, 1981, 1989). The significance is that in the event that more testosterone becomes available from the peripheral circulation, its action is amplified in androgen target cells by the increased production of behaviourally effective oestradiol. This steroid amplification system in the brain appears to occur widely, because similar testosterone-induced enzyme changes have now been shown to occur in other species of birds (Japanese quail: Schumacher & Balthazart, 1985) and mammals (e.g. the rat: Roselli, Horton & Resko, 1985). More recently we have found a further complexity in that aromatase activity is autocatalytically increased by the product of the reaction itself, oestradiol. This suggests that a positive feedback system may also exist (Hutchison & Steimer, 1984; Steimer & Hutchison, 1990).

The discovery that the intracellular activity of aromatase is not 'fixed' within brain cells, but depends on the internal hormonal environment, allows the behavioural action of androgen to be viewed differently. Metabolic activation of testosterone undoubtedly depends on regulation of genes coding for the enzyme protein and the way is now open for studies of the genetic mechanisms controlling the synthesis of this brain enzyme. However, our main interest has been to try to establish whether proximal, socio-sexual stimuli, such as those regulating interaction between the male and female during courtship, influence brain aromatase activity. A second major problem is whether seasonal factors such as day length also affect the brain aromatase. Both aspects are being studied, but I shall deal mainly with our work on the former problem. We designed an experiment to expose males to the sight and sound of courting pairs or only the sound of such pairs. Using this 'Voyeur' design in which one group was visually isolated, we found that formation of oestradiol in the preoptic area was higher in the 'Voyeur' males exposed to behavioural stimuli than in males that could hear but not see the stimulus pair of courting birds (Hutchison, 1990 for further discussion). Visual stimuli from courtship interactions appear, therefore, to influence preoptic aromatase activity. These stimuli have not yet been analysed in depth, but males 'prefer' to look at courting pairs rather than at either a single female or a dyad of sexually active females (Lovari and Hutchison, unpublished data). The special learning processes involved in making the preference (see Bateson, 1978, 1983; Domjan & Hall, 1986; Domjan, 1987; Domjan, Greene & Camille North, 1989 for discussion of learning in mate choice) may be important in changing enzyme activity and the rate of oestrogen formation. Since plasma testosterone increases rapidly during behavioural interactions, increased aromatase activity is likely to be due to the effects of testosterone on preoptic cells. We do not know yet whether behavioural stimuli have both indirect effects via changing testosterone level and other direct effects on preoptic neurones. However, socio-sexual stimuli derived from the courtship interaction evidently do have a profound effect on the formation of oestradiol formed locally in the brain, and this active metabolite appears to be essential for specific aspects of male courtship behaviour.

So far, I have mentioned in detail only one metabolic pathway involving aromatase activity. Other pathways, particularly those concerned with the catabolic inactivation of testosterone are also involved in adult behaviour (Hutchison & Steimer, 1984). The next question to be considered is whether they have a role in determining androgen involvement during brain development.

Behavioural development

Do sex hormones influence behavioural development and if so, where and how do they act, bearing in mind what is known about hormone action in the adult brain? The answer to the first question, based mainly on research into the mating behaviour of rats, is that sex hormones undoubtedly can influence behavioural development. Sufficient work has been done to know that part of the answer to the second question lies in understanding how developing brain cells are influenced by steroids. However, there are some theoretical considerations that complicate any discussion of the role of the sex hormones.

Current ideas on the developmental actions of hormones on behaviour are derived in part from embryological work (Jost, 1972). Sexually differentiated behaviour was thought to develop from an undifferentiated 'substrate' common to both genetic males and females. Behavioural differentiation was seen to occur along a masculine–feminine continuum which depended on hormone action. This led to the proposition of the classical 'organisational' hypothesis that androgens, acting immediately after birth in mammals, organise sexual behaviour to the male type irrespective of genetic sex. Organisation was believed to be irreversible and to occur at a 'critical' or time-limited 'window' in development. Both the suppression of feminine behaviour and enhancement of masculine behaviour were assumed to occur as a consequence of androgenic effects, suggesting a one-hormone process often described in the literature as 'hormonal imprinting'. Development of the feminine behavioural type was assumed to require no hormonal effect. The second assumption of this classical hypothesis was that in adulthood, hormones appropriate to the genetic sex of the individual 'activated' the behaviour (see reviews by Goy & McEwen, 1980; Yahr, 1988). Organisation and activation not only occurred at different stages of life, but were also assumed to be different processes. This theory has important implications, because the amount of androgen in the developing mammalian brain could determine the degree of behavioural masculinisation. In birds (specifically Japanese quail) the effects of steroids on behaviour appear to be the reverse of mammals (Adkins, 1975). Ovarian oestrogens, acting in early embryonic development, are thought irreversibly to feminise the brain. Therefore, the male can be demasculinised by oestrogen during critical periods of embryonic brain differentiation. The female is the sex which is actively differentiated and the male requires no hormone-dependent differentiating process. This finding has been linked to the fact that in birds, unlike mammals, the female is the heterogametic sex. In general the organisational effects of hormones on sex differentiation appear to be exerted on the heterogametic sex (Adkins, 1975). Hormones that are involved in the organisation of sex-typical behaviour also appear to activate the behaviour later in development (Goy & McEwen, 1980).

The basis of the organisational hypothesis has been questioned and it is interesting to consider this hypothesis in the light of ethological ideas on early development (e.g. sexual imprinting: Bateson, 1978, 1983, Chapter 3) which have dealt with similar conceptual problems relating to the temporal limits of 'critical periods'. One of the major difficulties is the supposition that sexual differentiation is a unitary event involving a 'one-hormone' androgenic effect. The 'orthogonal model' of sexual differentiation (Whalen, 1974) proposed, however, that in contrast to the one hormone theory, masculine and feminine aspects of sexual behaviour are probably differentiated at separate stages of development (heterochrony: see Yahr, 1988), and probably by different hormonal processes. A related difficulty with the organisational hypothesis is whether hormonal 'activation' of sexual behaviour in adulthood and 'organisation' during perinatal development are separable. The real difference between these processes was thought to lie in the transient nature of hormonal effects in the adult on mature neuro-endocrine mechanisms compared with the permanent effects of hormones early in life. A number of possibilities could, in theory, account for the physiological differences in hormone action. The sites of hormone action in the brain may differ between the infant and adult. The cellular mechanisms, including steroid metabolism may also differ. Thus steroids probably exert different actions depending on the maturational state of the target areas in the brain at the time of steroid exposure. Convincing arguments have been mounted against the rigid distinction between organisational and activational processes (Arnold & Breedlove, 1985). For example, although oestrogens may demasculine mechanisms underlying copulatory behaviour in female Japanese quail embryos, organising effects of oestradiol can be demonstrated even in adulthood (R. E. Hutchison, 1978). This finding suggests that the early sexually differentiating effects of oestrogen are not completed only during embryonic development. Therefore, an important aspect of the organisational hypothesis appears to be incorrect. The temporal limits for the differentiating effects of hormones are not well defined and certainly not limited to a simple 'critical' period (Hutchison & Hutchison, 1985; Schumacher & Balthazart, 1985).

Brain enzymes and development

Mechanisms that determine the developmental periods when the brain is sensitive to the organising effects of androgens are still virtually unknown. Brain cells involved in hormone action must have a role. If enzymes forming metabolites from androgen occur in the brain and are active during development, does steroid metabolism have similar regulatory roles to those in the adult brain? Are the same enzymes involved with an anatomical localization in the brain similar to that in the adult? These are important questions because the classical theory of development implies that organisational and activational effects of androgens differ. Perhaps embryonic or postnatal steroid metabolism and its regulatory mechanisms also differ from the adult. The effects of environmental stimuli on the ontogeny of androgen-metabolising enzymes in the mammalian brain are largely unknown. Only the brain aromatase has been studied in any detail (Weisz, Brown & Ward, 1982). One reason for this is that it is almost impossible to alter testosterone levels in the foetal brain of mammals directly due to the intervention of the foeto-placental endocrine unit. The effects of injection of androgen into maternal tissues are difficult to interpret because of peripheral and hepatic metabolism of testosterone in both the mother and the foetus.

An avian model, the quail embryo, provides an opportunity to study developing brain enzymes in the absence of maternal steroids. Oestrogen formation from testosterone occurs in the embryonic brain. During embryonic and post-hatching life, hypothalamic and preoptic localisation of the aromatase appears to be similar to that seen in the adult brain. In post-hatching quail chicks, testosterone enhances the activity of hypothalamic aromatase activity (Schumacher, Hutchison & Hutchison, 1988). The induction effects do not depend on the presence of gonadal hormones, since induction of aromatase activity occurs in the preoptic area of gonadectomised animals, nor are there sex differences in activity. This is of particular interest, because the aromatase induction effect is sexually dimorphic in adult quail (Schumacher & Balthazart, 1986). Therefore, enzyme activity in the developing brain differs fundamentally from the adult. Sexual differentiation of the aromatase system occurs at some as yet unspecified stage later in development. Using quail embryos we have also obtained an idea of when the capacity for induction of the enzyme first appears in the embryonic brain. Induction of aromatase activity by testosterone occurs as early as day 14 (hatching, day 21), but the effect obtained on the day after hatching is fourteen times greater than day 14 (Schumacher *et al.*, 1988). However, we found no increase in the aromatase activity of preoptic cells taken from day 10 embryos. At present it is difficult to understand why embryonic preoptic cells suddenly become sensitive to the inductive effects of testosterone. Does this involve the development of receptors to testosterone, removal of inhibitory factors affecting the enzyme, or perhaps the development of cells containing neurotransmitters which enhance aromatase activity? Alternatively, testosterone may activate genes coding for *de novo* synthesis of the enzyme at specific stages in development. None of these questions have been answered yet, but the techniques are available now to begin to explore them.

One aspect of sexual differentiation that has received considerable attention in recent years is whether 'protective' mechanisms exist which prevent the differentiation of the brain by active steroids circulating in genetic females. Steroids, particularly oestrogens, from the foeto-placental unit are available potentially to influence the brain. Circulating oestrogen concentrations are known to be high in male fetuses. The adrenals also secrete androgens which can be aromatised to oestrogens. Two basic types of protective mechanisms have been suggested: the first involves changes in the sensitivity of the brain cells to steroids which are determined by the presence or absence of steroid receptors, while the second mechanism is concerned with physiological 'protective' mechanisms that limit the effectiveness of steroids in the brain. Of these mechanisms, the latter has received the most serious consideration. The α-fetoprotein in neonatal rats, which specifically sequesters oestrogen in the plasma, may provide an example of a protective mechanism (Goy & McEwen, 1980), although the protein may have other functions (Toran-Allerand, 1984). By determining the active steroid environment of the developing brain, steroid-metabolising enzymes could also be part of a protective mechanism. In many species of birds, the major metabolites formed from testosterone are the 5β-reduced androgens (5β-androstanes). Although known to occur in the liver, very high levels of 5β-reductase activity appear to be a feature of the developing avian brain (see Hutchison & Steimer, 1984). Owing to the capacity for conversion of testosterone to inactive metabolites, 5β-reductase is likely to interfere with further metabolism and the binding of active steroids to the intracellular receptors. The 5β-reductase probably acts preferentially with the substrate (testosterone) entering the cells and competes with enzymes involved with alternative pathways (e.g. aromatase). Since the 5β-reduced androstanes are biologically inactive, and are also major products of hepatic catabolism, we have suggested that 5β-reduction is a pathway of androgen inactivation in the brain (Hutchison & Steimer, 1981). The 5β-reduction pathway in the avian brain could in theory provide such a protective mechanism. The activity of 5β-reductase in male and female ring dove chicks is higher by an order of magnitude than adult enzyme activity and, therefore, the half-life of testosterone in the preoptic area of the embryo and newly hatched chick is considerably shorter than in the adult (Schumacher *et al.*, 1988). Does this high level of 5β-reductase activity provide a protective mechanism in the embryonic brain?

There is one unique avian model for sexual differentiation which may throw some light on the functional role of the enzyme inactivation mechanism. The song control system in the telencephalic nuclei (RA, HVc) of the canary and the zebra finch are sexually dimorphic (Nottebohm & Arnold, 1976). Song occurs only in the male and is androgen-dependent. The differentiation of adult song patterns depends on oestrogen action during the post-hatching period. Structural differentiation of the song control nuclei to form the male type also depends on the action of oestrogen during the post-hatching period. This discovery by Gurney & Konishi (1980) represents the only example known of an early differentiating effect of an oestrogen on behaviour which can be related directly to structural changes in the brain. The source of the oestrogen required for brain differentiation in the zebra finch is not known. However, it appears likely that the oestrogen is derived from peripheral sources (e.g. the adrenals) in the male, since a massive surge of oestrogen occurs within the first 6 days of life only in the male (Hutchison, Wingfield & Hutchison, 1984). However, both male and female have high testosterone levels in the peripheral plasma during this period. The question that puzzled us is what prevents masculinisation of the female brain by oestrogens formed within the brain. As in other avian species, 5β-reduction is a major pathway of testosterone metabolism in the developing zebra finch brain (Vockel, Pröve & Balthazart, 1988). The aromatase system is also active. The 5β-reduction pathway could have a role in the sexual differentiation of the vocal control system, since there is no sex difference in plasma testosterone levels during post-hatching development. Both sexes have relatively high androgen concentrations in the blood which are likely to be inactivated rapidly by brain 5β-reduction. The surge in plasma oestradiol, unaffected by 5β-reductase activity during the early post-hatching period, would differentiate the male vocal control system (see Hutchison & Hutchison, 1985 for further discussion). Testosterone would be inactivated selectively in both male and female brains by 5β-reduction. The idea is speculative, but enzymes of steroid metabolism represent a group of factors that limit sensitive periods for the differentiating effects of androgens in the brain.

Conclusions

The effects of sex hormones on brain mechanisms of behaviour are influenced by environmental stimuli. But the physiological factors that control the timing and action of these hormones on the brain mechanisms of behaviour are poorly understood. With increasing interest in the interaction between environment, hormones and brain cells, a new approach has come to light. Instead of focusing exclusively on fluctuations in blood levels of steroid hormones, it has become essential to think about target tissues in the brain on which hormones are known to act. The crucial questions now are: does the sensitivity of brain cells to steroid sex hormones change in relation to the behavioural environment of the adult, or at certain stages of development, and what causes these changes?

This emphasis, and the new experimental data particularly from studies of the avian brain, are leading to attempts to unravel the cellular, molecular and genetic factors, including gene-coding of the expression of the cellular events within the brain which modulate androgen action. Steroid metabolising enzymes in brain cells have a functional role in determining active steroids available both for structural organisation of the brain in development and the integration of adult behaviour. The way in which these enzymes work in brain cells associated with behaviour is still not understood. However, work on the adult brain, mainly in avian species, has contributed some new ideas.

The first is that enzyme systems 'activate' and 'inactivate' androgens required for behaviour. Both types of metabolic pathway influence behaviourally effective levels of hormones in the brain. The second is that the balance between activation and inactivation of androgen in brain cells is influenced by both hormonal condition and environmental stimuli. Although speculative at present, these enzymatic processes are likely to contribute to the plasticity of hormone action on behavioural mechanisms in the brain.

Acknowledgements

I am grateful to Rosemary Hutchison, Pat Bateson and Robert Hinde for their comments and to Miss Helen Potter for typing the manuscript.

References

Adkins, E. K. (1975). Hormonal basis of sexual differentiation in the Japanese quail. *Journal of Comparative and Physiological Psychology*, **89**, 61–71.

Arnold, A. P. & Breedlove, S. M. (1985). Organisational and activational effects of sex steroids on brain and behavior: a reanalysis. *Hormones and Behaviour*, **19**, 469–98.

Bateson, P. (1978). Early experience and sexual preferences. In *Biological Determinants of Sexual Behaviour*, ed. J. B. Hutchison, pp. 29–55. Chichester: John Wiley.

Bateson, P. (1983). The interpretation of Sensitive Periods. In *The Behaviour of Human Infants*, ed. A. Oliverio and M. Zappella, pp. 57–70. New York: Plenum Press.

Baum, M. J. (1979). Differentiation of coital behaviour in mammals: A comparative analysis. *Neuroscience and Biobehavioral Reviews*, 3, 265–84.

Callard, G. V. (1984). Aromatization in brain and pituitary: An evolutionary perspective. In *Metabolism of Hormonal Steroids in the Neuroendocrine Structures*, ed. F. Celotti, pp. 79–101. New York: Raven Press.

Domjan, M. (1987). Photoperiodic and endocrine control of social proximity behavior in male Japanese quail (*Coturnix coturnix japonica*). *Behavioral Neuroscience*, 110, 385–92.

Domjan, M., Greene, P. & Camille North, N. (1989). Contextual conditioning and the control of copulatory behavior by species-specific sign stimuli in male Japanese quail. *Journal of Experimental Psychology: Animal Behavior Processes*. 15, 147–53.

Domjan, M. & Hall, S. (1986). Determinants of social proximity in Japanese quail. (*Coturnix coturnix japonica*): male behavior. *Journal of Comparative Psychology*, 100, 59–67.

Goy, R. W. & McEwen, B. S. (1980). *Sexual Differentiation of the Brain*. Cambridge, Mass.: MIT Press.

Gurney, M. E. & Konishi, M. (1980). Hormone-induced sexual differentiation of brain and behavior in zebra finches. *Science*, 208, 1380–2.

Hinde, R. A. (1955). A comparative study of the courtship of certain finches. *Ibis*, 97, 706–45.

Hinde, R. A. (1958). The nest-building behaviour of domesticated canaries. *Proceedings of the Zoological Society (London)*, 131, 1–48.

Hinde, R. A. (1960). Energy models of motivation. *Symposia of the Society for Experimental Biology*, 14, 199–213.

Hinde, R. A. (1965). Interaction of internal and external environments in integration of canary reproduction. In *Sex and Behavior*, ed. F. A. Beach, pp. 381–416. New York: John Wiley.

Hinde, R. A. (1970). *Animal Behaviour. A Synthesis of Ethology and Comparative Psychology*. New York: McGraw-Hill.

Hinde, R. A. (1987). *Individual Relationships and Culture*. Cambridge: Cambridge University Press.

Hinde, R. A. (1990). The interdependence of the behavioural sciences. Croonian Lecture. *Proceedings of the Royal Society of London, B* (in press).

Hinde, R. A. & Steel, E. A. (1964). Effect of exogenous hormones on the tactile sensitivity of the canary brood patch. *Journal of Endocrinology*, 30, 355–9.

Holman, S. D. & Hutchison, J. B. (1982). Precopulatory behaviour in the male Mongolian gerbil: II. Effects of post-castration sexual and aggressive interactions on responsiveness to androgens. *Animal Behaviour*, 30, 231–9.

Hutchison, J. B. (1978). Hypothalamic regulation of male sexual responsiveness to androgen. In *Biological Determinants of Sexual Behaviour*, ed. J. B. Hutchison, pp. 277–319. Chichester: John Wiley.

Hutchison, J. B. (1990). Androgen action in a changing behavioural environment: The role of brain aromatase. In *Hormones, Brain and Behaviour*, ed. J. Balthazart and R. Gilles. Karger (in press).

Hutchison, J. B. & Hutchison, R. E. (1985). Phasic effects of hormones on the avian brain during behavioural development. In *Neurobiology: Current Comparative Approaches*, ed. R. Gilles and J. Balthazart, pp. 105–20. Berlin: Springer-Verlag.

Hutchison, J. B., Joris, S., Hutchison, R. E. & Steimer, Th. (1989). Steroid control of sexual behavior and brain aromatase in the dove: Effects of nonaromatisable androgens, methyltrienelone (R1881) and 5α-dihydrotestosterone. *Hormones and Behavior*, **23**, 542–55.

Hutchison, J. B. & Lovari, S. (1976). Effects of male aggressiveness on behavioural transitions in the reproductive cycle of the Barbary dove. *Behaviour*, **59**, 296–318.

Hutchison, J. B. & Steimer, Th. (1981). Brain 5β-reductase: A correlate of behavioral sensitivity to androgen. *Science*, **213**, 244–6.

Hutchison, J. B. & Steimer, Th. (1984). Androgen metabolism in the brain: behavioural correlates. In *Sex Differences in the Brain*, ed. G. J. de Vries, J. P. C. de Bruin, H. B. M. Uylings and M. A. Corner. *Progress in Brain Research, Vol. 61*, pp. 23–51. Amsterdam: Elsevier.

Hutchison, J. B., Wingfield, J. C. & Hutchison, R. E. (1984). Sex differences in plasma concentrations of steroids during the sensitive period for brain differentiation in the Zebra finch. *Journal of Endocrinology*, **103**, 363–9.

Hutchison, R. E. (1978). Hormonal differentiation of sexual behaviour in Japanese quail. *Hormones and Behavior*, **11**, 363–87.

Hutchison, R. E., Hinde, R. A. & Bendon, B. (1968). Oviduct development and its relation to other aspects of reproduction in domesticated canaries. *Journal of Zoology (London)*, **155**, 87–102.

Jost, A. A. (1972). A new look at the mechanisms controlling sex differentiation in mammals. *Johns Hopkins Medical Journal*, **130**, 38–53.

Lehrman, D. S. (1965). Interaction between internal and external environments in the regulation of the reproductive cycle of the ring dove. In *Sex and Behavior*, ed. F. A. Beach, pp. 355–80. New York: John Wiley.

Lovari, S. & Hutchison, J. B. (1975). Behavioural transitions in the reproductive cycle of the Barbary dove (*Streptopelia risoria* L.). *Behaviour*, **53**, 126–50.

McGill, T. E. (1978). Genetic factors influencing the action of hormones on sexual behaviour. In *Biological Determinants of Sexual Behaviour*, ed. J. B. Hutchison, pp. 277–319. Chichester: John Wiley.

Nottebohm, F. & Arnold, A. P. (1976). Sexual dimorphism in vocal control areas of the song bird brain. *Science*, **194**, 211–13.

Roselli, C. E., Horton, L. E. & Resko, J. A. (1985). Distribution and regulation of aromatase activity in the rat hypothalamus and limbic system. *Endocrinology*, **117**, 2471–7.

Schumacher, M. & Balthazart, J. (1985). Sexual differentiation is a biphasic process in mammals and birds. In *Neurobiology*, ed. R. Gilles and J. Balthazart, pp. 203–19. Berlin: Springer-Verlag.

Schumacher, M. & Balthazart, J. (1986). Testosterone-induced aromatase is sexually dimorphic. *Brain Research*, **370**, 285–93.

Schumacher, M., Hutchison, R. E. & Hutchison, J. B. (1988). Ontogeny of testosterone-inducible brain aromatase activity. *Brain Research*, **441**, 98–110.

Steel, E. & Hutchison, J. B. (1987). The aromatase inhibitor, 1.4.6.-androstatriene 3,17-dione (ATD), blocks testosterone-induced olfactory behaviour in the hamster. *Physiology and Behaviour*, **39**, 141–5.

Steimer, Th. & Hutchison, J. B. (1981). Androgen increases formation of behaviourally effective oestrogen in the dove brain. *Nature*, **292**, 345–7.

Steimer, Th. & Hutchison, J. B. (1989). Is the androgen-dependent increase in preoptic estradiol-17β formation due to aromatase induction? *Brain Research*, **480**, 335–9.

Steimer, Th. & Hutchison, J. B. (1990). Is preoptic aromatase sexually differentiated in the avian and rodent brain? *Journal of Neurobiology*, **21**, 787–95.

Toran-Allerand, C. D. (1984). On the genesis of sexual differentiation of the central nervous system: Morphogenetic consequences of steroidal exposure and the possible role of α-fetoprotein. *Progress in Brain Research*, **61**, 63–98.

Vockel, A., Pröve, E. & Balthazart, J. (1988). Changes in the activity of testosterone-metabolising enzymes in the brain of male and female zebra finches during the post-hatching period. *Brain Research*, **463**, 330–40.

Weisz, J., Brown, B. L. & Ward, I. C. (1982). Maternal stress decreases steroid aromatase activity in brains of male and female rats fetuses. *Neuroendocrinology*, **35**, 374–9.

Whalen, R. E. (1974). Sexual differentiation: models, methods and mechanisms. In *Sex Differences in Behavior*, ed. R. C. Friedman, R. M. Richart and R. L. Van de Wiele, p. 467. New York: Wiley.

Wingfield, J. C. (1983). Environmental and endocrine control of reproduction: An ecological approach. In *Avian Endocrinology: Environmental and Ecological Aspects*, ed. S.-I. Mikami, S. Ishii and M. Wada, pp. 265–88. Tokyo: Japanese Scientific Society Press and Berlin: Springer-Verlag.

Wingfield, J. C., Hegner, R. E., Dufty, A. M. & Ball, G. F. (1990). The 'Challenge Hypothesis': Theoretical implications for patterns of testosterone secretion, mating systems and breeding strategies of birds. *American Naturalist* (in press).

Wingfield, J. C. & Moore, M. C. (1986). Hormonal, social and environmental factors in the reproductive biology of free-living male birds. In *Psychobiology of Reproductive Behavior: An Evolutionary Perspective*, ed. D. Crews, pp. 149–75. New York: Prentice-Hall.

Yahr, P. (1988). Sexual differentiation of behavior in the context of developmental psychobiology. In *Handbook of Behavioral Neurobiology 9*, ed. E. M. Blass, pp. 197–243. New York: Plenum Press.

—7—

Testosterone, attention and memory

R. J. Andrew

Robert Hinde taught me how to study the causation of behaviour. I began work at Madingley as his student, convinced that the main goal of such work was to construct a grand unifying theory which would explain behaviour. I slowly learned from Robert that the task was quite different; it was far more difficult than I had thought, and far more interesting. The right strategy was to seize hold of promising novel phenomena, to study them with the best tools which physiology or other disciplines could provide and to allow the phenomena themselves to instruct you step by step in the way in which behaviour is organised. Whilst using other disciplines, it was always necessary to remember that the main concern of the ethologist was the rigorous definition and exploration of behavioural mechanisms.

I describe here a programme of work in which I have tried over the years to apply these principles. It owes much to my collaborators, in particular to Lesley Rogers, Peter Clifton and Richard Klein.

Gonadal steroids are well known to affect aggressive, sexual and parental behaviour. Robert himself played an important part in showing the multiplicity of routes by which a particular hormone might facilitate or depress such specific systems of responses. I describe here, in contrast, effects which are not specific to a particular system of responses. The effect with which I chiefly deal involves the stabilisation of attention. As a result, stimuli other than the type of stimulus to which attention is currently directed, tend to be ignored; patterns of search, ease of distraction and the kind of information which is accepted for storage in memory all reveal the effect.

Other such effects are now coming to light. That just mentioned is produced by oestrogens (which may be metabolites of testosterone). A second effect, this time caused by androgens, increases the effort put into overcoming obstacles. Both effects have very short latencies, and so probably

171

do not depend upon the classic route of changes in the rate of gene transcription. Instead they may result from binding of particular steroids to specific receptor sites in the cell membrane of neurones.

The effects of testosterone on behaviour: an introduction

The possibility that testosterone might cause changes in the way in which domestic chicks attended to the environment was first suggested by changes in their behaviour following injection, which seemed to have nothing to do with fighting, copulating or crowing. Testosterone-treated chicks appeared to sustain attention for longer on some interesting or novel stimulus; they would then suddenly break off such attention, often with head or body shakes, almost as though detaching themselves forcibly. They also behaved differently when placed in some entirely novel place: untreated chicks would persistently and mechanically scan the environment, giving distress calls, whereas such behaviour appeared to be less common and less markedly developed following testosterone.

Effects of testosterone on attention in chicks were formally demonstrated in search tests (Andrew & Rogers, 1972). Work which developed out of this finding identified short latency oestrogenic effects of testosterone, whose action on mechanisms affecting attention is now quite well defined at the behavioural level. At present, particular interest attaches to the possible involvement of these effects in memory formation.

Hormonal effects on attention, memory formation and retrieval are best known from the classic work of de Wied and his associates: a recent review (de Wied & Jolles, 1982) listed such effects of adrenocorticotropic hormone (ACTH) and related peptides as including 'reduced or increased fear, facilitated motivation and vigilance, enhanced concentration and (visual) attention, promoted learning and stimulated memory-retrieval processes'. A central aim of this very extensive body of work has been to attempt to exclude peripheral routes of action by central application of smaller peptides, consisting of parts of the larger ACTH molecule, and lacking most or all of its peripheral effects. This is important, since in at least one case, that of vasopressin (which has been shown to have many of the effects of ACTH), effects of injection following learning or before test, have been argued to be due to aversive and inhibitory effects of peripheral blood pressure rises (Van Haaren, van Zanten & van de Poll, 1986).

The hypothesis that the effects of ACTH listed above represent a functional grouping is strengthened by the fact that in general all are opposed by oxytocin. Ermisch, Landgraf & Mobius (1986) found that when rats were sorted into high and low performers on a brightness discrimination task, the former had significantly higher levels of oxytocin in septum and striatum but lower in the hippocampus, together with higher levels of arginine vasopressin in septum and striatum: they argue that this suggests a central and physiological route of action for these hormones.

The evidence for production of a very similar range of effects by systemic administration of ACTH is also extensive. It is not clear how far circulating ACTH could affect the central nervous system directly; perhaps the most reasonable hypothesis is that ACTH of pituitary origin acts in parallel with central release of ACTH (or central activation of appropriate peptidergic systems).

It is in the peripheral route of action that testosterone enters the story. (It should be remembered in what follows that testosterone may give rise to oestradiol intracellularly, so that either hormone may be involved in the effects of testosterone secretion.) Two quite different patterns of endocrine activity accompany ACTH secretion or administration. In the initial acute response to ACTH in male mammals (such as rabbit and pig) there is a marked rise in circulating levels of both corticosteroids and testosterone (Faulborn *et al.*, 1979; Hahmeier *et al.*, 1980); such rises appear within 20 minutes and may last for up to an hour or so. The testosterone is largely or entirely testicular in origin. ACTH also causes comparable rises when given centrally, apparently by causing LH release (Haun & Haltmeyer, 1975); here it is known that in females a corresponding effect causes a rise in progesterone.

Natural changes of this sort have been described for the male Japanese quail (Ramenofsky, 1985), a close relative of the domestic fowl. Here, birds removed from their home quarters and placed in a different compartment showed a rise in circulating testosterone within half a minute and a somewhat later rise in corticosterone. Both changes were affected if birds were introduced in pairs, so that a fight resulted: testosterone levels were depressed, but less in winners than losers, whilst corticosterone levels rose to above central levels after some minutes but in winners only.

Longer and chronic secretion or administration of ACTH leads to depression of circulating testosterone levels in male mammals (Faulborn *et al.*, 1979). It is this pattern of endocrine activity with high ACTH, vasopressin, and corticosteroids, but low testosterone, which has been considered as possibly affecting memory formation (Roche & Leshner, 1979; Leshner, 1980). However, the evidence cited here suggests that the initial phase when both ACTH and testosterone levels are high, may be more important.

At least one effect of ACTH in the male rat, delayed extinction of a conditioned taste aversion, is blocked by castration and can be produced by testosterone alone (Chambers, 1980). This finding is particularly instructive in that an ACTH fragment (ACTH 4–10), as well as ACTH, has also been

173

shown to delay extinction of an aversion when given centrally (Smotherman, 1985), suggesting that delayed extinction may be promoted by both peripheral and central actions of ACTH with the former (but not necessarily the latter) involving testosterone secretion.

A common central site of action of ACTH and testosterone is suggested by evidence from a quite different behaviour effect (Rodriguez-Sierra *et al.*, 1981). A characteristic pattern of stretching and yawning is produced by ACTH given into the cerebral ventricle in some male mammals; a lower-intensity form of the behaviour (yawning alone) is facilitated by testosterone given subcutaneously. When the two treatments are combined the incidence of the full pattern is greatly increased.

Some involvement of testosterone in at least some of the effects associated with ACTH is thus likely in male mammals. Whether there is any equivalent involvement of androgens or oestrogens with ACTH in females is an entirely open question; it will be seen later that in both mammals and the chick androgens and oestrogens given systemically do affect, respectively, extinction and (in the chick at least) attention in females as well as males.

At least three patterns of action are possible: androgens and oestrogens, on the one hand and ACTH, on the other, may act synergistically; or one may substitute for the other (so that similar effects are produced by either); or ACTH may act by causing testosterone secretion; perhaps all three patterns occur.

There is considerable variation in the hypotheses advanced to explain the effects of pituitary peptide hormones on behaviour. This is partly because it is not clear how far a number of separate effects are under study; de Wied himself has argued for a single basic change underlying at least most of them (de Wied & Jolles, 1982). At the same time it has been suggested that different hormones are most effective at different points in learning and retrieval: thus α-MSH (melanocyte stimulating hormone) may chiefly affect attention or trial-to-trial memory, vasopressin long-term memory processes and ACTH retrieval (de Wied & Jolles, 1982).

A striking example of the difficulties which remain in the interpretation of the effects of these hormones and their fragments is provided by recent work with the ACTH analogue ORG 2766. This agent might be expected to have a restricted set of effects since it lacks or has much reduced peripheral action (including reduced steroidogenesis). It has many of the effects of ACTH of interest here: it delays extinction of active avoidance, facilitates passive avoidance and acts on processes following learning and on retrieval (Fekete & de Wied, 1982a). Nevertheless, it has proved necessary to postulate in addition that ORG 2766 increases arousal in a dose-related way (Fekete & de Wied, 1982b) and that it 'affects integration of sensory stimuli' (Wolterink & Van Ree, 1987).

There is thus considerable advantage in turning to the corresponding effects of testosterone and its metabolites in order to complement the work on pituitary peptide hormones. First, although testosterone too has a wide range of effects, these are relatively well known, and are very different from those of (say) ACTH, with the exception of the effects under discussion. Secondly, it will be shown here that it is possible to exclude most of the other effects of testosterone on behaviour by (for example) studying only effects following immediately on injection. Thirdly, the work on the cognitive effects of testosterone in the chick has from the start been concerned with overt effects on behaviour. Thus, effects on attention have been measured by recording at what the chick looks or which stimuli it selects out of an array. As a result, it has been possible to establish in some detail the nature of the attentional mechanisms which are affected by testosterone, and to show that this effect differs from all other effects of testosterone so far studied in a combination of properties: namely that it has very short latency (*c.* 15 min), occurs in both sexes (unlike long latency facilitation of copulation and attack) and depends upon oestrogenic metabolites of testosterone.

In this latter feature it differs from a second short latency effect which does not involve particular species-specific behaviour patterns; namely, delay of extinction. This was first demonstrated in the chick for extinction of a conditioned taste aversion, but it has now been shown in a range of different tests (below) to be quite separate from the oestrogenic effect on attention. It remains to be seen whether different peptides (perhaps fragments of ACTH) also separately give the two effects.

Finally, it is important to stress the significance of the short latency of the effects under discussion. Long latency (2–4 days) effects of androgens and oestrogens are well known in the chick. These may be androgenic (facilitation of aggressive pecking) or oestrogenic (facilitation of copulation); crowing requires both androgenic and oestrogenic effects if it is to occur (Clifton & Andrew, 1981, 1989). It is almost certain that these effects depend upon the classical route of action of steroids, which involves changes in the rates of gene transcription. In contrast, effects with latencies as short as 15 minutes are probably due to action at the neuronal membrane.

There is in fact direct evidence of such action by steroids. The best-understood example is provided by the specific binding of a group of pregnane steroids (including naturally occurring metabolites of deoxycorticosterone and progesterone) to the GABA receptor complex (Harrison *et al.*, 1987). As a result GABA-mediated inhibitory postsynaptic currents are greatly prolonged.

It remains to be seen whether the short-latency effects of oestrogens and androgens also involve effects on receptor complexes or act by other routes. This is likely to be a fruitful field of research in the next few years.

Effects of testosterone which are not specific to particular systems of behaviour

Delay of extinction (androgenic, both sexes; short latency)

Delay of extinction of a conditioned taste aversion by testosterone was described for both male and female rats by Chambers (1976). It was subsequently shown to be androgenic (Early & Leonard, 1979; Chambers, 1980). Early & Leonard (1979) argued that a mechanism like that responsible for attentional changes in the chick might be involved. However, it is not obvious how this could explain delay of extinction produced by testosterone given well after extinction but before the beginning of extinction trials (Chambers & Sengstake, 1979).

The matter has been resolved, for the chick at least, by the demonstration (Clifton & Andrew, 1987) of an androgenic effect on extinction, which is thus likely to be independent of oestrogenic effects on attention and memory formation (below).

A conditioned aversion was induced by the method of Gaston (1977): following consumption of water of characteristic appearance and taste aversion was induced by injection of lithium chloride. Extinction of the aversion was then followed over a series of trials (making impossible accurate measurement of latency of the effects of the hormone). Since the hormone was given well after the acquisition of the aversion (e.g. 6 h), it is unlikely to have affected memory formation; since testosterone and 5α-HDT (de-hydroxytestosterone) were effective but oestradiol was not, the effect is androgenic.

Testosterone was already known also to oppose extinction of approach to food at the end of a runway. Two procedures were used to demonstrate the effect. In one (Archer, 1974) the food dish was empty (and could be seen to be so from a distance); in the other (Klein, 1983) the dish contained food under a transparent cover. Under neither condition did testosterone affect the rate at which latency to reach the dish increased during extinction. When food could be seen, testosterone increased the time spent in the goal area. Under both conditions, testosterone increased the time looking and pecking into the dish. When food could be seen, testosterone caused a series of forceful pecks to be given; when the dish was empty, pecks were often combined with scratching with the feet at the dish, suggesting attempts to uncover food.

Recently (R. J. Andrew and R. M. Klein, unpublished data) we have shown that these changes are due to a combination of the oestrogenic effect on attention and an androgenic effect. Oestradiol increased the time spent beside and looking in the dish, without changing other patterns of behaviour:

176

attention thus appeared to be locked on the dish. In contrast, 5α-DHT facilitated vigorous pecking and scratching. This was not apparently attributable to a decrease in the aversive effects of failure to obtain food: strikingly, in the midst of vigorous pecking, loud distress calls would occur. Such behaviour never occurred in either controls or chicks receiving other hormones. Speed of running to the food dish was also sustained at very high values by 5α-DHT, in contrast to controls. Taken together, the behavioural changes produced by 5α-DHT suggest that the androgenic effect directly sustains the vigour and likelihood of repetition of the motor responses which previously resulted in access to feeding.

In the runway test, then, opposition of extinction of response is specifically androgenic. Oestrogens have an effect, but on attention; the next section will give other examples of this. The androgenic effect may be responsible for sustaining response in other tests. Testosterone causes escape jumps to be continued in a series rather than to be given singly (open field tests: Archer, 1973; home cage after introduction of small novel object: Clayton & Andrew, 1979). In both cases, the proportion of birds showing escape responses was unchanged by testosterone.

Effects on attention and recognition (oestrogenic, short latency: both sexes)

The term attention is usually restricted to the processes which allow an animal or human being to select particular stimuli out of an array of possible targets for examination and response. The oestrogenic short latency effect of testosterone (OSLE) affects attention by stabilising in use the information used in such selection (Andrew, 1972, 1983); evidence for this is reviewed later. However, a crucial feature of the OSLE is that it also affects processes not usually considered in discussion of attention, even though they are central to the working of attentional mechanisms. These involve the use of centrally held information to recognise and interpret a stimulus after attention has been focused on it (competition tests: below).

Three main experimental procedures are considered below.

1. *Distraction tests.*   Discussion of effects on attention will begin with tests of distractibility, since it has now been demonstrated that the action of testosterone here is oestrogenic, of short latency (and present in both sexes: R. J. Andrew and R. M. Klein, unpublished data).

In the standard form of the distractibility test (Archer, 1974) chicks which have been trained to traverse a runway in order to feed from a dish at its other end, are presented with conspicuous change either in the walls half-way down the runway (resulting from the introduction of panels) or in the dish itself. Testosterone decreases the delay in reaching the dish and beginning to feed which is caused by the panels, but increases that due to change in the dish. This pattern of effects cannot be explained by an overall increase or decrease in the effectiveness of conspicuous changes in disturbing behaviour. As hunger increases, the duration of delay due to both types of change decreases (Klein & Andrew, 1986); the effects of testosterone are shown at all deprivation levels. Testosterone thus does not appear to act by changing motivation to reach the food.

The two kinds of conspicuous change will be considered in turn. Change in the dish affects behaviour only when the chick (still running at high speed) is almost at the dish: if the chick responds, then it suddenly checks its approach, often swerving or leaping over the dish (Klein & Andrew, 1986). Untreated chicks commonly reach the dish and begin feeding without any such response. A comparable effect can be seen when food dishes are presented for the first time in alcoves half-way down the runway as well as at its end (Klein & Andrew, 1986): testosterone greatly increases the proportion of chicks which swing to one side and feed in an alcove. Untreated chicks pass the alcoves at full speed to continue as usual to the end of the runway.

In both this instance, and response to change in the dish, a decision has to be made very soon after perception: a decision which requires comparison between what is perceived and a centrally held description of the appearance of the food dish. If such comparison falters or is interrupted, then a few steps will take the chick beyond the point at which response is possible: in the case of change in the dish, the food will become visible and available, so that feeding is likely to be irresistible. Stabilisation of the description of the food dish, it is here argued, allows comparison to proceed to a point at which response can begin, before it is too late.

The effects of testosterone in the panel test are complicated by the fact that they affect attention both to the panels and to the food dish. As a result, changes in the overall pattern of behaviour with increasing dosage (and so with increasing stabilisation) are marked (unlike the case of response to change in the dish). In early studies (Klein, 1983; Andrew, 1983) dosages ran from 800 μg to 12.5 mg testosterone oenanthate; injection was 48 hours before test, so that even the highest dose is likely to have resulted in circulating levels lower than adult (Andrew, 1983).

At the higher doses the full sequence of response to the panels in treated chicks begins with a momentary examination. This, which may be no more than a turn of the head whilst running, represents a brief forced shift of attention to the conspicuous and novel panel. It is here argued that the ability of treated chicks to continue on their way depends on the stabilisation of information which specifies the food dish as the current point of attention.

Such stabilisation allows return of attention to the food dish, after the brief shift and then holds it there, so that the run continues. However, information about the panels is retained, and does affect attention subsequently. After some time feeding, such birds return to examine the panels. This occurs even if the panels cannot be seen from the food dish; the birds behave as though they have two stably specified points of attention, dish and panels, between which they alternate. Comparable behaviour is quite absent in untreated birds (Klein & Andrew, 1986).

At the lowest dose (800 μg), a quite new pattern was seen. The chicks commonly passed the panels, as with higher doses, but then turned (without reaching the dish) and came back to inspect the panels. This suggests that information derived from examination of the panels is sufficiently stabilised in temporary storage, in which it is available for continuing analysis, to allow the decision to be taken to return. It has further to be assumed that, at this near-threshold dose, over the same period of time the record of the food dish as the current object of attention is lost.

The effects of increasing stabilisation thus appear to be as follows: in untreated birds, shift of attention to the panels is accompanied by loss of the food dish as a point of attention; delay is often long and the bird may leave the panels and wander back along the runway as though it has forgotten what it had intended to do. With minimal stabilisation, the bird is able to bring attention back to the food dish and pass the panels but then, as processing information about the panels is sustained, attention is not held on the food dish, but returns to the panels. With fuller stabilisation, such return is not seen until after feeding, when establishment of two points of attention becomes clear.

Most, at least, of these effects of testosterone are due to the oestrogenic route of action. Clifton, Andrew & Brighton (1988) used a range of doses of oestradiol dipropionate, given 30 minutes before test: 10 ng was below, and 1 μg was close to threshold. The standard pattern (with delay at the dish increased by comparison with untreated birds, and delay at the panels decreased) was obtained at 5 μg, whilst a new one appeared at 100 μg: delay in the dish test was even higher than usual but accompanied by equally long delay because of the panels. At this very high dose stabilisation is apparently so great that, once shifted to the panel, attention is held there for some time.

2. *Competition test.* In this test, the chick is allowed to peck a red bead on two successive occasions. At the first presentation the red bead is clean, but at the second it tastes unpleasant. As a result the two experiences give contradictory information about the bead: which is the more effective is revealed by a final test with a clean red bead. Normally, experience of the ill-tasting bead depresses rates of pecking at a red bead in the final test to very

low levels. However, if testosterone is acting, and the interval between the presentations is either very short or falls within certain well defined windows of time (see below), then the effectiveness of the first experience in competing with the second is greatly enhanced. This effect of testosterone was first discovered by Messent (1973) at Sussex, using very short intervals. In the absence of a first experience with a bead, testosterone has no effect (Andrew, Clifton & Gibbs, 1981); testosterone thus does not directly interfere with the effects of training with an ill-tasting bead.

There are differences between the outcome of competition with very short intervals and with longer intervals. The most important for present purposes is that with longer intervals the second experience is temporarily effective in changing subsequent behaviour: inhibition of pecking persists for at least 30 minutes, but disappears progressively thereafter (Clifton, Andrew & Gibbs, 1982). In contrast, with intervals up to about 2 minutes in length there is no evidence that information about the bad taste is ever associated with seeing and pecking the red bead: even with test as close to training as 5 minutes, the red bead is pecked (Clifton *et al.*, 1982). In this section, I shall be concerned only with short intervals; longer intervals are considered later.

Two experiences with a bead, which are separated by a minute or so are in many ways comparable with the search tests which are discussed later. During search, testosterone makes it more likely that the chick will continue, in the presence of alternative targets, to select only food grains of an appearance similar to that which it was taking at the beginning of the test. It is argued here that this results from the stabilisation in use in the selection of stimuli of a record of the type of stimulus to which attention is currently directed.

In competition tests, the second experience may be compared with a single examination of a target during search. It seems likely that a record of the first experience is used to recognise and evaluate the bead at its second appearance. Testosterone makes it less likely that new and discrepant features of the second experience will be incorporated into memory (or, if incorporated, ensures that they will not be associated with seeing and pecking the bead). This can be explained by stabilisation of the record which is being used to evaluate the second experience, if it is assumed that change in, or clearance of this record is necessary, before new and discrepant information to the bead can be accepted. Note that, before the bead is pecked and the bad taste is detected, the bead is presumably judged to be identical with that seen at the first experience; a reversal of a judgement of identity is thus required before what is held in memory relating to the red bead can be changed.

Competition tests were the first to be used to demonstrate the oestrogenic character of effects of testosterone on attentional mechanisms (Rainey, 1983;

Table 1. *Thresholds for effects on memory formation*

Sex	Hormones	Free steroid	Propionate
Female	Oestradiol	100 pg	–
	Testosterone	10 ng	–
Male	Oestradiol	1 ng	100 ng
	Testosterone	100 ng	*c.* 100 μg
	Progesterone	500 ng	–
	5α-DHT	*c.* 5 μg*	Not found (> 1 mg)
	Corticosterone	*c.* 5 μg*	–
	Cholesterol	Not found	

Free steroids were administered in dimethylacetamide (Andrew, 1983), propionates in oil (Clifton *et al.*, 1986). *, appearance of effect with increasing dose so gradual and irregular that no clear threshold could be established.

Andrew, 1983; Clifton, Andrew & Rainey, 1986). When the induction of competition by injection just before the first presentation is used as a measure, female chicks prove to be more sensitive than males by a factor of 10; both sexes show a similar ratio between the thresholds for oestradiol and testosterone of about 100 (Table 1). 5α-DHT is almost ineffective, as is corticosterone, a result of interest in view of effects of glucocorticoids on memory formation in rodents (Flood *et al.*, 1978).

A 10 μg dose of free testosterone (about 100-fold above threshold) results initially in plasma levels somewhat above those usual in adult cocks; these fall in 5–10 minutes to adult levels and remain somewhat elevated for somewhat more than 60 minutes (Andrew, 1983). It is thus likely that at the threshold doses shown in Table 1 adult levels are reached only briefly, if at all.

The measurement of the latency of action of testosterone using the competition procedure is complicated by the fact that the hormone also affects memory formation when given following learning (below). Uncertainty as to the time of action can be reduced to a minimum by using a very short interval (10 seconds) between the two presentations. It is likely that competition (due to the OSLE) occurs at and just after the second presentation: in any case, since loss of memory of unpleasant taste is marked within 5 minutes, estimates of latency derived in this way are at the most 5 minutes too short. Action is within about 15 minutes (Clifton *et al.*, 1982), a strikingly short time, particularly when time for entry into the bloodstream, and probably for aromatisation is taken into account.

Teyler *et al.* (1980) describe a change in the excitability of hippocampal pyramidal cells within less than 20 minutes of the application of gonadal steroids: oestradiol (but not testosterone) was effective in males, whereas in females testosterone (but not oestradiol) had effects, which differed with phase of oestrus. Teyler *et al.* doubt whether RNA synthesis can be involved.

3. *Searching tests.*   Effects of testosterone on attention were first discovered during food search (Andrew & Rogers, 1972; Andrew, 1976). Information relating to both position and type of sought after food appears to be stabilised. Changes attributable to testosterone in the way in which chicks use information about the position(s) in which food has been found, have been most fully explored in a test in which black food grains are presented singly on occasional black squares of a large chequerboard (Rogers & Andrew, 1989). Video recordings of locomotion and head position revealed two types of effect. First, testosterone-treated birds adopted a strategy of moving to search one of the black squares neighbouring that which they had just searched; they rarely detected grains at a greater distance or grains situated in the lateral visual fields. Untreated birds, in contrast, commonly did both, first turning the head to fixate the new target binocularly, and then changing route in order to run to it.

Secondly, treated, but not untreated chicks often returned to squares on which they had previously found food, much as treated birds in the runway would return to view the panels. However, in the case of the chequerboard, there were so many black squares which might have been searched, that guidance by recently acquired information about the exact position of the area visited was much clearer.

In search over floors which are lightly scattered with food grains of two types, testosterone stabilises both the area of search and the type of food sought. This can be well seen if the food is arranged in clumps. Treated birds not only search more persistently within a clump, but when the type of food which they have been selecting is largely or entirely consumed within a particular clump, they may peck at a grain of another type, before moving to a new clump. They then return at once to selection of the first type of food. In untreated birds, in contrast, once a second type of food is taken, then at least a short run of selection of such food follows. Untreated birds thus show full shifts of attention between types of food. This is even clearer when search occurs amongst a distracting background of pebbles. Here untreated birds shift repeatedly and readily between two types of food, whereas testosterone-treated birds stick to one type or the other.

More persistent specification of type of food is almost certainly attributable to the oestrogenic effect on attention. However, sustained search in an area where the type of object sought has become rare or has disappeared could also reflect resistance to extinction. The resemblance to extinction tests is even higher in tests where chicks were faced with groups of light caps, each covering a depression in which food might or might not be present (Messent, 1973). Testosterone caused chicks to turn over more caps without finding food, before moving.

It is thus possible that the short latency androgenic effect also affects search. The only direct evidence so far available is that provided by Young & Rogers (1978) who found, in an experiment where chicks receiving testosterone showed the expected increased persistence of choice of one of the two available types of food, that 5α-DHT had the reverse effect: it increased the number of shifts between the two types.

Young & Rogers (1978) argued that 5α-DHT might lower endogenous levels of testosterone by depressing gonadotrophin secretion. It is more likely that 5α-DHT acts to sustain pecking in an area where the previously chosen type of food is becoming exhausted, and so forces pecks at the second type of food. In the absence of oestrogenic stabilisation of information specifying the type of food to be selected, this might result in the acceptance of whatever food was present in the area of search.

Finally, testosterone affects search in female chicks as well as males (Zappia & Rogers, 1987).

Effects of testosterone on memory formation

In the chick testosterone is known to affect memory formation in much the same way as do pituitary peptide hormones. Further, these effects are much more clearly tied to processes integral to memory formation than is yet possible to demonstrate for hormones in the rat, in that in the chick the hormones are known to act upon specific events in memory formation (Andrew, 1980, 1985).

In the case of testosterone, evidence is accumulating that action occurs at the time of one or other of a series of brief periods of food retrieval, which are associated with the left hemisphere (Andrew & Brennan, 1985; Andrew, 1991a). These 'retrieval events' repeat with a period of about 16 minutes. In competition experiments (above), in which the interval between the first experience with a clean red bead, and the second with an unpleasant tasting red bead, is systematically varied, competition occurs when the second experience coincides with food retrieval of the first (i.e. with a retrieval event). This is so far shown for the first two left hemisphere events (at about 16 and 32 minutes after learning). Competition is present even in controls at these times, and is enhanced by testosterone. A corresponding series of retrieval events is associated with the right hemisphere, but with a different period: no competition occurs at the first of these (about 25 minutes after learning), at least.

When the intervals between the first and second experiences are long (e.g.

120 minutes), a final route of action of testosterone can be demonstrated. Testosterone then produces competition when given up to about 30 minutes after the first experience, but not later (Clifton *et al.*, 1982); here the change in memory formation which makes the record of the first experience effective in producing competition evidently occurs well before the second experience. This is important because in all the other cases, enhancement of competition could be due entirely to various effects of testosterone on learning associated with the second experience. All could stem from stabilisation of the record used to assess the second experience; differences between the outcome at different intervals between the experiences would then be due to differences in the information available to be stabilised. Action on purely central processes cannot be so explained; however, it remains possible that action on the same or similar mechanisms is still involved. Since the argument is complicated, I set it out in steps:

(a) In the chick the two hemispheres appear to be specialised in somewhat different ways for the analysis of information (review in Andrew, 1987; and below). As a result, they are likely initially to hold somewhat different versions of an experience like pecking a bead.

(b) At 50 minutes after learning, changes occur in memory formation in the chick which have long been identified as in some way responsible for the appearance of the final version of a memory (Gibbs & Ng, 1977). Amongst the dramatic changes which result at this time from the much earlier application of amnestic procedures (at or just after learning), are the abrupt disappearance of memory, or its sudden reappearance after temporary amnesia (Allweis *et al.*, 1984).

Both these phenomena require the existence of two versions of the learning event, only one of which is disrupted by the amnestic procedure. One version must be predominantly responsible for the control of behaviour up to 50 minutes, so that if it is disturbed, there is no effective memory available to retrieval until that time. At about 50 minutes some mechanism must reverse the consequences of the amnestic procedure.

(c) I have argued elsewhere (Andrew, 1991a) that independent records in right and left hemisphere provide exactly what is needed to explain these striking and complex phenomena. One hemisphere must be assumed to be in predominant control of response; there is evidence that this is likely to be the left hemisphere in the case of the bead task (Andrew, 1991b), so this will be assumed here for the sake of exposition. It is also necessary that amnestic procedures should chiefly affect sometimes the right and sometimes the left hemisphere: there is now evidence for this (Andrew & Brennan, 1985; Patterson *et al.*, 1986).

At 50 minutes after learning, for the first time, retrieval events occur coincidentally in both hemispheres. If, as a result, there is the opportunity for information transfer, then the reappearance or disappearance at this time of access to a memory which is effective in causing the inhibition of pecking, can be explained. After loss of memory effective in controlling response, due to disturbance of the left hemisphere record, a surviving right hemisphere record would allow reinstatement of an effective left hemisphere record by information transfer. Disturbance of the right hemisphere record would have no immediate effect, but later transfer of degraded information would result in disturbance of the left hemisphere record also. Note that both effects require that the important transfer at 50 minutes after learning should be from the right to the left hemisphere.

(d) In normal memory formation, also, there may be sharp changes at about 50 minutes after learning: after training with diluted aversant, Gibbs (Crowe, Ng & Gibbs, 1990) has found that inhibition of pecking disappears suddenly at 50 minutes.

This can be explained on the present hypothesis, if specific assumptions are made about the differences between the records in right and left hemispheres. Let us suppose that the left hemisphere record clearly associates seeing and pecking the bead with the subsequent taste, but (under these circumstances, when the taste is only marginally unpleasant) the right hemisphere record does not. Information transfer at 50 minutes after learning would then result in reduced effectiveness of the left hemisphere trace in the inhibition of pecking. These assumptions are at least consistent with evidence as to the specialisation of right and left hemispheres for analysis of information (Andrew, 1987, 1991b). The right hemisphere appears to be especially concerned with the unique combination of visual properties associated with a particular object; this might make a series of 'snapshot' records more likely (here: appearance of bead; after-taste). The left hemisphere appears to be especially concerned with the assignment of stimuli to categories, using selected cues, so that response can be appropriate and rapid; such analysis seems likely to need to take into account the consequences of response.

(e) The fact that, when the interval between the first and second experiences is systematically varied from very short to beyond half an hour, testosterone is effective in enhancing competition only when the second experience coincides with a left hemisphere retrieval event (above), suggests that it is the left hemisphere record that must be protected from change if competition is to be observed.

The final step in this argument is to suppose that testosterone does the same at 50 minutes after learning, but here by affecting information transfer between the hemispheres. Evidence that testosterone does indeed act at about 50 minutes is reviewed elsewhere (Andrew, 1991a); note that such a timing of action is consistent with the ending of the effectiveness of testosterone injections at around 30 minutes after learning.

Testosterone might act on information transfer as follows: information which has been accessed at the time of a retrieval event in the left hemisphere, as a part of internally initiated processes, would be held in a temporary store and used to find and assess corresponding material in the right hemisphere. Stabilisation of such information in its temporary storage by testosterone would then make acceptance of new and discrepant information from the right hemisphere less likely, much as stabilisation of the description held by attentional mechanisms makes more likely rejection of information from stimuli which do not match the description. In this particular case, change of the left hemisphere record by right hemisphere material would be opposed, leading to enhanced competition when later there is training with an ill-tasting bead.

Conclusion

Considerable evidence suggests that testosterone and pituitary peptide hormones have effects on attention in mammals very like the short latency oestrogenic effects described here for the chick. Reduction by testosterone of distractibility by irrelevant stimuli has been demonstrated in tests directly modelled on those used in work on chick, in both mouse (Archer, 1977) and rat (Thompson & Wright, 1979). ACTH reduces lapses of attention in sustained human performance (review: Gaillard, 1981): comparable effects have been reported for testosterone (Klaiber, Broverman & Kobayashi, 1967). In both rat and human studies ACTH 'focuses' attention, improving performance when intradimensional shifts are required during learning but worsening it for extradimensional shifts (review: Sandman & Kastin, 1977). Finally, increased stability of short-term storage due to ACTH has been found in human studies (van Praag & Verhoeven, 1980).

It is then likely that in both mammals and birds testosterone and pituitary peptide hormones have linked or common routes of action on attention. Such action may occur in males in association with the physiological rises in ACTH and testosterone which follow exposure to novel, frightening (or perhaps also highly valent) stimuli. As a result, attention is more likely to be sustained on, and returned to such stimuli. In the chick, a limit of 1–2 minutes is set on such stabilisation by testosterone at least under the simplest condition, when the stimulus is presented briefly and then withdrawn; this may allow extreme stabilisation of attention in the short term without maladaptive extension for long periods of time, when appropriate stimuli are no longer to be found.

In the chick such effects of testosterone are produced by a short-latency oestrogenic route. The discovery of an androgenic effect, which increases resistance to extinction, suggests that testosterone may act to sustain behaviour against obstacles and distraction by at least two routes. The OSLE affects attention, whilst the androgenic effect has an immediate facilitatory effect on the motor pattern which is in use. Of course, in social interaction classic effects of testosterone, such as the specific facilitation of aggressive responses, will also play a part. Testosterone thus produces a cocktail of different central effects which complement each other when, for example, the animal is faced with some check or obstacle. The androgenic effect sustains repeated performance of the motor sequence which has been successful in previous experience. The oestrogenic effect on attention postpones shift of attention to other stimuli, and so opposes change to other types of behaviour. If the obstacle is another animal, then classic effects of testosterone on aggressive behaviour may result in attack being used as a way of removing the obstacle.

I believe that the changes produced by the short-latency oestrogenic route have the most interesting implications for further research. Current evidence suggests that these arise from stabilisation of information in a working memory, which affects the first moments of recognition and interpretation of a stimulus. The same store allows attention to be returned to a stimulus after shifts of duration varying from a moment to many seconds. The information held within it may be assembled from, on the one hand, immediately previous experiences and, on the other, long-established rules for the selection of stimuli of known importance. In human terms, an effect of this sort would both hold attention for longer on particular types of objects in the outside world and sustain a particular interpretation through protracted attempts to make it fit the circumstances.

It is the possible role of the OSLE in processes entirely internal to memory formation which is potentially the most novel. I have speculated here that similar or the same mechanisms may be involved in search and assessment of the external world and search for and assessment of information held in memory. I was led to this idea by the accumulating resemblances between the way in which testosterone affects attention and the way in which it acts at the time of retrieval events in memory formation. The speculation has the merit that the attentional processes affected by testosterone are relatively well understood; the predictions which follow from the hypothesis that they are also important in memory formation are thus potentially specific and detailed.

References

Allweis, C., Gibbs, M. E., Ng, K. T. & Hodge, R. J. (1984). Effects of hypoxia on memory consolidation: implications for a multistage model of memory. *Behavioural Brain Research*, **11**, 117–22.

Andrew, R. J. (1972). Recognition processes and behaviour, with special reference to effects of testosterone on persistence. *Advances in the Study of Behaviour*, **4**, 175–208.

Andrew, R. J. (1976). Attentional processes and animal behaviour. In *Growing Points in Ethology*, ed. P. P. G. Bateson and R. A. Hinde, pp. 95–133. Cambridge: Cambridge University Press.

Andrew, R. J. (1980). The functional organisation of phases of memory consolidation. *Advances in the Study of Behaviour*, **11**, 337–67.

Andrew, R. J. (1983). Specific short-latency effects of oestradiol and testosterone on distractibility and memory formation in the young domestic chick. In *Hormones and Behaviour in Higher Vertebrates*, ed. J. Balthazart, E. Pröve and R. Gilles, pp. 463–73. Berlin: Springer-Verlag.

Andrew, R. J. (1985). The temporal structure of memory formation. *Perspectives in Ethology*, **6**, 219–59.

Andrew, R. J. (1987). The development of visual lateralisation in the domestic chick. *Behavioural Brain Research*, **29**, 201–9.

Andrew, R. J. (1991a). Cyclicity in memory formation. In *Neural and Behavioural Plasticity*, ed. R. J. Andrew. Oxford: Oxford University Press.

Andrew, R. J. (1991b). The nature of behavioural lateralisation in the chick. In *Neural and Behavioural Plasticity*, ed. R. J. Andrew. Oxford: Oxford University Press.

Andrew, R. J. & Brennan, A. (1985). Sharply timed and lateralised events at time of establishment of long term memory. *Physiology and Behavior*, **34**, 547–56.

Andrew, R. J., Clifton, P. G. & Gibbs, M. E. (1981). Enhancement of effectiveness of learning by testosterone in domestic chicks. *Journal of Comparative and Physiological Psychology*, **95**, 406–17.

Andrew, R. J. & Rogers, L. J. (1972). Testosterone, search behaviour and persistence. *Nature*, **237**, 343–6.

Archer, J. (1973). A further analysis of response to a novel environment by testosterone-treated chicks. *Behavioral Biology*, **8**, 389–96.

Archer, J. (1974). The effect of testosterone on the distractibility of chicks by irrelevant and relevant novel stimuli. *Animal Behaviour*, **22**, 397–404.

Archer, J. (1977). Testosterone and persistence in mice. *Animal Behaviour*, **25**, 479–88.

Chambers, K. C. (1976). Hormonal influence on sexual dimorphism in the rate of extinction of a conditioned taste aversion in rats. *Journal of Comparative and Physiological Psychology*, **90**, 851–6.

Chambers, K. C. (1980). Progesterone, estradiol, testosterone and dihydrotestosterone: Effects on rate of extinction of a conditioned taste aversion in rats. *Physiology and Behavior*, **24**, 1061–5.

Chambers, K. C. & Sengstake, C. B. (1979). Temporal aspects of the dependency of a dimorphic rate of extinction on testosterone. *Physiology and Behavior*, **22**, 53–6.

Clayton, D. A. & Andrew, R. J. (1979). Phases of inhibition and response during investigation of stimulus change by the domestic chick. *Behaviour*, **69**, 36–56.

Clifton, P. G. & Andrew, R. J. (1981). A comparison of the effects of testosterone on aggressive responses by the domestic chick to the human hand and to a large sphere. *Animal Behaviour*, **29**, 610–20.

Clifton, P. G. & Andrew, R. J. (1987). Gonadal steroids and the extinction of conditioned taste aversion in young domestic fowl. *Physiology and Behaviour*, **39**, 27–31.

Clifton, P. G. & Andrew, R. J. (1989). Contrasting effects of pre- and post-hatch exposure to gonadal steroids on the development of vocal, sexual and aggressive behaviour of young domestic fowl. *Hormones and Behavior*, **23**, 572–89.

Clifton, P. G., Andrew, R. J. & Brighton, L. (1988). Gonadal steroids and attentional mechanisms in young domestic chicks. *Physiology and Behavior*, **43**, 441–6.

Clifton, P. G., Andrew, R. J. & Gibbs, M. E. (1982). Limited period of action of testosterone on memory formation in the chick. *Journal of Comparative and Physiological Psychology*, **96**, 212–22.

Clifton, P. G., Andrew, R. J. & Rainey, C. R. (1986). Effects of gonadal steroids on attack and on memory processing in the domestic chick. *Physiology and Behavior*, **37**, 701–7.

Crowe, S. F., Ng, K. T. & Gibbs, M. E. (1989). Memory formation processes in weakly reinforced learning. *Pharmacology, Biochemistry and Behavior*, **33**, 881–7.

de Wied, D. & Jolles, J. (1982). Neuropeptides derived from pro-opiocortin: behavioural, physiological and neurochemical effects. *Physiological Reviews*, **62**, 976–1059.

Early, C. J. & Leonard, B. E. (1979). Effects of prior experience on conditioned taste aversion in the rat: Androgen and estrogen dependent events. *Journal of Comparative Physiological Psychology*, **93**, 793–805.

Ermisch, A., Landgraf, R. & Mobius, P. (1986). Vasopressin and oxytocin in brain areas of rats with high or low behavioural performance. *Brain Research*, **379**, 24–8.

Faulborn, K. W., Fenske, M., Pitzel, L. & Konig, A. (1979). Effects of an intravenous injection of tetracosactid on plasma corticosteroid and testosterone levels in unstressed male rabbits. *Acta Endocrinologica*, **91**, 511–18.

Fekete, M. & de Wied, D. (1982a). Potency and duration of action of the ACTH 4–9 analog (ORG 2766) as compared to ACTH 4–10 and [D-Phe^7] ACTH 4–10 on active and passive avoidance behaviour of rats. *Pharmacology, Biochemistry and Behavior*, **16**, 387–92.

Fekete, M. & de Wied, D. (1982b). Dose-related facilitation and inhibition of passive avoidance behaviour by the ACTH 4–9 analog (ORG 2766). *Pharmacology Biochemistry and Behavior*, **17**, 177–82.

Flood, J. F., Vidal, D., Bennett, E. L., Orme, A. E., Vasquez, S. & Jarvik, M. E. (1978). Memory facilitating and anti-amnesic effects of corticosteroids. *Pharmacology, Biochemistry and Behavior*, **8**, 81–7.

Gaillard, A. W. K. (1981). ACTH analogs and human performance. In *Endogenous Peptides and Learning and Memory Processes*, ed. J. L. Martinez, R. A. Jensen, R. B. Messing, H. Rigter and J. L. McGaugh, pp. 181–96. London: Academic Press.

Gaston, E. E. (1977). An illness-induced conditioned aversion in domestic chicks: One trial learning with a long delay of reinforcement. *Behavioral Biology*, **20**, 441–53.

Gibbs, M. E. Ng, K. T. (1977). Psychobiology of memory: towards a model of memory formation. *Biobehav. Rev.* **1**, 113–36.

Hahmeier, W., Fenske, M., Pitzel, L., Holtz, W. & Konig, A. (1980). Corticotropin- and lysine-vasopressin-induced changes of plasma corticosteroids and testosterone in the adult male pig. *Acta Endocrinologica*, **95**, 518–22.

Harrison, N. L., Majewska, M. D., Harrington, J. W. & Barker, J. L. (1987). Structure–activity relationships for steroid interaction with the γ-aminobutyric acid$_A$ complex. *Journal of Pharmacology and Experimental Therapeutics*, **241**, 346–53.

Haun, C. K. & Haltmeyer, G. C. (1975). Effects of an intraventricular injection of synthetic ACTH on plasma testosterone, progesterone and LH levels, and on sexual behaviour in male and female rabbits. *Neuroendocrinology*, **19**, 201–13.

Klaiber, E. L., Broverman, D. M. & Kobayashi, Y. (1967). The automatization cognitive style, androgens and monoamine oxidase. *Psychopharmacology*, **11**, 320–36.

Klein, R. M. (1983). Stabilization of attention by testosterone. DPhil thesis, University of Sussex.

Klein, R. M. & Andrew, R. J. (1986). Distraction, decisions and persistence in runway tests using the domestic chick. *Behaviour*, **99**, 139–56.

Leshner, A. J. (1980). The interaction of experiences and neuroendocrine factors in determining adaptation to aggression. *Progress in Brain Research*, **53**, 427–38.

Messent, P. R. (1973). Distractibility and persistence of chick. DPhil thesis, University of Sussex.

Patterson, T. A., Alvarado, M. O., Warner, I. T., Bennett, E. L. & Rosenzweig, M. R. (1986). Memory stages and brain asymmetry in chick learning. *Behavioral Neuroscience*, **100**, 850–9.

Rainey, C. R. (1983). Steroid specificity and memory in the chick. DPhil thesis, University of Sussex.

Ramenofsky, M. (1985). Acute changes in plasma steroids and agonistic behaviour in male Japanese Quail. *General and Comparative Endocrinology*, **60**, 116–28.

Roche, K. E. & Leshner, A. I. (1979). ACTH and vasopressin treatments immediately after a defeat increase further submissiveness in male mice. *Science*, **204**, 1343–4.

Rodriguez-Sierra, J. F., Terasawa, E., Goldfoot, D. A. & de Wied, D. (1981). Testosterone potentiation of the effectiveness of ACTH[1–24] in the induction of the stretch–yawning syndrome (SYS) in male guinea pigs. *Hormones and Behavior*, **15**, 77–85.

Rogers, L. J. & Andrew, R. J. (1989). Changes in the relative use of frontal and peripheral visual fields following treatment of chicks with testosterone. *Animal Behaviour*, **38**, 394–405.

Sandman, C. A. & Kastin, A. J. (1977). Pituitary peptide influences on attention and memory. In *Neurobiology of Sleep and Memory*, ed. R. R. Drucker-Colin and J. L. McGaugh, pp. 347–60. London: Academic Press.

Smotherman, W. P. (1985). Glucocorticoid and other hormonal substrates of conditioned taste aversion. *Annals of the New York Academy of Science*, **443**, 126–44.

Teyler, T. J., Vardaris, R. M., Lewis, E. & Rawitch, A. B. (1980). Gonadal steroids: effects on excitability of hippocampal pyramidal cells. *Science*, **209**, 1017–19.

Thompson, W. R. & Wright, J. S. (1979). 'Persistence' in rats: effects of testosterone. *Physiol. Psychol.* **7**, 291–4.

van Haaren, F., van Zanten, S. & van de Poll, N. E. (1986). Vasopressin disrupts radial-maze performance in rats. *Behavioral and Neural Biology*, **45**, 350–7.

van Praag, H. M. & Verhoeven, W. M. A. (1980). Neuropeptides. A new dimension in biological psychiatry. *Progress in Brain Research*, **53**, 123–40.

Wolterink, G. & Van Ree, J. M. (1987). The ACTH 4–9 analog ORG 2766 'normalizes' the changes in the motor activities of rats elicited by housing and test conditions. *Brain Research*, **421**, 41–7.

Young, C. E. & Rogers, L. J. (1978). Effects of steroidal hormones on sexual, attack, and search behaviour in the isolated male chick. *Hormones and Behavior*, **10**, 107–17.

Zappia, J. V. & Rogers, L. J. (1987). Sex differences and reversal of brain asymmetry by testosterone in chickens. *Behavioral and Brain Research*, **23**, 261–7.

—8—
A psychobiological approach to maternal behaviour among the primates

Jay S. Rosenblatt

Introduction

Progress in the psychobiological study of maternal behaviour among the non-primate mammals, especially among the rodents and ungulates, has been considerable. The hormones and other neuroactive substances which stimulate the onset of maternal behaviour are known in part for several species, the neural substrates on which they act are increasingly becoming known, and the conditions under which maternal behaviour, once initiated, is maintained after parturition and retained for some time afterward even in the absence of the performance of maternal care, are also being revealed in recent studies. There has been considerably less progress in the study of these aspects of maternal behaviour among primates. In part this is attributable to the practical difficulties and barriers to this kind of study among the primates. More important may be the different approach which has been adopted in primate studies of maternal behaviour, including studies of human maternal behaviour. This approach is no less 'biological' than that described above but it has emphasised psychosocial aspects of maternal behaviour, i.e. the individual and social features that play such a large role in primate social interactions.

Robert Hinde (Hinde and Stevenson-Hinde, 1976; Hinde, 1987) has not neglected the role of psychobiological factors in maternal behaviour among the primates. This approach would be in the forefront of his thinking because of his own background in the study of the neuroendocrine basis of reproduction in the canary (Hinde, 1965). Together with D. S. Lehrman, who did similar studies on ring dove reproductive behaviour (Lehrman, 1965), he did much to establish the psychobiological approach to reproduction in these particular species and reproductive behaviour in general among animals. Moreover, his scheme of levels of analysis of social relationships includes as a basic level the psychobiological factors underlying interactions between the mother and her offspring.

Does the progress made in the study of maternal behaviour among the lower mammals using the psychobiological approach have value for the study of primate maternal behaviour? The aim of the present article is to examine some links between the two. I shall review basic findings derived from several lines of investigation of maternal behaviour among non-primate mammals. With these findings in mind I will then turn to studies of the primates to see whether a similar analysis can be pursued.

Reviews adopting the psychobiological approach to maternal behaviour among the primates (Capitanio, Weissberg & Reite, 1985; D. A. Goldfoot, L. J. Swanson, D. A. Neff and L. Leavitt, unpublished data) and several reviews with evolutionary and psychobiological perspectives on maternal behaviour among the non-human primates and humans (Kaufman, 1970) have appeared. Fleming & Corter (1988) and Trevathan (1987) have explicitly approached the study of human maternal behaviour from the background of studies on lower mammals.

The sudden onset of maternal behaviour at parturition among the lower mammals correlated with hormonal changes has proved an important indicator of the hormonal basis of this behaviour and has helped to identify the hormones which stimulate the onset of maternal behaviour (Rosenblatt, Mayer & Giordano, 1988). This analysis has been extended backward into the period of pregnancy and prepartum, when it has been found in several species that maternal responsiveness increases and aspects of maternal behaviour may appear spontaneously (e.g. nest-building, maternal aggression toward conspecific adults). Following the onset of maternal behaviour the question of what maintains these activities emerges as a separate issue. We have proposed that the immediate postpartum period is one of transition in which the hormonal stimuli wane and new kinds of stimuli, namely those arising during interaction with the newborn, become the basis for the maintenance of maternal behaviour (Rosenblatt, Siegel & Mayer, 1979). Immediate postpartum maintenance of maternal behaviour may provide the basis for long-term retention of maternal responsiveness. At later times, therefore, multiparous females may initiate maternal behaviour even when not exposed to the hormones which originally stimulated such behaviour in primiparous females.

Psychobiology of maternal behaviour: non-primate mammals

Development of maternal responsiveness during pregnancy
and in the prepartum period

In several species of *non-primate mammals* elements of maternal behaviour appear spontaneously during pregnancy (nest-building and maternal aggression in mice: Lisk, 1971; Svare, Miele & Kinsley, 1986), while in others an increase in maternal responsiveness can be shown experimentally by exposing females to young and observing shortened latencies, compared with non-pregnant females, for the appearance of maternal behaviour (e.g. retrieving, licking young, adopting a nursing position over them, inhibition of aggression towards young, and exhibiting maternal aggression towards intruding animals; Rosenblatt *et al.*, 1988). In the rat and mouse, latencies to the onset of maternal behaviour can be reduced to less than two days if females are hysterectomised after mid-pregnancy (Rosenblatt & Siegel, 1975; Hauser & Gandelman, 1985; Svare *et al.*, 1986).

The beginnings of maternal behaviour in females of a number of non-primate species more often are seen shortly before delivery of their own young rather than during pregnancy. Females of several species engage in nest-building (rabbit, mouse, rat, hamster), others inhibit any aggression they may have shown earlier towards newborn, and still others, exposed to young, exhibit the full pattern of maternal behaviour. Among sheep and goats prepartum females are attracted to young being cared for by other mothers (Poindron & Le Neindre, 1980).

The termination of pregnancy and the hormonal changes which accompany it are gradual processes which accelerate as parturition nears. It is during this period that the hormonal conditions which stimulate the onset of maternal behaviour arise, enabling the female to respond positively to the newborns when they appear. Behaviour patterns preparatory to the appearance of the newborns (e.g. nest-building, maternal aggression towards intruders of the nestsite) may appear but others await their appearance although they may be elicited prematurely by providing the female with substitute newborns.

The decline in circulating levels of progesterone and the rise in oestradiol during the last several days of pregnancy have pointed to these hormones as central to the onset of maternal behaviour in the rat. This pattern of hormonal changes is common to many but not all mammals (e.g. the hamster and rhesus monkey are exceptions), with differences among species in the timing of these changes in relation to parturition (Rosenblatt & Siegel, 1981). Many studies have now confirmed that both of these changes are essential for stimulating the onset of maternal behaviour in the rat: the withdrawal of the inhibitory effect of progesterone enables rising levels of oestradiol to stimulate maternal behaviour (Rosenblatt *et al.*, 1979; Bridges, 1984; Giordano, Siegel & Rosenblatt, 1989).

The pituitary hormone prolactin has recently been implicated in the action of oestradiol on the onset of maternal behaviour. Several studies using hypophysectomised females that are unable to secrete prolactin and females treated with bromocriptine to block the release of prolactin have shown that this hormone (or a similar, lactogenic hormone secreted by the placenta during pregnancy) plays an important role in the onset of maternal behaviour (Bridges *et al.*, 1985). Nest-building in the rabbit and in the mouse are also stimulated by prolactin and this hormone has been shown to stimulate maternal behaviour and maternal aggression in hamsters.

Oxytocin, a hormone known for its action on smooth muscles of the uterus during parturition and the mammary gland during lactation, has also been found to stimulate maternal behaviour (Pedersen & Prange, 1979; Pedersen *et al.*, 1982; Fahrbach, Morrell & Pfaff, 1984). It does not act alone, however, since oestrogen priming is necessary for oxytocin to be effective. Oxytocin also inhibits the pup-killing which occurs during pregnancy in wild house mice simulating the effects of parturition and it stimulates maternal behaviour as well (McCarthy, Bare & Vom Saal, 1986).

It is among sheep that perhaps the strongest evidence for a role for oxytocin in the onset of maternal behaviour has been found (Kendrick, Keverne & Baldwin, 1987; Keverne, 1988). Vaginal–cervical stimulation during delivery in the ewe stimulates the release of oxytocin which in turn plays a role in initiating maternal behaviour toward the newborn lamb (Poindron *et al.*, 1988). A peridural anaesthetic administered to primiparous ewes at the start of parturition prevents the reflex release of oxytocin and thereby prevents the onset of maternal behaviour (Krehbiel *et al.*, 1987). Replacement of oxytocin by injection into the intracerebral ventricles overcomes this inhibition (F. Lévy, personal communication). Oxytocin may act in part by altering the ewe's aversive response to newborn odours derived from the amniotic fluid, enabling her to react positively to them (Lévy, Poindron & Le Neindre, 1983; Lévy & Poindron, 1984, 1987).

The onset of maternal behaviour at parturition

The mother's first responses to her young occur during parturition in the non-primate mammals as in all mammals. Detailed descriptions of parturition in the rat and cat depict the interplay of physiological and behavioural processes which initially focus the female's licking on her vaginal–genital region and increasingly on the newborns and placentas when they emerge (Rosenblatt & Lehrman, 1963; Schneirla, Rosenblatt & Tobach, 1963). In all but the pig among nesting species, the female licks the amniotic fluid from the body of the newborn, stimulates them to breathe, and deposits them in the nest or carries them to it and consumes the placentas when they emerge. These constitute the main items of parturition behaviour. In species with precocial newborn, such as among the ungulates, and in a few smaller mammals with precocial young, parturition behaviour consists of licking the newborn and some forms of stimulus interchange (e.g. vocalisation, body rubbing) occur (Rosenblatt & Siegel, 1981). The moose cow's behaviour towards its calf at parturition has been described by Bogomolova & Kurochkin (1984) as follows:

The birth . . . markedly changes the mother's reactivity to certain environmental stimuli so that its behavior becomes directed towards the calf. After the birth only, it manifests a positive reaction to small moving objects, smell of amniotic fluid, squeak of the newborn and the aggressive reaction to the approach of another cow or a man.

Female rats and cats assist the delivery of the newborn by postural changes in response to uterine contractions which facilitate passage of the foetuses through the birth canal, and often by the use of forepaws and mouth to assist in the final emergence of the newborn from the vaginal opening. Among the large ungulates less direct contact with the foetus occurs while it emerges from the vulva but adjustments are made (Kristal & Noonan, 1978). After the newborn has emerged, moreover, the mother turns to it and licks its head and body as mother and young engage in their first extended behavioural interaction.

Multiple births during delivery among the lower mammals, especially those with altricial young, but also among those with precocial young that give birth to twins, is undoubtedly an important factor in the establishment of maternal behaviour and mother–young interaction. During the several deliveries the mother's attention is repeatedly focused on the newborns, and to the extent that stimulation of birth canal by the passage of the foetuses potentiates maternal responsiveness (see Yeo & Keverne, 1986; Poindron *et al.*, 1988) this occurs repeatedly and over a longer period in these species.

Characteristically, parturition is followed by a period of intense interaction between the mother and her newborns during which the first nursing may occur and the young are gathered at the nest or home region where the mother remains with them. Activity gradually subsides as the female enters the 'postpartum resting interval'. The mother usually falls asleep in the nest or at the parturition site with her newborns huddled against her, the young often attached to her nipples, suckling. Among the ungulates the mother often lies down with her young.

In the rat, virgins show an initial aversive response to both newborn and slightly older pups and may cannibalise them (Fleming & Rosenblatt, 1974a; Fleming & Luebke, 1981). This is based in part upon the pups' odours since anosmic virgins are highly responsive to pups and exhibit maternal behaviour quite readily (Fleming & Rosenblatt, 1974b, c). Non-pregnant females are more fearful than lactating females and less able to deal with anxiety-provoking conflict situations in which approach responses are pitted against avoidance responses (Mayer *et al.*, 1987). The prepartum female undergoes a change in her response to nest and pup odours (Bauer, 1983) and is attracted to them (perhaps based upon the prepartum rise in circulating levels of β-endorphin: Mayer *et al.*, 1985; Kinsley & Bridges, 1989) and the lactating female has reduced fear responses to novel stimuli, menacing conspecifics, and loud noises (Härd & Hansen, 1985; Hansen & Fereira, 1986; Fereira *et al.*, 1989).

Prepartum females are more responsive to pup distress calls than non-pregnant and early pregnant females (Koranyi *et al.*, 1976) and seek out the pups. During pregnancy and lactation they employ their increased sensitivity to thermal stimuli to avoid overheating while in contact with the pups (Wilson & Stricker, 1979; Woodside & Jans, 1988). Moreover, mothers are highly responsive to tactile stimuli around the snout region during the licking of pups: this increased snout sensitivity is based upon the action oestradiol and is instrumental in retrieving pups and in other aspects of the female's maternal behaviour (Bereiter & Barker, 1975; Stern & Kolunie, 1990; Stern & Johnson, 1990).

In the ewe the onset of maternal behaviour at parturition is based upon an attraction to amniotic fluid bathing the newborn lamb which is in contrast to the repulsion produced by this fluid even as late as 2 hours before parturition (Levy & Poindron, 1984, 1987; Lévy *et al.*, 1983).

Mother–young relationship in the postpartum period

In the rat the hormonal stimulus for maternal behaviour wanes shortly after parturition and, as the residual hormonal effects decline, pup stimulation maintains the behaviour on a non-hormonal basis (Rosenblatt *et al.*, 1979). A similar situation pertains in the ewe; and in the hamster maternal behaviour wanes if pups are removed after 24 hours but not if they are removed after 48 hours. It is important, therefore, that the mother establish a behavioural relationship with her young while her maternal behaviour is under hormonal influence so that when this declines, stimulation by the young is able to maintain her maternal responsiveness.

In nesting species of small mammals (e.g. rats) the relationship between the mother and the young is exhibited during frequent daily periods in the nest, starting during the postpartum resting interval when the exhausted mother remains in the nest and the young initiate suckling. During these contacts the mother is stimulated by the suckling of the young, by the thermal stimuli while in contact with them, and by their tactile and olfactory properties. During the first week distant contacts are initiated by the mother but, while in contact, the young may initiate suckling, and huddling with the mother (Rosenblatt & Lehrman, 1963).

Among species with precocial young that do not nest (the ungulates include both species with an early nesting period and species in which the newborn follow the mother immediately postpartum) the young follow the mother from the beginning (Lent, 1974). The relationship is based upon the exchange of olfactory and auditory stimulation between mother and young and the extensive licking of the young by the mother during parturition. The mother initiates the interactions but the young play an active role when near her (Poindron & Le Neindre, 1980).

Contact with the newborn during and immediately after parturition, when the mother is under strong hormonal stimulation and highly aroused, is most effective for the maintenance of maternal responsiveness (Bridges, 1975; Fleming, 1990). In the rat the amount of contact the female has with pups during parturition, which may last less than an hour, by itself enables her to maintain her responsiveness for at least 25 days (Bridges, 1975). Contact during parturition is not essential, however, because Caesarean-section delivered females allowed contact with pups for 2 hours starting 36 hours after delivery are able to maintain their responsiveness for at least 10 days (Bridges, 1977; Orpen & Fleming, 1987).

During contact with their pups, female rats, following Caesarean delivery, undergo a special kind of learning different from that which occurs at other times as, for example, learning the spatial characteristics of their environment (Malenfant, Fleming & Kucera, 1990). Their retention of maternal behaviour 10 days later is based upon the long-term memory of this earlier contact and can be inhibited by agents which prevent memory consolidation by blocking CNS protein synthesis (A. S. Fleming, U. S. Cheung and M. Barry, unpublished data). The learning is enhanced by hormonal stimulation and is more difficult to establish without it.

It has been proposed that the onset of maternal behaviour around parturition is stimulated by hormones but that its maintenance is based upon sensory stimuli provided by the young. Considerable evidence supporting this proposal has been reviewed elsewhere (Rosenblatt *et al.*, 1979). The transition from hormonal to non-hormonal regulation of maternal behaviour in the rat occurs soon after parturition and may begin during contact with pups at delivery. Formation of a relationship with the young is essential if the mother's responsiveness is to be maintained. Anything that promotes this relationship therefore plays a role in maternal behaviour. However, the female's maternal responsiveness is vulnerable during this period since failure to progress from the hormonal to non-hormonal regulation of maternal behaviour results in its waning. Either inadequate hormonal stimulation or interference with responses to the newborn for any reason may, therefore, result in the failure of the maintenance of maternal care of the young.

Psychobiology of maternal behaviour: primates

The study of maternal behaviour among the primates has grown enormously over the past 25 years and the large literature will not be reviewed here. I am concerned only with the psychobiology of maternal behaviour. Most research on primate maternal behaviour, including that which deals with problems of ecological adaptation and evolution, has been guided by the psychosocial approach.

Since no single primate species has been studied intensively from a psychobiological point of view as, for example, the rat, mouse and ewe have been among the non-primates, we must rely upon studies scattered over several primate species to find answers to questions that were dealt with above with respect to the non-primate mammals. Where experimental studies do not exist I shall use descriptive studies or observations to answer certain questions about maternal behaviour among the primates.

Maternal behaviour during parturition

Observations of parturition among the primates are rare and most often take place among animals held in captivity in zoos or laboratories (which is true also for non-primate mammals with the addition of farms and homes): this introduces the possibility that any abnormalities can be attributed to the conditions of captivity.

Despite evidence of cannibalism during parturition in captive tree shrews (Kaufman, 1965; Conaway & Sorenson, 1966), and of ignoring the newborn in these species (Brandt & Mitchell, 1971) and even among gorillas (Nadler, 1974) and humans, the evidence points overwhelmingly to the immediate onset of maternal behaviour towards the newborn during parturition. Although parturition is brief among the tree shrews, as it is among most prosimians, in *Tupaia belangeri* Martin (1966) described the behaviour of the female in the natal nest in terms that could be applied to many nesting non-primate mammals with altricial newborn: 'In the course of 1–2 hours the female gives birth, disposes of the embryonic membranes and umbilical cord and suckles the young until the stomachs are fully distended' (p. 1403).

Parturition has been described in greater detail in the lesser bushbaby (*Galago senegalensis moholi*) (Doyle, Pelletier & Bekker, 1967) and bears out the similarity with the non-primate mammals noted above. Parturition was initiated by the female carrying and manipulating nest material without constructing a nest and in her avoidance of other animals. This was followed by her entering the nestbox occupied by other animals and beginning to focus her activity on her genital region which she groomed intensely while adopting a head-between-the-legs position. During delivery, which lasted 30 seconds for each of the two newborns, the mother licked the infant's head as it emerged. This was followed by grooming the infants, carrying and handling them, and examining her own genitals. Following the last delivery the mother ate the afterbirths, and she gradually became less active and settled down to sleep with her infants (i.e. postpartum resting interval). The mother nursed the infants during the first hour after birth. Equally vivid are reports of lesser bushbabies in captivity ignoring their newborn or cannibalising them after birth (Doyle *et al.*, 1967).

Descriptions of parturition among the lemurs are fragmentary but sufficient to establish that the mother, among several species (*Lemur variegatus*, *L. catta*, *L. fulvus*, and *Propithecus verreauxi*), engages in nestbuilding up to the start of parturition, is immediately attentive to the infant when it emerges and grabs her own ventral hair, licks it extensively, eats the placenta and cuts the cord, and engages in maternal aggression against conspecific intruders (Petter-Rousseaux, 1964; Klopfer & Klopfer, 1970; Brandt & Mitchell, 1971). An exception to the preparatory behaviour shown above is the report by Richard (1976) which describes a female (*P. verreauxi*) that gave birth during foraging: she moved to the end of a branch and began to lick her ano-genital region, sitting with her legs stretched out in front of her, and within 40 minutes was seen with a newborn clinging to her ventrum headed for the nipples under the armpits.

Although they are less secretive and more accessible in the wild than the prosimians, the simians and apes are nevertheless elusive particularly with respect to parturitive behaviour and until recently there were few descriptions of parturition. These descriptions too are largely of captive animals, although a few are of animals in the wild.

Parturition in the patas monkey (*Erythrocebus patas*) is typical of many other species of monkey (Goswell & Gartlan, 1965). It was anticipated by the female's increasing attention to her vulval region: she touched it frequently with her finger then brought her finger to her nose. Movements of the foetus within the abdomen focused the female's attention to that region and she laid her hand on it. When the birth began, which lasted about $3\frac{1}{2}$ hours, the female exhibited many postural changes in response to abdominal contractions, and when water was expelled she reached down, pulled mucus from the vagina and ate it. When the infant's head emerged the female gripped the long hairs on the head to help in removing it from the vagina, all the while licking fluid from her hand. She stood to facilitate passage of the infant from the vagina, expelled the infant's body, and in response to its squeaking and screaming, she licked the infant's head region for several minutes.

Goswell & Gartlan (1965) describe what followed: '...the infant grabbed the mother's fur with both hands. ...The mother licked its face, then pressed it to her chest, continuing to lick it but now concentrating on the hands' (p. 194). Shortly afterward '...the mother stood up and the infant clung to her fur with its hands but was unable to support itself, the mother supporting it by putting her left arm round its neck. She sniffed at its ano-genital region' (p. 194). Two minutes after birth the infant reached for the teat with its mouth and at 4 minutes it located the teats and took one in its mouth and sucked. Following delivery of the placenta and eating it, the mother again turned her attention to the infant '...she held the infant's head against the lower part of her abdomen and supporting it under the tail with her right hand, she lifted up its leg with her left hand and licked all around the ano-genital area and the base of the tail' (p. 195).

As parturition progressed, note that the female's attention shifted from her own body to her vulval region and then to the emerging infant. The sequence was paced by the organic events of parturition and mediated by the profusion of somatic, olfactory, gustatory, visual and auditory stimuli to which she was exposed. This is similar in many respects to parturitive behaviour among lower mammals as described earlier. What differs is the use of the hands and arms to explore her own body, to assist in the birth, and to hold the infant against her body and support it while it reaches for the nipple. Pook (1975) described parturition in Goeldi's monkey (*Callimico goeldii*) in a zoo in terms similar to those found in the above description.

The single field observation of parturition in a multiparous female rhesus monkey (*Macaca mulatta*) describes how the female separated herself from the troop and 5 minutes later, grasped the arm of the infant protruding from the vulva and pulled it towards her at the same time that the rest of the infant was delivered (Teas *et al.*, 1981). The infant cried once but the mother ignored it and groomed herself as the infant clung to her abdomen; not until she had cleaned herself and eaten the placenta did she begin to clean the infant, nearly half an hour after birth. Gibber (1986) described, by contrast, the laboratory births of seven primiparous rhesus monkeys in which the mothers picked up the infants as soon as they emerged and licked them while holding them in both arms. Other mothers licked their infants as they lay on the floor and it was the infants that reached up and climbed on to the mothers ventrum as they bent over them, an action which the mothers accepted. Still others, however, did not allow ventral contact until 2 hours after parturition and one mother completely ignored her infant.

Similarly, field observation of parturition in the howler monkey (*Alouatta seniculus*) also described two precipitous births by multiparous females in which there was no prior behaviour directed at the vulva before the infant's head emerged and shortly afterward the infant emerged (Sekulic, 1982).

Bowden, Winter & Ploog (1967), on the other hand, reported observations of two prolonged live deliveries in captive squirrel monkeys (*Saimiri sciureus*). In both deliveries the females climbed perches at the start of uterine contractions. These were few during the initial stage of delivery (i.e. initiation of contractions to the first appearance of the foetus) and in both deliveries they occurred over periods of 40–60 minutes at infrequent intervals. The two females differed widely in the performance of genital inspection and licking, scratching, and rubbing the vulva but both their postural adjustments and rubbing the perineum against the perch indicated that they were focusing increasingly on the vulval region from which was discharged a large amount of mucus. Actual deliveries occurred rapidly requiring only 63 seconds in one female and 14 minutes in the other. During both parturitions, after their emergence from the birth canal the infants were supported by the mothers' arms while they grasped her fur and began to climb, reaching the nipple region and attaching within a short time with no additional help from the mother.

The parturition of a free-living Gelada baboon (*Theropithecus gelada*) observed by Dunbar & Dunbar (1974) was abrupt. In the midst of grooming another adult female on the ground '...she suddenly stood up in a half crouching position, staccato coughed (a vocalization of fear threat) and gave birth, the neonate falling onto the ground beneath her' (p. 186). The infant was immobile for about 8 minutes during which the mother picked it up and began to lick it, then sat down and intermittently licked the infant and herself but she provided little help to the infant in its eventual grasping of the nipple and suckling.

Gillman & Gilbert (1946, cited in Nash, 1974) described the prolonged birth of a captive chacma baboon (*Papio ursinus*) during which the mother pulled the baby as it emerged from the vulva. In a field observation of parturition of a Hamadryas baboon (*P. hamadryas*) reported by Abegglen & Abegglen (1976) labour was brief. The female was first observed already in a squatting position on the ground undergoing labour contractions; within 5 minutes the foetus's head became visible and 20 minutes later, after intensive contractions, the infant was born. Even so the female frequently touched her vulva and licked her hand during the contractions. Later the mother held the infant to her belly, licked it as it screamed, and continued to clean it.

Turning to the Hominoidea (gibbons, orang utan, chimpanzee, gorilla and human) Ibscher (1967) described the parturition of a captive gibbon (*Hylobates lar* L.). Labour contractions were prolonged for several hours but once the foetus's head emerged it was only 10 minutes before the entire foetus was expelled with the help of the female grasping the infant's head. Soon afterward the mother held the infant against her body, cradling it and licking it.

Two orang utan births in free-living animals (Galdikas, 1982) are notable in that both females delivered their infants in nests perched high in trees. The onset of one of the deliveries interrupted foraging and was accompanied by the female building a nest. Graham-Jones & Hill (1962) have provided complete and detailed observations on parturition in a captive zoo Bornean orang utan. The first signs of abdominal contractions were accompanied by manual investigation of the vulva, followed in 20 minutes by the emergence of the foetus's head. With manual assistance by the mother the infant was expelled completely almost immediately. The mother then alternated in her attention to her vulva and the umbilical cord, and the infant, cradling the infant in her arms and licking it while examining its hands. An hour after delivery, the infant was suckling at the mother and crying.

Parturition in captive chimpanzees (*Pan troglodytes schweinfurthii*) has been reported several times (Tinklepaugh, 1932; Nissen & Yerkes, 1943) and once in a free-living animal (Goodall & Athumani, 1980). In a summary report on 49 parturitions in captive chimpanzees the period from onset of uterine contractions to emergence of the foetus's head in the birth canal varied from 40 minutes to 8 hours, during which manual vulval exploration occurred. Birth was completed in 4 minutes in all but one female in which it required 22 minutes (Nissen & Yerkes, 1943). Primiparous females responded with fear and avoidance of their infants at parturition while multiparous females, even those with little experience with their first infants, showed an immediate strong attachment and were protective of it.

A multiparous female was observed during parturition in the single free-living chimpanzee reported (Goodall & Athumani, 1980). In contrast to the births in captive females, the birth took place in a tall tree. Abdominal contractions were first observed about 2 hours before the infant's head was visible inside the vagina. During this period the female placed her hand over the vaginal opening and then sniffed her finger; later she did this again when amniotic fluid was discharged. The infant was delivered 4 minutes later and was soon licked by the mother and carried to another tree where she made a new nest and lay down, licking the infant and feeding on the placenta. In the final stages of the delivery the female took the infant's head in her hands and tried to pull it while bearing down during uterine contractions.

Thomas (1958) described parturition in a primiparous captive lowland gorilla (*Gorilla gorilla gorilla*) in which the entire sequence from the start of contractions to delivery occurred in 20 minutes. An equally rapid delivery in a captive primiparous lowland gorilla was described by Beck (1984). The total time for delivery from the appearance of a mucous exudate from the vulva to delivery of the infant was 28 minutes. During the first 21 minutes the female continually touched the vulva then sniffed and licked her fingers: in the moments before delivery, she reached back with her right hand, ruptured the sac with her index finger and supported the infant's head in her right hand. One minute later she reached back and caught the infant as it was delivered, she held it in her hand and licked birth fluids from its body. She inserted her tongue deeply into the infant's mouth and nostrils. The female alternated between licking the umbilical cord, eating the placenta, and handling the infant, including thoroughly licking its body. Within 10 minutes of birth the female held the infant in a ventral–ventral contact position and cuddled it close to her chest. About half an hour after delivery, the mother lay down and began to sleep with the infant lying alongside her and tightly grasping her fur.

Nadler's (1974) description of parturition in a primiparous captive lowland gorilla is quite similar to that of Beck (1984). However, in the hour that followed delivery, the female initially ignored the infant, manipulating it occasionally and mainly licking her own hands. Gradually she began to lick the infant and brought it into ventral–ventral support and it became the focus of her attention until she fell asleep.

Several authors have noted that observations of human delivery comparable to those of non-human primates are rare or non-existent (Brandt & Mitchell, 1971; Trevathan, 1987). It has been argued, however, that the mode of presentation of the human infant (occiput anterior) precludes delivery by the mother alone and necessitates help by others (Trevathan, 1987). Natural delivery cannot therefore be compared directly to that of non-human primates in which delivery is exclusively by the mother alone (except for a midwife delivery observed in one squirrel monkey in which the infant was in an abnormal rotated position (occiput anterior) that prevented the mother from delivering it by herself: Kirkendall, 1979).

My interest is in the onset of maternal behaviour during parturition and immediately afterward. Unaided parturitions would provide the best opportunity to observe how the mother responds to the infant but even when parturitions are done with aid, the mother's initial responses during the delivery when the infant is given to her would provide an indication of her responsiveness to it. It is interesting, however, that those who describe the physiological aspects of parturition (Trevathan, 1987, Ch. 3) or its cultural determinants (Jordan, 1980) in humans often do not describe the mother's initial responses to the infant *during parturition*.

Perhaps closest to natural parturition is that described by Odent (1984). Odent has developed the practice of allowing mothers complete freedom to undergo delivery fully awake and without modern obstetrical assistance except for the presence of a midwife, husband, or passively attending physician. Under these conditions the mother is immediately maternal towards her infant and exhibits holding it to her breast, often allowing it to suckle quite soon after delivery, adopting the *en face* position and touching it, talking to it, and caressing it. One sees, therefore, the full range of maternal behaviour during parturition as in other primates and in non-primate mammals.

Similar observations were made in a study by Trevathan (1982) in which mothers were encouraged to complete the delivery of their own child after the head and shoulders had been delivered by reaching down between their legs and bringing the infant up to their chest. Although the author's interest was in investigating laterality in the mother's initial positioning of the infant against her body, she found, as others before her had reported, that mothers, regardless of their own handedness, preferentially held their infants on their left side; she reported that they also patted their infants, rocked them, talked to them, stroked their faces, rubbed and massaged the infants with their hands, and held them in their arms against their bodies. An important behavioural response shown by mothers is the specialised visual attentiveness to the infant labelled *en face* in which the mother aligns her face in the same vertical plane as the infant's face and looks at the open eyes of her infant for prolonged periods, about 40% of the time during the first hour after birth (Trevathan, 1983). *En face* behaviour during the first hour after parturition was most often associated with talking to the infant. When permitted, nursing was initiated by the mother within the first half hour after parturition (Trevathan, 1987).

Although less attention has been paid to maternal responses to infant odours than to visual, auditory, and somatosensory stimuli, these are present and mothers initiate the process of recognising their infants by odour received during close contact and kissing in the first hours after birth (Schaal *et al.*, 1980; Porter, Cernock & McLaughlin, 1983).

Jordan (1980) described a midwife delivery in Mexico; although the mother plays a rather passive role apart from her efforts to expel the foetus, she is made to focus her attention on the foetus by the midwife. 'Birth talk' by the midwife keeps the mother informed about the foetus and the progress of the delivery. Immediately postpartum the mother is allowed brief visual contact with the infant which is placed on her abdomen or held up in front of her then the infant is swaddled tightly and is laid in her arms. For the next 7 days mother and infant remain alone, the mother does only limited household chores, and spends most of her time with the infant.

Absent from human maternal responses during parturition are manual investigation of the vulva, assisting breaking of the amniotic sac, licking and eating the placenta, and severing the umbilical cord. Although they use different means to become focused on the forthcoming birth and the newly born infant than other non-primate mothers, nevertheless the appearance of the infant triggers a fairly reliable range of maternal responses in human mothers.

Maternal responsiveness during pregnancy and prepartum

The most systematic study of maternal responsiveness during pregnancy and the prepartum, which was done in the rhesus monkey, revealed no regular increase in responsiveness (i.e. picking up and remaining in contact with a 1- to 15-day-old infant) in primiparous females (Gibber, 1986). The pregnant females did, on occasion, score highly in these tests. This never occurred in nulliparous females (Holman & Goy, 1980; Gibber & Goy, 1985). Cross & Harlow (1963) presented similar results using a preference viewing situation and multiparous pregnant females. These findings contrast with those of Tinklepaugh & Hartman (1930) who reported that a rhesus female 3 days from parturition licked amniotic fluid from a neighbouring female in labour, and ate some of the afterbirth that was within her reach; 36 days earlier this female showed no interest in newborn. Rosenblum (1972) tested female squirrel monkeys for retrieval, contact, or simply approaching and exploring a $2\frac{1}{2}$–$3\frac{1}{2}$ week infant. Pregnant females within the last 2 weeks of pregnancy (i.e. 22–24 weeks pregnant) were more responsive in all three measures than were females between 4 and 21 weeks of pregnancy and these were no more responsive than non-pregnant females.

Many non-human primate species exhibit non-specific changes in behaviour during pregnancy that undoubtedly reflect their hormonal condition. A patas monkey alternated between cringing fearfulness/ nervousness and strong aggression 2 weeks before delivery and had to be separated from cagemates (Goswell & Gartlan, 1965). During pregnancy in the squirrel monkey sleep, activity, drinking and eating patterns changed; restlessness during the night time appeared 4 weeks before parturition accompanied by short periods of separation from the social group (Bowden *et al.*, 1967). There are scattered reports that females withdraw from other animals shortly before parturition and give birth in relative solitude. However, females of several species are reported to give birth in the midst of a group of juveniles and adults, several assisting in the delivery or examining the female and infant very closely (Kirdendall, 1979).

Among the prosimians in which there are two basic patterns of maternal care, either depositing young in the nest or carrying young which cling to the mother, prepartum preparation differs accordingly. Doyle *et al.* (1967) described the lesser bushbaby's increasing aggressiveness toward male attempts to mate as parturition nears, their increased nest-building at various sites, and the prepartum onset of maternal behaviour shown by the attention paid to young of other females including attempts to pick them up. Similar maternal behaviour prepartum was reported by Lowther (1940) for this same species with more details concerning nest-building. Among the lemurs nests are built by the smaller species (*L. microcebus, L. variegatus*) and young cling to the mother in the larger ones (*L. catta, L. fulvus, Propithecus verreauxi*). In species that build nests, nest material may be gathered from the vicinity or, as in *L. variegatus*, hair may be pulled from the flank on the day before parturition and used to line the nest. Nest-building before parturition is prevalent among the shrews (*T. belangeri, T. montana, T. tana*) and the nest is built by the male in *T. glis*. Other behavioural changes have been described during later pregnancy including decreased activity and antisocial aggressiveness which declines at parturition.

Fleming & Corter (1988), in their excellent review of human maternal responsiveness, found no clear evidence of the expression of maternal behaviour during pregnancy when the opportunity presented itself or when pregnant women were exposed to infants, but the mother's relationship to the foetus changes. Feldman & Nash (1978) found that pregnant primiparae were no more responsive to a baby than non-pregnant women. Bleichfeld & Moely (1984) used the ingenious technique of recording heart rate responses to an infant's pain cry in non-pregnant, pregnant, and recently postparturient women. Although all responded to the cry and not to a control auditory stimulus, the pregnant women responded more like the non-pregnant women than the postparturient mothers.

During pregnancy, on the other hand, women become increasingly aware of the infant they are carrying and begin to develop a relationship with it especially when it begins to move in the womb (Fleming & Corter, 1988). In Jordan's (1980) description of the actions of the midwife in a Mexican village during a prenatal visit we see the role of the midwife in making the mother aware of the child she is carrying. As Jordan described it, 'They discuss how the woman has been feeling and talk about the expected date of birth. Then as Dona Juana probes a little deeper to determine the baby's position, she explains to the woman where she feels the head and reassures her that everything looks good for the birth' (pp. 20–21). It is the midwife who examines the vaginal area rather than the mother who explores it as in non-human primates; nevertheless the mother's attention is focused on this region.

Brandt & Mitchell (1971) describe the prenatal precautions concerning the welfare of the foetus practiced among the Flathead Indians of Montana.

These arrangements prepare the mother for care of the infant. Similar precautions about the welfare of the foetus were impressed upon African women in Uganda before the European influence and served to establish a caring relationship between the mother and the foetus.

Fleming & Corter (1988) used a questionnaire to determine the degree of attachment to the foetus during gestation and reported a rise from the 14th to the 20th–24th week, which could be attributed to the 'quickening', when the mother first feels foetal movement, and again after the 40th week when the mother gives birth.

Hormonal basis of maternal behaviour

Although circulating levels of ovarian/placental steroids, chorionic gonado-trophin and prolactin have been measured in many species of non-human primates (for a sample see Rosenblatt & Siegel, 1981) few attempts have been made to relate these findings to the onset of maternal behaviour in these species. In one recent study in the red-bellied tamarin (*Saguinis labiatus*: Pryce *et al.*, 1988) good mothers (i.e. labelled good because their young survived for at least a week after parturition) had significantly higher urinary levels of oestradiol at 4–5 weeks prepartum and maintained higher levels during the last week prepartum than poor mothers (labelled poor because their young died during the first week) who had lower levels of oestradiol earlier and in whom levels declined significantly during the last week. During a 2-hour observation shortly after parturition good mothers exhibited significantly higher levels of carrying, licking and cleaning, and nursing the newborns whereas poor mothers exhibited significantly higher levels of pushing or rubbing the infant off and consequently the infants spent more time off the mother. These infants died during the first day.

An unusual correlation was found between *male parental behaviour* in the common marmoset (*Callithrix jacchus*) and circulating levels of prolactin (Dixson & George, 1982). What was particularly interesting was that only the presence of females with infants aged 10–30 days and not the presence of pregnant females alone was effective in increasing male plasma prolactin levels and then only when the male had been carrying an infant immediately prior to blood sampling. In this species in which females have twins, the male carries the young after the first week while the female only nurses them.

The same pattern of hormonal changes at the end of pregnancy and the onset of maternal behaviour occurs among most non-human primates as among non-primate mammals. Oestradiol levels increase or remain high while progesterone levels decline and prolactin levels also increase (Hodgen *et al.*, 1972; Reyes *et al.*, 1975; Weiss *et al.*, 1976; Winterer *et al.*, 1985; Diamond *et al.*, 1987). We have every reason to believe that these hormones are involved in the onset of maternal behaviour in the non-human primates as they are in the lower mammals.

The endocrine regulation of pregnancy shifts from the maternal pituitary and ovaries to the foetal placenta in non-human primates as it does in humans (Heap & Flint, 1986). Smith's (1954) finding that hypophysecto-mising rhesus monkeys between the first and fifth month (shortly before parturition) does not prevent completion of pregnancy is, therefore, not surprising. What is interesting, however, is that those hypophysectomised females who gave birth normally also exhibited maternal behaviour and '...zealously guarded their babies against having them removed' (p. 658).

Endocrine secretions during pregnancy in women have been reported extensively and several reviews have focused specifically on the hormonal control of parturition (Fuchs & Fuchs, 1984; Itskovitz & Hodgen, 1988). Fleming & Corter (1988) have reported plasma levels of oestradiol, progesterone, testosterone, cortisol, β-endorphin, and prolactin in primi-parae throughout most of pregnancy and the first 6 weeks postpartum and have attempted to correlate these with measures of maternal responsiveness in the same woman. They found no correlation between the varying levels of the different hormones during pregnancy and changes in the mothers' feelings towards their foetuses; the hormone levels did not correlate with positive or negative feelings towards the foetuses. In their own words,

Although both mothers' attachment to their fetuses/babies and concentrations of the different hormones showed overall increases across pregnancy, no direct significant relationship could be found between changes in the different hormones and changes in mothers' attachment to the fetus. Moreover, there were no obvious differences in the hormonal profile between the few women who, during the first trimester, expressed negative feelings toward the fetus and those who did not' (p. 197)

It should be noted that the difficulty of correlating hormone levels and behaviour in individual women also exists in the area of sexuality: chronic low sexual desire among women was not found to correlate during the menstrual cycle with altered levels of testosterone, oestradiol, progesterone, prolactin, luteinising hormone, or sex hormone-binding globulin (Schreiner-Engel *et al.*, 1989).

In the immediate *postpartum period*, when concentrations of various hormones declined gradually, Fleming & Corter (1988) were able to correlate levels of cortisol with maternal behaviour in new mothers whose behaviour towards their babies was observed directly. High cortisol levels taken on day 3 postpartum correlated positively with the mother's level of maternal approach responses and these were accompanied by positive maternal attitudes both at the time of the observations and earlier in pregnancy. The authors propose that the high level of cortisol on day 3 might indicate a high level of arousal, the particular behavioural expression of which would be positive if the mother's attitude towards the baby had been positive and remained so, but negative if the mother's attitude were negative.

Other factors in relation to maternal behaviour

A number of additional factors have been studied in relation to maternal behaviour among the primates that bear on issues raised in the study of maternal behaviour among the non-primate mammals. In non-primate mammals (rat, ewe, goat) Caesarean-section deliveries are followed by the display of maternal behaviour immediately upon awakening from the anaesthetic used during surgery or within 24 h (Rosenblatt & Siegel, 1981; J. S. Rosenblatt, unpublished data). While this does not indicate that contact between mother and young during parturition is unimportant for establishing maternal behaviour, it does suggest that as long as hormonal influences are still strong, as they are immediately following Caesarian section the mother will respond to her young.

In monkeys (*Macaca mulatta* and *M. fascicularis*), by contrast, females usually refuse to accept their own infants after Caesarean section. As cited by Lundblad & Hodgen (1980) only 7 of 211 females accepted their infants after Caesarean section. Either the mother's maternal responsiveness is deficient following Caesarean section delivery or Caesarean-section delivered infants are less able to attract the mother. Lundblad & Hodgen (1980) proposed that vaginal secretions of near-term parturient mothers on the infant's fur are crucial for the mother's attraction for her newborn. This was confirmed when the application of these secretions to newborn delivered by Caesarean section resulted in all five infants being nursed by their mothers. Among 11 others without these secretions only one was accepted and nursed by the mother.

A study by Meier (1965) raises the issue of whether the onset of maternal behaviour in laboratory-reared female rhesus monkeys is particularly vulnerable to Caesarean-section delivery resulting in the failure of mothers to respond to their young. He found that they ignored their approaches, and avoided them when they were presented to them on three occasions starting soon after delivery. Feral-reared monkeys also showed some effects of the Caesarean-section delivery: more than half did not accept the infant during the first test but they did accept them on the second test one day later. All of these feral-reared mothers showed normal aggressive responses towards the experimenter when he presented or removed the infants. Laboratory rearing may impose social isolation on the mothers which interferes with the development of their maternal responses. A similar effect of social isolation on gorilla maternal responsiveness was reported by Rock (1978) based upon studies by Nadler.

These findings do point to parturition as a narrow window during which the mother establishes her initial maternal responses towards her newborn but they also indicate that as long as the hormonal stimulation persists, which may be for several days postpartum, even Caesarean-section mothers can compensate for the loss of the opportunity during parturition.

I am not aware of any reports of difficulties encountered in the acceptance of their infants by women who have been delivered by Caesarean section. It is not clear, however, that this has been investigated with techniques subtle enough to reveal any difficulties should they exist. Also, the procedure following normal births of withholding the infant from the mother for several hours in many instances may reduce any differences in the behaviour of Caesarian-section mothers who may be forced by the effects of the surgery to delay their initial contact with their infants.

In the rat retention of maternal responsiveness has been studied in two contexts, short-term and long-term: the first is in the postpartum female whose young have been removed at birth and the second is in the female who has given birth and reared her young through weaning or some shorter period. In the former, females are tested to determine how long the effects of hormones last which stimulate the onset of maternal behaviour and this has been found to be about 7 days (Orpen & Fleming, 1987). In the latter case, females may be tested after any interval provided they exhibit oestrous cycles (and, therefore, are not pregnant) or are ovariectomised to remove the possible effects of the steroid hormones which originally stimulated their maternal behaviour. Long-term retention requires that the mother have postpartum experience with her young; even a brief experience will suffice for retention over 10 days to 4 weeks, becoming fixed in long-term memory for use during subsequent exposure to new young (Bridges, 1975, 1977; Orpen & Fleming, 1987). Retention of maternal responsiveness in this context has been reported over several months and may be for life.

Among non-human primates Holman & Goy (1980) reported that in a group of 19 multiparous rhesus females either cycling, menopausal, or ovariectomised, 90 % of the females immediately adopted infants younger than 2 weeks old, retrieved and held them, and refused to give them up at the end of testing. These females did as well as the multiparous females studied by Deets & Harlow (1974) who were separated from their own infants within hours of parturition for periods of 1–12 days, all of whom immediately and completely adopted foster infants under 10 days of age. The behaviour of these experienced females contrasted with that of nulliparous females, who showed only minimal interest in the infants and did not adopt them. Among the multiparous females a milky fluid could be expressed from their nipples after one week of exposure to the infants even though they had not received sucking stimulation by the infants. Hansen (1966) observed two multiparous rhesus females, 9 months after separation from their last infant, which in one case immediately adopted an infant and in the other a $2\frac{1}{2}$-month-old monkey.

Cross & Harlow (1963) also found that multiparous rhesus mothers 2–4 months after their previous delivery, when they had been without their infants for that period, were, nevertheless, highly responsive to 10–40-day infants viewed in a visual exploration apparatus but were unresponsive to a 1-year-old monkey. They viewed the infants for longer durations and more frequently than either nulliparous non-pregnant females, pregnant females or even postparturient females 3 weeks after delivery. Gibber (1981) found that multiparous rhesus females were more responsive to the infants than either nulliparous females or males and in addition they usually picked up the infant immediately and held it ventrally, whereas nulliparous females and males usually only positioned themselves to permit the infant to initiate ventral–ventral contact. In Sackett's (1970) test of maternal responsiveness in which animals expressed their preference for a 30-day-old infant over older animals by the amount of time they spent in front of it, multiparous females, not rearing infants, ranked higher than primiparous mothers and nulliparous females.

Among women, Bleichfeld & Moely (1984) found that recently delivered multiparous mothers showed a greater cardiac acceleration in one phase of the response to an infant's pain cry than primiparous mothers. Also Boukydis & Burgess (1982) found that multiparous parents were less responsive (i.e. exhibited lower levels of cardiac activity) to normal levels of hunger crying and were more responsive to extremes of crying than primiparous parents and in this respect were similar to non-parents. Sagi (1981) also found that experienced mothers, compared with infant caretakers that had not themselves been mothers, were better able to identify the different types of infant cries, including hunger, pain and pleasure cries.

Discussion

In non-primate mammals the onset of maternal behaviour at parturition is based upon hormonal secretions which, in turn, are associated with the termination of pregnancy and the process of delivery itself (i.e. vaginal–cervical stimulation). The hormones of pregnancy and parturition produce motivational/emotional changes, perceptual changes and changes in response patterns. The mother's behaviour is selectively directed at the newborn, she is less fearful than earlier and able to resolve conflicts between her fear and her attachment to her young by remaining with the young and fending off intruders. Her responses to the newborns require her to overcome an aversion to their odours from amniotic fluid. She is especially sensitive to auditory, tactile, and visual stimuli from the newborn.

Among the primates similar behavioural changes probably occur at parturition, rather abruptly, as we have seen, although in individuals of several species that have been studied responses to newborn appear to be weak, absent, or even negative. In general prosimian mothers are immediately attentive to their newborns, even responding to their appearance at the vulval opening by beginning to focus their attention on them and assisting in their expulsion with their hands, followed by licking, grooming, handling, and assisting them to grasp the mother's fur, and in climbing her body to reach the nipples and suckle. These observations certainly point to the likelihood that the behavioural changes at parturition are hormonally induced. The parallels are even greater in nesting species among both the non-primate mammals and the prosimians. Those prosimians which carry their newborn, largely through the infant's ability to cling to the mother's fur, are somewhat like the ungulates in which following the mother is mainly the responsibility of the newborn although the mother may induce the young to follow at times.

It is among the nesting species of prosimians that we find evidence of prepartum maternal behaviour: in several prosimian species the mother begins to build a nest several days before parturition and this continues sporadically until delivery begins. At this time she may already be responsive to young. In the monkeys and great apes, mainly observed in captive animals, birth is characterised by the abruptness of the onset of delivery and the speed with which the actual expulsion of the newborn occurs. This is confirmed in the few observations of free-ranging animals. The period of abdominal/uterine contractions may be extended but the actual expulsion of the newborn often takes only a few minutes or even seconds. Earlier we presented Travathan's (1987) proposal that parturition in non-human primates is facilitated by the mode of presentation of the foetus. In the single reported case of a squirrel monkey receiving help during parturition, the foetus was delivered in an abnormal position (Kirkendall, 1979).

Prepartum behavioural changes in these species consist of increasing irritability, immobility, and, as delivery approaches, some degree of social isolation from the troop, but not complete separation as is often seen in the non-primate mammals (see summary table in Brandt & Mitchell, 1971). Even on the day of birth the female travels with the troop and engages in foraging. The female receives little advance notice that delivery is imminent though once abdominal contractions begin there may be a prolonged period before the infant emerges.

In these troop-living primates, females, for their safety and sense of security, must remain in contact with the foraging troop members while at the same time they often seek some degree of social isolation in order to give birth undisturbed by group members. Jolly (1972) has considered the conflicting demands made upon the parturitive female by this situation. It may be that one adaptation to this situation is the abrupt nature of delivery and the few specifically maternal behaviour items which primate females exhibit prepartum. Chism, Olson & Rowell (1983) have also noted the influence of possible predation on parturition in the free-living patas monkey females and have accounted for the predominance of daytime births at specific times by the need to remain in contact with their social group and avoid predation. The duration of parturition and lack of prepartum preparation might also be influenced by these factors. Among herd-living moose and elk Altman (1963) has noted that the same problem exists but parturitive females provide mutual protection from predators by remaining behind the migrating herd as a group to give birth, which is a consequence of synchronised mating during the previous fall. Among nesting species of primates where there is no requirement to keep up with the foraging social group prepartum maternal behaviour is more common.

Despite the abruptness of the beginning and later phases of parturition, the female's attention is gradually focused on the emerging infant and she is introduced to the odours and tastes of the fluids adhering to the infant, the umbilical cord and the placenta. Almost universal among these primate species is manual investigation of the vulval region, and licking of the hand brought to the mouth. The hand is often used to rupture the membranes surrounding the infant and both hands are used to pull the infant from the birth canal, while the female licks its protruding head. In the short period between emergence of the infant's head and its complete expulsion, the female exhibits the beginnings of maternal care but often the infant emerges and must cling to the mother before she begins to support it and lick it. Too often, as described in several births of chimpanzees, primiparous mothers are unable to respond to the infant with anything but fear and they abandon the infant, while in other instances the infant may lie on the floor where it was born for a prolonged period (i.e. up to 2 hours) before the mother attends to it.

As we have noted, little note has been taken of the importance of single births, as the rule, among most non-human primates for the onset of maternal behaviour. Since the birth is completed fairly rapidly and there has been little or no preparation for it, the female has little time to become habituated to the newborn during parturition. Even when maternal behaviour is not successfully initiated by primiparous females after parturition, females who give birth are more successful in their second pregnancies indicating that the repetition has some value in promoting the onset of maternal behaviour. In species with single births the immediate postpartum period is of crucial importance since it provides the mother with the opportunity to establish her maternal behaviour.

Among the smaller mammals with altricial young, as we have noted, birth is a repeated event lasting up to an hour with the cumulative effect of the foetuses emerging at intervals, and placentas expelled between births, almost ensuring that the female will have initiated maternal care repeatedly during parturition. In species with precocial young, repeated births may also occur but although single or twin births are frequent in most ungulates the pace of delivery and the isolation of the mother from the social group, as well as her tendency to remain with the young at the parturition site, ensure that maternal care will begin. Among sheep the mother spends a long time immediately postpartum licking her newborn systematically from front to back (McGlone & Stobart, 1986); during this period in both the ewe and goat the mother responds to the odour on the kid and this forms the basis for her individually specific maternal behaviour towards her young (Klopfer & Klopfer, 1968; Alexander *et al.*, 1986). Whether among non-human primates the initial licking of the infant by the mother serves a similar function has not yet been studied.

It is in this context that the important studies of Klaus & Kennell (1976) on the beneficial effects of allowing mothers extensive physical contact with their infants immediately postpartum should be viewed. This extends the period during which mothers can initiate their maternal behaviour and further strengthens their maternal responsiveness. There is general agreement that this increasingly widespread practice has immediate positive effects on the mother–infant relationship which may last as long as one month (Fleming & Corter, 1988). By then mothers who have not had this additional postpartum contact with their infants have compensated for it in their daily homecare of their infants. What has been disputed about their findings is the extent and significance of long-term effects of this postpartum contact (Trevathan, 1987; Fleming & Corter, 1988).

There is little evidence, therefore, that hormones increase maternal responsiveness among non-human primates during pregnancy. *Whatever effects hormones have emerge as specific behavioural changes during parturition itself and in the immediate postpartum period.* Exceptions are, of course, in stationary nest-building species in which maternal responsiveness does appear before parturition and nestbuilding is also initiated early.

Maternal behaviour among women also seems to have an abrupt onset at parturition. Parturition itself is drawn out over many hours if its beginning is timed from the start of regular and vigorous uterine contractions. The process of focusing on the infant begins long before parturition is imminent in several cultures. Whether this indicates that hormones are acting during pregnancy to stimulate maternal responsiveness is difficult to determine because their emotional/cognitive abilities enable women to become attached to their foetuses on a fantasy level and this is strongly supported by social conventions and specific practices. In practice, women are often not given the opportunity to respond to their infants during parturition and even immediately after delivery. When permitted to do so they exhibit a stereotyped pattern of tactile exploration and visual fixation as well as cuddling and vocalisations which express their feelings towards the infant and their efforts to attract its attention to them (Trevathan, 1981, 1982, 1983; Odent, 1984).

The few studies of Caesarean-section delivery among non-human primates indicate that their maternal behaviour, even in multiparous females, is highly vulnerable to deprivation of the opportunity to initiate maternal behaviour at parturition. The usual parturitional hormonal changes probably occur either in advance of Caesarean section or as a consequence of it. However, the opportunity for the Caesarean-section mother to compensate for the loss of parturitional contact by promoting postpartum contact with the young by applying vaginal fluid to the coat of the newborn and introducing it to the mother when she awakens from the surgery indicates that maternal responsiveness persists at least for a short period following the surgery (Lundblad & Hodgen, 1980)

Studies are needed of non-human primates and women who have aborted their pregnancies before term to determine whether there is a rise in maternal responsiveness that can be correlated with the hormonal changes accompanying the pregnancy termination.

The maintenance of maternal behaviour postpartum in the presence of the young among primates is self-evident but this does not necessarily show that it is non-hormonally based as we believe is the case in several lower mammals. That responsiveness requires continual stimulation from the young is a first step in testing this possibility.

The study of adoptive mothers of newborn infants would provide another test of this hypothesis by measuring changes in their maternal responsiveness over the first few months. If it included measurements of any possible hormonal changes this would add to the test of this hypothesis. The work of David & Appell (1961) indicates that although adoptive mothers show appropriate maternal behaviour almost from the start, they experience a lack of strong motivation. Several weeks later they report a change and become strongly motivated in their responses to their infants.

Among the many problems faced by women giving birth prematurely, until recently, has been the required separation from the newborn and its effect upon their maternal responsiveness. The increasingly prevalent practice of allowing mothers of premature infants into the nursery in this country and in Europe, or of treating them at home, testifies to the recognition that the mother is in danger of reduced maternal responsiveness if she is kept separated from her newborn, especially since she often has not been allowed even to hold the infant at delivery (Klaus & Kennell, 1976).

Acknowledgements

The research reported in this paper was done under NIMH grant MH-08604 to JSR. I am indebted to many students who contributed to this research and in particular to my Research Associate Anne D. Mayer who for the past 17 years has played the major role in this research. This is publication number 501 from the Institute of Animal Behavior. My appreciation to Winona Cunningham for typing this paper.

References

Abegglen, H. & Abegglen, J. J. (1976). Field observation of a birth in hamadryas baboons. *Folia Primatologica*, **26**, 54–6.

Alexander, G., Poindron, P., Le Neindre, P., Stevens, D., Lévy, F. & Bradley, L. (1986). Importance of the first hour post-partum for exclusive maternal bonding in sheep. *Applied Animal Behaviour Science*, **16**, 295–300.

Altman, M. (1963). Naturalistic studies of moose and elk. In *Maternal Behavior in Mammals*, ed. H. L. Rheingold, pp. 233–53. New York: John Wiley.

Bauer, J. H. (1983). Effects of maternal state on the responsiveness to nest odors of hooded rats. *Physiology and Behaviour*, **30**, 229–32.

Beck, B. B. (1984). The birth of a lowland gorilla in captivity. *Primates*, **25**, 378–83.

Bereiter, D. A. & Barker, D. J. (1975). Facial receptive fields of trigeminal neurons: increased size following estrogen treatment in female rats. *Neuroendocrinology*, **18**, 115–24.

Bleichfeld, B. & Moely, B. E. (1984). Psychophysiological responses to an infant cry: comparison of groups of women in different phases of the maternal cycle. *Developmental Psychology*, **20**, 1082–91.

Bogomolova, E. M. & Kurochkin, Ju. A. (1984). Moose cow delivery: behavior of the cow and the newborn calf. *Zoologicheskii Zhurnal*, **63**, 1713–24.

Boukydis, C. F. Z. & Burgess, R. L. (1982). Adults physiological response to infant cries: effects of temperament of infant, parental status, and gender. *Child Development*, **53**, 1291–8.

Bowden, D., Winter, P. & Ploog, D. (1967). Pregnancy and delivery behavior in the squirrel monkey (*Saimiri sciureus*) and other primates. *Folia Primatologica*, **5**, 1–42.

Brandt, E. M. & Mitchell, G. (1971). Parturition in primates: behavior related to birth. In *Primate Behavior: Developments in Field and Laboratory Research*, ed. L. A. Rosenblum, pp. 177–223. New York: Academic Press.

Bridges, R. S. (1975). Long-term effects of pregnancy and parturition upon maternal responsiveness in the rat. *Physiology and Behaviour*, **14**, 245–9.

Bridges, R. S. (1977). Parturition: its role in the long term retention of maternal behavior in the rat. *Physiology and Behaviour*, **18**, 487–90.

Bridges, R. S. (1984). A quantitative analysis of the roles of dosage, sequence, and duration of estradiol and progesterone exposure in the regulation of maternal behavior in the rat. *Endocrinology*, **114**, 930–40.

Bridges, R. S., Loundes, D. D., DiBase, R. & Tate-Ostroff, B. A. (1985). Prolactin and pituitary involvement in maternal behavior in the rat. In *Clinical Correlates*, ed. R. M. MacLeod, M. O. Thorner and U. Scapagnini. *Fidia Research Series*, *Vol. 1*, pp. 591–9. Padua: Liviana.

Capitanio, J. P., Weissberg, M. & Reite, M. (1985). Biology of maternal behavior: recent findings and implications. In *The Psychobiology of Attachment and Separation*, ed. M. Reite and T. Field, pp. 41–91. New York: Academic Press.

Chism, J., Olson, D. K. & Rowell, R. E. (1983). Diurnal births and perinatal behavior among wild patas monkeys: evidence of an adaptive pattern. *International Journal of Primatology*, **4**, 167–84.

Conaway, C. H. & Sorenson, M. W. (1966). Reproduction in tree shrews. *Symposia of the Zoological Society of London*, **15**, 471–92.

Cross, H. A. & Harlow, H. F. (1963). Observations of infant monkeys by female monkeys. *Perceptual and Motor Skills*, **16**, 11–15.

David, M. & Appell, G. (1961). A study of nursing care and nurse–infant interaction. In *Determinants of Infant Behavior*, ed. B. M. Foss, London: Methuen.

Deets, A. C. & Harlow, H. F. (1974). Adoption of single and multiple infants by rhesus monkey mothers. *Primates*, **15**, 192–203.

Diamond, E. J., Aksel, S., Hazelton, J. M., Wiebe, R. H. & Abee, C. R. (1987). Serum oestradiol, progesterone, chorionic gonadotrophin and prolactin concentrations during pregnancy in the Bolivian squirrel monkey (*Saimiri sciureus*). *Journal of Reproduction and Fertility*, **80**, 373–81.

Dixson, A. F. & George, L. (1982). Prolactin and parental behavior in a male New World primate. *Nature*, **299**, 551–3.

Doyle, G. A., Pelletier, A. & Bekker, T. (1967). Courtship, mating and parturition in the lesser bushbaby (*Galago senegalensis moholi*) under semi-natural conditions. *Folia Primatologica*, **7**, 169–97.

Dunbar, R. I. M. & Dunbar, P. (1974). Behaviour related to birth in wild gelada baboons (*Theropithecus gelada*). *Behaviour*, **50**, 185–91.

Fahrbach, S. E., Morrell, J. I. & Pfaff, D. W. (1984). Oxytocin induction of short-latency maternal behavior in nulliparous, estrogen-primed female rats. *Hormones and Behaviour*, **18**, 267–86.

Feldman, S. S. & Nash, S. C. (1978). Interest in babies during young adulthood. *Child Development*, **49**, 617–22.

Ferreira, A., Hansen, S., Nielsen, M., Archer, T. & Minor, B. G. (1989). Behavior of mother rats in conflict tests sensitive to antianxiety agents. *Behavioral Neuroscience*, **103**, 193–201.

Fleming, A. S. (1990). Factors influencing post-partum retention of maternal behavior. *Conference on Reproductive Behavior*, *Abstract*, p. 42.

Fleming, A. S. & Corter, C. (1988). Factors influencing maternal responsiveness in humans: usefulness of an animal model. *Psychoneuroendocrinology*, **13**, 189–212.

Fleming, A. S. & Luebke, C. (1981). Timidity prevents the virgin female rat from being a good mother: emotionality differences between nulliparous and parturient females. *Physiology and Behavior*, **27**, 863–8.

Fleming, A. S. & Rosenblatt, J. S. (1974a). Maternal behavior in the virgin and lactating rat. *Journal of Comparative and Physiological Psychology*, **86**, 957–72.

Fleming, A. S. & Rosenblatt, J. S. (1974b). Olfactory regulation of maternal behavior in rats: I. Effects of olfactory bulb removal in experienced and inexperienced lactating and cycling females. *Journal of Comparative and Physiological Psychology*, **86**, 221–32.

Fleming, A. S. & Rosenblatt, J. S. (1974c). Olfactory regulation of maternal behavior in rats: II. Effects of peripherally induced anosmia and lesions of the lateral olfactory tract in pup-induced virgins. *Journal of Comparative and Physiological Psychology*, **86**, 233–46.

Fuchs, A.-R. & Fuchs, F. (1984). Endocrinology of human parturition: review. *British Journal of Obstetrics and Gynaecology*, **91**, 948–67.

Galdikas, B. M. F. (1982). Wild orangutan birth at Tanjuing Puting Reserve. *Primates*, **23**, 500–10.

Gibber, J. F. (1981). Infant directed behaviour in male and female rhesus monkeys. Unpublished doctoral dissertation, University of Wisconsin-Madison.

Gibber, J. R. (1986). Infant-directed behaviour of rhesus monkeys during their first pregnancy and parturition. *Folia Primatologica*, **46**, 118–24.

Gibber, J. R. & Goy, R. W. (1985). Infant-directed behavior in young rhesus monkey: sex differences and effects of prenatal androgens. *American Journal of Primatology*, **8**, 225–37.

Gillman, J. & Gilbert, C. (1946). The reproductive cycle of the Chacma baboon (*Papio ursinus*) with special reference to the problem of menstrual irregularities as assessed by the behavior of sex skin. *South African Journal of Medical Science, Biology Supplement*, **11**, 1–54.

Giordano, A. L., Siegel, H. I. & Rosenblatt, J. S. (1989). Nuclear estrogen receptor binding in the preoptic area and hypothalamus of pregnancy-terminated rats: correlation with the onset of maternal behavior. *Neuroendocrinology*, **50**, 248–58.

Goodall, J. & Athumani, J. (1980). An observed birth in a free-living chimpanzee (*Pan troglodytes schweinfurthii*) in Gombe National Park, Tanzania. *Primates*, **21**, 545–49.

Goswell, M. J. & Gartlan, J. S. (1965). Pregnancy, birth, and early infant behaviour in the captive patas monkey, *Erythrocebus patas*. *Folia Primatologica*, **3**, 189–200.

Graham-Jones, O. & Hill, W. C. O. (1962). Pregnancy and parturition in a Bornean orangutan. *Proceedings of the Zoological Society of London*, **139**, 503–10.

Hansen, E. W. (1966). The development of maternal and infant behavior in the rhesus monkey. *Behaviour*, **27**, 107–49.

Hansen, S. & Ferreira, A. (1986). Food intake, aggression, and fear behavior in the mother rat: control by neural systems concerned with milk ejection and maternal behavior. *Behavioral Neuroscience*, **100**, 64–70.

Härd, E. & Hansen, S. (1985). Reduced fearfulness in the lactating rat. *Physiology and Behaviour*, **35**, 641–3.

Hauser, H. & Gandelman, R. (1985). Lever pressing for pups: evidence for hormonal influence upon maternal behavior of mice. *Hormones and Behavior*, **19**, 454–68.

Heap, R. B. & Flint, A. P. F. (1986). Pregnancy. In *Hormonal Control of Reproduction*, 2nd edition, ed. C. R. Austin and R. V. Short, pp. 153–93. Cambridge: Cambridge University Press.

Hinde, R. A. (1965). The integration of internal and external factors in integration of canary reproduction. In *Sex and Behavior*, ed. F. A. Beach, pp. 381–415. New York: John Wiley.

Hinde, R. A. (1987). *Individual Relationships and Culture*. Cambridge: Cambridge University Press.

Hinde, R. A. & Stevenson-Hinde, J. (1976). Towards understanding relationships: dynamic stability. In *Growing Points in Ethology*, ed. P. P. G. Bateson and R. A. Hinde. Cambridge: Cambridge University Press.

Hodgen, G. D., Dufau, M. L., Catt, K. J. & Tullner, W. W. (1972). Estrogens, progesterone and chorionic gonadotrophin in pregnant rhesus monkeys. *Endocrinology*, **91**, 896–900.

Holman, S. D. & Goy, R. W. (1980). Behavioral and mammary responses of adult female rhesus to strange infants. *Hormones and Behavior*, **14**, 348–57.

Ibscher, Von L. (1967). Geburt und Fruhe Entwicklung Zweier Gibbons (*Hylobates lar* L.). *Folia Primatologica*, **5**, 43–69.

Itskovitz, J. & Hodgen, G. D. (1988). Endocrine basis for the initiation, maintenance, and termination of pregnancy in humans. *Psychoneuroendocrinology*, **13**, 155–70.

Jolly, A. (1972). Hour of birth in primates and man. *Folia Primatologica*, **18**, 108–21.

Jordan, B. (1980). *Birth in Four Cultures*. Montreal: Eden Press Women's Publications.

Kaufman, I. C. (1970). Biologic considerations of parenthood. In *Parenthood: Its Psychology and Psychopathology*, ed. E. J. Anthony and T. Benedek, pp. 3–56. Boston, Mass: Little Brown & Co.

Kaufman, J. H. (1965). Studies of the behavior of captive tree shrews. *Folia Primatologica*, **3**, 50–74.

Kendrick, K. M., Keverne, E. B. & Baldwin, B. A. (1987). Intracerebroventricular oxytocin stimulates maternal behaviour in sheep. *Neuroendocrinology*, **46**, 56–61.

Keverne, E. B. (1988). Central mechanisms underlying the neural and neuroendocrine determinants of maternal behaviour. *Psychoneuroendocrinology*, **13**, 127–41.

Kinsley, C. H. & Bridges, R. S. (1989). Morphine treatment and reproductive condition alter olfactory preferences for pup and adult male odors in female rats. *Developmental Psychobiology*, **23**, 331–47.

Kirkendall, M. (1979). Midwife behavior in captive Bolivian squirrel monkeys. *Primate News*, **17**, 6–8.

Klaus, M. H. & Kennell, J. H. (1976). *Maternal–Infant Bonding*. St Louis, Mo.: Mosby Company.

Klopfer, P. H. & Klopfer, M. S. (1968). Maternal imprinting in goats: fostering of alien young. *Zeitschrift für Tierpsychologie*, **25**, 862–6.

Klopfer, P. H. & Klopfer, M. S. (1970). Patterns of maternal care in Lemurs: I. Normative description. *Zeitschrift für Tierpsychologie*, **27**, 984–96.

Koranyi, L., Lissak, K., Tamasy, V. & Kamaras, L. (1976). Behavioral and electrophysiological attempts to elucidate central nervous system mechanisms responsible for maternal behavior. *Archives of Sexual Behavior*, **5**, 503–10.

Krehbiel, D., Poindron, P., Lévy, F. & Prud'Homme, M. J. (1987). Peridural anesthesia disturbs maternal behavior in primiparous and multiparous parturient ewes. *Physiology and Behavior*, **40**, 463–72.

Kristal & Noonan (1978). Perinatal maternal and neonatal behaviour in the captive reticulated giraffe. *South African Journal of Zoology*, **14**, 103–7.

Lehrman, D. S. (1965). Interaction between internal and external environments in the regulation of the reproductive cycle of the ring dove. In *Sex and Behavior*, ed. F. A. Beach, pp. 355–80. New York: John Wiley.

Lent, P. C. (1974). Mother–infant relationships in ungulates. In *The Behaviour of Ungulates and Its Relation to Management*, Vol. 1, ed. V. Geist and F. Walther, pp. 14–55. IUCN Publications New Series No. 24.

Lévy, F. & Poindron, P. (1984). Influence du liquide amniotique sur la manifestation du comportement maternel chez la brébis parturiente. *Biology of Behavior*, **9**, 65–88.

Lévy, F. & Poindron, P. (1987). Importance of amniotic fluids for the establishment of maternal behaviour in relation with maternal experience in sheep. *Animal Behaviour*, **35**, 1188–92.

Lévy, F., Poindron, P. & Le Neindre, P. (1983). Attraction and repulsion by amniotic fluids and their olfactory control in the ewe around parturition. *Physiology and Behavior*, **31**, 687–92.

Lisk, R. D. (1971). Oestrogen and progesterone synergism and elicitation of maternal nestbuilding in the mouse (*Mus musculus*). *Animal Behaviour*, **19**, 606–10.

Lowther, F. De (1940). A study of the activities of a pair of *Galago senegalensis moholi* in captivity, including the birth and postnatal development of twins. *Zoologica*, **25**, 433–59.

Lundblad, E. G. & Hodgen, G. D. (1980). Induction of maternal–infant bonding in rhesus and cynomologous monkeys after caesarean delivery. *Laboratory Animal Science*, **30**, 913.

Malenfant, S. A., Fleming, A. S. & Kucera, C. (1990). Maternal and sexual experience effects are not blocked by MK-801, an *N*-methyl-D-aspartate antagonist. *Conference on Reproductive Behaviour, Abstract*, p. 90.

Martin, R. D. (1966). Tree shrews: unique reproductive mechanism of systematic importance. *Science*, **152**, 1402–4.

Mayer, A. D., Faris, P. L., Komisaruk, B. R. & Rosenblatt, J. S. (1985). Opiate antagonism reduces placentophagia and pup cleaning by parturient rats. *Pharmacology, Biochemistry and Behavior*, **22**, 1035–44.

Mayer, A. D., Reisbick, S., Siegel, H. I. & Rosenblatt, J. S. (1987). Maternal aggression in rats: changes over pregnancy and lactation in a Sprague–Dawley strain. *Aggressive Behavior*, **13**, 29–43.

Mayer, A. D. & Rosenblatt, J. S. (1987). Hormonal factors influence the onset of maternal aggression in laboratory rats. *Hormones and Behavior*, **21**, 253–67.

McCarthy, M. M., Bare, J. E. & vom Saal, F. S. (1986). Infanticide and parental behavior in wild female house mice: effects of ovariectomy, adrenalectomy and administration of oxytocin and prostaglandin F2 alpha. *Physiology and Behavior*, **36**, 17–23.

McGlone, J. J. & Stobart, R. H. (1986). A quantitative ethogram of behavior of yearling ewes during two hours post-parturition. *Animal Behaviour Science*, **16**, 157–64.

Meier, G. W. (1965). Maternal behavior of feral and laboratory-reared monkeys following the surgical delivery of their infants. *Nature*, **206**, 492–3.

Nadler, R. D. (1974). Periparturitional behavior of a primiparous lowland gorilla. *Primates*, **15**, 55–73.

Nash, L. T. (1974). Parturition in a feral baboon (*Papio anubis*). *Primates*, **15**, 279–85.

Nissen, H. W. & Yerkes, R. M. (1943). Reproduction in the chimpanzee: report on forty-nine births. *Anatomical Record*, **86**, 567–78.

Odent, M. (1984). *Birth Reborn*. New York: Pantheon.

Orpen, B. G. & Fleming, A. S. (1987). Experience with pups sustains maternal responding in postpartum rats. *Physiology and Behavior*, **40**, 47–54.

Pedersen, C. A., Ascher, J. A., Monroe, Y. L. & Prange, A. J., Jr (1982). Oxytocin induces maternal behavior in virgin female rats. *Science*, **216**, 648–50.

Pedersen, C. A. & Prange, A. J., Jr (1979). Induction of maternal behavior in virgin rats after intracerebroventricular administration of oxytocin. *Proceedings of the National Academy of Sciences (USA)*, **76**, 6661–5.

Petter-Rousseaux, A. (1964). Reproductive physiology and behavior of the Lemuroidea. In *Evolutionary and Genetic Biology of the Primates, Vol. 2*, ed. J. Buettner-Janush, pp 91–132. New York: Academic Press.

Poindron, P. & Le Neindre, P. (1980). Endocrine and sensory regulation of maternal behavior in the ewe. In *Advances in the Study of Behavior, Vol. 11*, ed. J. S. Rosenblatt, R. A. Hinde, C. G. Beer and M.-C. Busnel, pp. 75–119. New York: Academic Press.

Poindron, P., Lévy, F. & Krehbiel, D. (1988). Genital, olfactory, and endocrine interactions in the development of maternal behavior in the parturient ewe. *Psychoneuroendocrinology*, **13**, 99–125.

Pook, A. G. (1975). Breeding Goeldi's monkey. *Jersey Wildlife Preservation Trust. 12th Annual Report*, pp. 17–20.

Porter, R. H., Cernock, J. M. & McLaughlin, F. J. (1983). Maternal recognition of neonates through olfactory cues. *Physiology and Behavior*, **30**, 151–4.

Pryce, C. R., Abbott, D. H., Hodges, J. K. & Martin, R. D. (1988). Maternal behavior is related to prepartum urinary estradiol levels in red-bellied tamarin monkeys. *Physiology and Behavior*, **44**, 717–26.

Reyes, F. I., Winter, J. S. D., Faiman, C. & Hobson, W. C. (1975). Serial serum levels of gonadotrophins, prolactin, and sex steroids in the nonpregnant and pregnant chimpanzee. *Endocrinology*, **96**, 1447–55.

Richard, A. F. (1976). Preliminary observations on the birth and development of *Propithecus verreauxi* to the age of six months. *Primates*, **17**, 357–66.

Rock, M. A. (1978). Gorilla mothers need some help from their friends. *Smithsonian*, **9**, 58–62.

Rosenblatt, J. S. & Lehrman, D. S. (1963). Maternal behavior of the laboratory rat. In *Maternal Behavior in Mammals*, ed. H. L. Rheingold, pp. 8–57. New York: John Wiley.

Rosenblatt, J. S., Mayer, A. D. & Giordano, A. L. (1988). Hormonal basis during pregnancy for the onset of maternal behavior in the rat. *Psychoneuroendocrinology*, **13**, 29–46.

Rosenblatt, J. S. & Siegel, H. I. (1975). Hysterectomy-induced maternal behaviour during pregnancy in the rat. *Journal of Comparative and Physiological Psychology*, **89**, 685–700.

Rosenblatt, J. S. & Siegel, H. I. (1981). Factors governing the onset and maintenance of maternal behavior among nonprimate mammals: the role of hormonal and nonhormonal factors. In *Parental Care in Mammals*, ed. D. J. Gubernick and P. H. Klopfer, pp. 13–76. New York: Plenum Press.

Rosenblatt, J. S., Siegel, H. I. & Mayer, A. D. (1979). Progress in the study of maternal behavior in the rat: hormonal, nonhormonal, sensory, and developmental aspects. In *Advances in the Study of Behavior, Vol. 10*, ed. J. S. Rosenblatt, R. A. Hinde, C. G. Beer and M.-C. Busnel, pp. 225–311. New York: Academic Press.

Rosenblum, L. A. (1972). Sex and age differences in response to infant squirrel monkeys. *Brain, Behavior and Evolution*, **5**, 30–40.

Sackett, G. P. (1970). Unlearned responses, differential rearing experiences and development of social attachments by rhesus monkeys. In *Primate Behavior: Developments in Field and Laboratory Research*, ed. L. A. Rosenblum. New York: Academic Press.

Sagi, A. (1981). Mothers' and non-mothers' identification of infant cries. *Infant Behavior and Development*, **4**, 37–40.

Schaal, B., Montagner, H., Hertling, E., Bolzoni, D., Moyse, A. & Quichon, R. (1980). Les stimulations olfactives dans les relations entre l'enfant et la mère. *Reproduction, Nutrition, Développement*, **20**, 843–58.

Schneirla, T. C., Rosenblatt, J. S. & Tobach, E. (1963). Maternal behavior in the cat. In *Maternal Behavior in Mammals*, ed. H. Rheingold. New York: John Wiley.

Schreiner-Engel, P., Schiavi, R. C., White, D. & Ghizzani, A. (1989). Low sexual desire in women: the role of reproductive hormones. *Hormones and Behavior*, **23**, 221–34.

Sekulic, R. (1982). Birth in free-ranging howler monkeys *Alouatta seniculus. Primates*, **23**, 580–2.

Smith, P. E. (1954). Continuation of pregnancy in rhesus monkeys (*Macaca mulatta*) following hypophysectomy. *Endocrinology*, **55**, 655–64.

Stern, J. M. & Johnson, S. K. (1990). Perioral somatosensory determinants of nursing behavior in Norway rats. *Journal of Comparative Psychology* (in press).

Stern, J. M. & Kolunie, J. M. (1990). Perioral anesthesia disrupts maternal behavior during early lactation in Long-Evans rats. *Journal of Comparative Psychology* (in press).

Svare, B., Miele, J. & Kinsley, C. (1986). Progesterone stimulates aggression in pregnancy-terminated females. *Hormones and Behavior*, **20**, 194–200.

Teas, J., Taylor, H. G., Richie, T. L., Shrestha, R. D., Turner, G. K. & Southwick, C. H. (1981). Parturition in rhesus monkeys (*Macaca mulatta*). *Primates*, **22**, 580–6.

Thomas, W. D. (1958). Observations on the breeding in captivity of a pair of lowland gorillas. *Zoologica*, **43**, 95–104.

Tinklepaugh, O. L. (1932). Parturition and puerperal sepsis in a chimpanzee. *Anatomical Record*, **53**, 193–205.

Tinklepaugh, O. L. & Hartman, C. G. (1930). Behavioral aspects of parturition in the monkey (*Macacus rhesus*). *Comparative Psychology*, **11**, 63–98.

Trevathan, W. R. (1981). Maternal touch at first contact with the newborn infant. *Developmental Psychobiology*, **14**, 549–58.

Trevathan, W. R. (1982). Maternal lateral preference at first contact with her newborn infant. *Birth*, **9**, 85–90.

Trevathan, W. R. (1983). Maternal *en face* orientation during the first hour after birth. *American Journal of Orthopsychiatry*, **53**, 92–9.

Trevathan, W. R. (1987). *Human Birth: An Evolutionary Perspective.* New York: Aldine De Gruyter.

Weiss, G., Butler, W. R., Hotchkiss, J., Dierschke, D. J. & Knobil, E. (1976). Periparturitional serum concentrations of prolactin, the gonadotrophins, and the gonadal hormones in the rhesus monkey. *Proceedings of the Society for Experimental Biology and Medicine*, **151**, 113–6.

Wilson, N. E. & Stricker, E. M. (1979). Thermal homeostasis in pregnant rats during heat stress. *Journal of Comparative and Physiological Psychology*, **93**, 585–94.

Winterer, J., Palmer, A. E., Cicmanec, J., Davis, E., Harbaugh, S. & Loriaus, D. L. (1985). Endocrine profile of pregnancy in the patas monkey (*Erythrocebus patas*). *Endocrinology*, **116**, 1090–3.

Woodside, B. & Jans, J. E. (1988). Neuroendocrine basis of thermally regulated maternal responses to young in the rat. *Psychoneuroendocrinology*, **13**, 79–98.

Yeo, J. A. G. & Keverne, E. B. (1986). The importance of vaginal–cervical stimulation for maternal behaviour in the rat. *Physiology and Behavior*, **37**, 23–6.

Note added in proof

An excellent review covering many of the issues presented in this article was recently published (Coe, 1990). Data are presented describing changes during pregnancy in chimpanzees which include social interactions, feeding, and activity.

Coe, C. L. (1990). Psychobiology of maternal behavior in nonhuman primates. In *Mammalian Parenting: Biochemical, Neurobiological, and Behavioral Determinants*, ed. N. A. Krasnegor and R. S. Bridges, pp. 157–83. New York: Oxford University Press.

Commentary

—2—

When John Fentress was at Madingley, his PhD work was with the vole, one of the smallest British mammals, and in his spare time he hand-reared a wolf. He has continued to work with small mammals and wolves ever since. His initial finding – that the response of voles to a fear-provoking stimulus depended on what they had been doing previously – has formed the basis for nearly all he has done since. His highly original chapter points to a new era in the study of brain–behaviour relations, and I found it extraordinarily stimulating. It would not surprise him to know that, as I read what he wrote about items of behaviour and behaviour systems, I was applying the principles he described to the manner in which 4-year-olds behave differently according to the social context, to the well-known poor cross-situational consistency of personality traits, and to the view of the family as a system.

Fentress's thesis insists that we move backwards and forwards between behavioural and physiological levels of analysis. A similar theme occurs in all other chapters in this section, but perhaps especially in the work of Gabriel Horn – a friend and colleague over many years. The unique, highly original and crucially important project on imprinting in which he (with Pat Bateson) has been involved for more than twenty years started with behavioural data; involved localisation of a particular brain region; returned to behavioural data to eliminate alternative interpretations; proceeded from brain regions to cells, synapses, and parts of synapses and thence to a biochemical level; and returned to a behavioural level because of effects described at the neural level. It is because Horn has moved backwards and forwards between levels in this way that his work has been so much more fertile than most work with simpler systems, and provides a splendid lead that further studies on brain–behaviour relations must follow. For a similar reason, with the

223

phenomenon of habituation (to which Horn, e.g. 1970, has also made major contributions), I believe that studies of relatively simple systems can throw only limited light on habituation in higher vertebrates: it may or may not be that habituation in some invertebrates can be accurately described as the simple waning of a response, but in birds and mammals it is inseparable from associative learning, and involves interacting incremental and decremental effects. Unfortunately this isn't always recognised, and generalisations about habituation as a simple dropping out of responses persist.

As I mentioned earlier, when W. H. Thorpe started the Madingley laboratory, he set it up as an Ornithological Field Station because he believed that birds, with their stereotyped motor patterns and marked learning abilities, provided the ideal material for studying the relations between learning and instinct. John Hutchison has shown that they also provide very favourable opportunities for studying endocrine–behaviour relations – again in part because of their easily identifiable and quantifiable behaviour patterns, but also because they are primarily visual animals and the difficulties of working with olfaction are avoided. A friend and colleague for around twenty-five years now, John Hutchison first came to Madingley to do a PhD when he already had one to his credit. (In this respect he resembled Peter Marler.) His work also moved from behavioural and hormonal to intracellular enzyme levels, the latter studies maintaining a behavioural end point. Identifying two components of ring dove courtship, he showed that they were related to different hormones and then investigated the mechanisms by which the effectiveness of the hormones is regulated. His finding that the behavioural effectiveness of hormones on male courtship is affected by external stimuli (day length, courtship) is of special interest to me. It resembles a similar finding by Elizabeth Steel (another valued colleague) and myself with the nest-building behaviour of female canaries (Hinde & Steel, 1978), but the mechanism discovered by Hutchison for the ring dove must be different from that (as yet uninvestigated) in canaries. Like that of Gabriel Horn, John Hutchison's work shows how identifying a particular problem, and then sticking with it persistently, with first one technique and then another, can yield golden results.

Richard Andrew, one of the first graduate students at Madingley, demonstrates the crucial importance of detailed behavioural data in work on the effects of hormones on the brain. For instance, before Andrew, most runway tests merely measured time from release to goal. The highly original findings which have come from his painstaking work, and that of his colleagues, depend on much more than that – on detailed attention to how and where the chick hesitates, and where it looks as it traverses the runway. Without such close observation the differences between the oestrogenic effects of testosterone (on attention) and its androgenic effects (on vigour) would not have been discovered. (There are interesting parallels here with John Hutchison's demonstration that one type of the courtship of male doves is under oestrogenic control, the other under androgenic.) Another general issue emerging from Richard Andrew's work is the crucial importance of studying hormonal effects on males and females separately. This was previously neglected in much work with chicks, which are not easy to sex anyway. But it is a lesson that comes up repeatedly in many of the chapters in this volume, whether they are concerned with birds, monkeys or humans.

Jay Rosenblatt, a friend of longer standing than perhaps any other, has discussed a line of research that he and another friend – the late Danny Lehrman – initiated in the 1950s (Lehrman, 1965). The course of reproductive development, previously ascribed to a series of presumed endogenous hormonal changes, can be understood only when the importance of the subtle interplay between the animal and its environment is taken fully into account. (Conceptually, the issue is closely related to the general problem of development discussed by Bateson.) Here the interplay is complicated by the fact that the animal actively changes its environment, and comes to perceive its environment differently because of (partially) environment-induced changes in its own endocrine state. Danny Lehrman took up this issue with the reproductive behaviour of the ring dove; I, attempting rather unsuccessfully to investigate the role of goal-direction in canary nest-building, got drawn into a similar problem; and Jay Rosenblatt has persistently tackled a similar issue centring on the initiation of maternal behaviour. I think all three of us were encouraged and helped by the kindly interest and friendship of Frank Beach and W. C. Young, and we were working in a fortunate era when we could study closely similar problems without competing for funds or recognition, and meet frequently on one side of the Atlantic or the other to discuss progress. Danny died too young, but his work has been continued at the Institute of Animal Behaviour in New Jersey by Mei Cheng and others under Jay Rosenblatt's general direction. In Chapter 8 Jay Rosenblatt demonstrates the value of a comparative approach for the study of maternal behaviour, the chapter making use of data from one species to suggest lines of research in others, while at the same time never neglecting species differences.

References

Hinde, R. A. & Steel, E. A. (1978). The influence of daylength and male vocalizations on the estrogen-dependent behavior of female canaries and budgerigars, with discussion of data from other species. *Advances in the Study of Behavior*, **8**, 39–73.

Horn, G. (1970). Changes in neuronal activity and their relationship to behaviour. In *Short-term Changes in Neural Activity and Behaviour*, ed. G. Horn and R. A. Hinde, pp. 567–606. Cambridge: Cambridge University Press.

Lehrman, D. (1965). Interaction between internal and external environments in the regulation of the reproductive cycle of the ring dove. In *Sex & Behavior*, ed. F. A. Beach. New York: John Wiley.

R.A.H.

IV
Social organisation

—9—

The evolution of sex differences and the consequences of polygyny in mammals

T. H. Clutton-Brock

Introduction

It was a cold November day in 1968. Cambridge rain pattered on Robert Hinde's window. Outside, the Soay sheep huddled in the shelter of the Sub-Department of Animal Behaviour at Madingley. I was just off to Tanzania for two years, to investigate the social organisation and ecology of redtail monkeys. Over the past three months, Robert had emphasised the need to integrate studies of primate ecology with the far more advanced work then available on birds (Kear, 1962; Newton, 1967). He had shown me the importance of collecting precise, quantitative information in the field as well as the laboratory; and he had stressed the need to understand the behavioural mechanisms underlying differences in behaviour, rather than merely describing their pattern. His parting advice was characteristic: 'Don't be afraid to concentrate on some particular aspect of behaviour', he emphasised, 'the way they eat a particular food may be the key to understanding their feeding behaviour – and their social organisation as well. That may be worth any number of glib generalisations.' Three years later I remembered his advice when I eventually realised that the striking differences in social organisation between black and white colobus and the red colobus monkeys that I eventually worked on were largely attributable to the former's ability to eat mature leaves (Clutton-Brock, 1974).

All three themes that Robert stressed to his students – the need to integrate research on different groups of animals; the importance of collecting precise standardised data so that it was possible to measure how often individuals did *not* do things as well as how frequently they did; and the need to understand the dynamics of behaviour, especially social behaviour, in order to appreciate why animals did things – recur through his early work on the

229

function and evolution of behaviour (Hinde, 1955, 1956, 1958, 1975a) as well as that of his students (see Hinde, 1983). It is easy to forget that, in the 1960s, all three points were novel, if not revolutionary. Little attempt was then being made to integrate research on mammals with studies of birds, fish and invertebrates. Field studies seldom collected systematic, quantitative data – guided by Robert, I believe that I was one of the first primate fieldworkers to use check sheets in the field. And we are still, today, learning the dangers of ignoring the mechanisms responsible for differences in behaviour and, in particular, the importance of understanding the dynamics of relationships in order to appreciate the functional significance of social behaviour (Kummer, 1978; Dunbar, 1983; Goldizen, 1987; Brown, 1987; T. H. Clutton-Brock, 1991).

Though Robert himself was only indirectly involved in field studies during the 1960s and 1970s, he exerted an influence both on the development of quantitative techniques for fieldwork and on the questions being asked that extended far beyond his own students and research associates. As well as supervising many of the most important primate field studies himself (Goodall, 1968; Seyfarth, 1976, 1977; Harcourt, 1979a, b; Wrangham, 1979; Lee, 1981; Fossey, 1983), he had an important influence on research on many other mammals, including elephants (Douglas Hamilton, 1972; Poole, 1982), deer (Clutton-Brock, Guinness & Albon, 1982) and carnivores (van Lawick & van Lawick-Goodall, 1970; Moehlmann, 1983). Largely as a result of his guidance, field studies of primates rapidly surpassed research on most other animal groups in the precision of the questions asked and the sophistication of the quantitative techniques being used (see Hinde, 1983; Smuts *et al.*, 1987).

The rest of this chapter examines our current understanding of a topic tangential to Robert's main interests – the evolution of sex differences. Yet here, too, his emphasis on integrating studies of different animals, on firm quantification and on understanding the behavioural mechanisms underlying differences in behaviour are important.

In contrast to birds, where over 95 % of species are typically monogamous, the males of more than 90 % of mammalian species are habitually polygynous while females may either be monogamous or polyandrous (Kleiman, 1977; Rutberg, 1983). Types of polygyny found among mammals include species where males wander widely in search of oestrous females (Geist, 1971; Mackinnon, 1974; Ramsay & Stirling, 1986), species where males occupy independent ranges or territories overlapping the ranges of several females with whom they mate in the breeding season (e.g. Kawata, 1985), species where males defend mating access to temporary or permanent groups of females (Armitage & Downhower, 1974; Hrdy, 1977; Clutton-Brock *et al.*, 1982; Franklin, 1983), species where breeding groups include several reproductively active males (Sinclair, 1977; Packer, 1979a, b) and a small number of species where males defend very small territories in clusters on traditional mating grounds or leks (Leuthold, 1966; Bradbury, 1981; Gosling, 1986a). Female mating systems include promiscuity, serial monogamy, life-long monogamy and serial and life-long polyandry.

The form of male and female mating systems affects the selection pressures operating on the two sexes and thus on their morphological, physiological and behavioural characteristics. These, in turn, have important consequences for sex differences in energetics, demography and population structure. In this chapter, I briefly describe some of the consequences of polygyny for the form and intensity of selection pressures operating on males and females and their relationship to sex differences in morphology, physiology, behaviour and ecology.

Polygyny and the distribution of reproductive success in males and females

Where males breed monogamously and the frequency of extra-pair copulations is low, the reproductive rate of males is likely to be constrained by that of their partners, with the result that variation in breeding success is usually approximately similar in both sexes (Trivers, 1972; Payne, 1979; Clutton-Brock, 1988). No studies of monogamous mammals other than humans have yet measured variation in lifetime breeding success in both sexes but studies of long-lived monogamous birds confirm that variation in breeding success is similar in the two sexes (Clutton-Brock, 1988).

In contrast, where males breed polygynously, variation in breeding success is usually larger in males than females, both within breeding seasons (Trivers, 1972) and across the lifespan (Clutton-Brock, 1983), and the relative variance in breeding success in males and females increases as the sex ratio of breeding females to breeding males becomes progressively imbalanced (Figure 1). Though it is clear that sex differences in the variability of lifetime breeding success are usually greater in polygynous mating systems than in monogamous ones, we know little about the magnitude of these differences across different types of polygynous mating systems (Clutton-Brock, 1988). Moreover, it is unsafe to assume that species which show the greatest variation in male mating success within particular breeding seasons necessarily show the greatest variation in lifetime mating success (see below).

Mating systems also affect the relative importance of different components of breeding success. Variation in lifetime breeding success is composed of variation in four main components: survival to breeding age; longevity after reaching breeding age, average annual fecundity (females) or mating rate

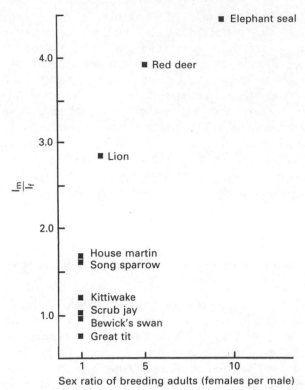

Figure 1. Ratios of the standardised variance in lifetime reproductive success in males and females reaching breeding age in different vertebrates, plotted on the sex ratio of breeding adults in each population (from Clutton-Brock *et al.*, 1988).

(males), and offspring survival (Clutton-Brock, 1988). In several species, it is now clear that environmentally acquired parental characteristics can influence the breeding success of grandoffspring and even great-grand-offspring (Huck, Labov & Lisk, 1987; Albon & Clutton-Brock, 1988). Where males are monogamous, the relative importance of the four main components of breeding success in contributing to individual differences in lifetime breeding success is usually similar in males and females (Clutton-Brock, 1988). In contrast, where males breed polygynously, the relative contributions of the different components of breeding success usually differ between the sexes. For example, among red deer reaching breeding age, over half the variance in lifetime breeding success among females is caused by differences in juvenile survival and individual differences in fecundity are relatively small while, among males, individual differences in mating rate are

Table 1. *Percentage contributions of those components of reproductive performance (Reproductive Lifespan (RLS), Average Annual Fecundity (FEC), Mating Success (MS), and Percentage Survival of Offspring (OS) and their covariances (values off the diagonal) to Variation in Lifetime Reproductive Success (LRS) (= the number of offspring reared to sexual maturity), in samples of 33 female and 31 male red deer that reached breeding age on the Isle of Rhum (Clutton-Brock* et al., *1988)*

	Hinds		
Component	RLS	FEC	OS
Reproductive lifespan (RLS)	26·5		
Fecundity (FEC)	−3·1	7·7	
Offspring survival (OS)	9·9	1·8	57·4
Three way contribution −0·2			
	Stags		
Component	RLS	FEC	OS
Reproductive lifespan (RLS)	6·8	6	
Mating success (MS)	25·82	31·73	
Offspring survival (OS)	−0·90	6·76	19·56

responsible for much of the variation in lifetime breeding success (see Table 1).

The intense competition between males often associated with polygyny affects the age distribution of mating success. In many polygynous species, males are excluded from breeding until they reach full adult size and their reproductive lifespans are relatively short. For example, longitudinal studies of elephant seals show that effective reproduction in males is commonly limited to 3–4 years between the ages of 9 and 13 while the breeding lifespans of females may be three times as long (LeBoeuf & Reiter, 1988: see Figure 2). Interspecific comparisons suggest that the extent to which the effective breeding lifespans of males are compressed increases with the degree of polygyny (Dunbar, 1988). However, the compression of male reproductive lifespans is also affected by other aspects of the breeding system. For example, in primates living in multi-male troops, males commonly assist each other in competition for females and a male's status and breeding success may be strongly influenced by the rank of the males with which he has developed a reciprocal cooperative relationship (Witt, Schmidt & Schmidt, 1981; de Waal, 1982; Strum, 1982; Smuts, 1985). In these species, male breeding success appears to be less affected by increasing age than in harem-forming mammals, like red deer or elephant seals, where a male's mating success depends directly on his fighting ability. Indeed, in some polygynous

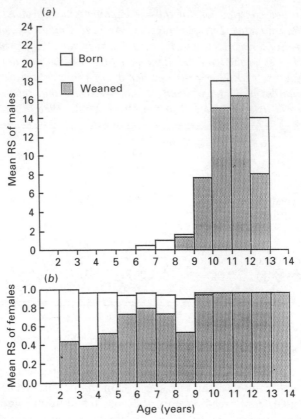

Figure 2. Mean reproductive success of (*a*) male and (*b*) female elephant seals at different ages. □, pups born; ▩, pups weaned (from Le Boeuf *et al.*, 1988).

human societies the breeding success of males apparently increases into old age as a result of the accumulation of wealth and wives (Borgerhoff Mulder, 1988).

It is important to appreciate that variation in breeding or mating success does not measure the intensity of selection or sexual selection in either sex (Clutton-Brock, 1983; Endler, 1986; Grafen, 1988) for a substantial proportion of variation in reproductive success may arise by chance (Sutherland, 1985) or by environmental factors unrelated to phenotype (Clutton-Brock, 1983). It does, however, set an upper limit to the intensity of selection (Arnold, 1986) though this may seldom be reached. In addition, it can be useful in suggesting where selection pressures may be particularly strong (Clutton-Brock, 1988).

One result of the compression of breeding lifespans in males of polygynous species is that a substantial proportion of the variation in breeding success among breeding males at a single point in time is usually caused by differences in age. Consequently, estimates of variation in male breeding success calculated across males of unknown age usually overestimate variation in lifetime success, in some cases by as much as an order of magnitude (Clutton-Brock, 1983, 1988). If the effects of age on reproductive success are ignored, estimates of the effects of age-related characters, such as body size, on reproductive success may also be exaggerated (Clutton-Brock, 1983).

Polygyny and selection pressures on males and females

Where individual males can monopolise breeding access to several females, there is commonly intense direct competition between males for access to females or to resources which attract them (Trivers, 1972). Though females do compete for access to males in some mammals (Wasser, 1983) the potential benefits of success are likely to be smaller than in males and success in mating competition will usually be weaker in females than males. In contrast, in monogamous species, selection pressures on traits favouring competitive success are likely to be more similar in males and females, though they will not necessarily be identical, especially where one sex plays a greater part in defence of territory or progeny (see Scott, 1988).

While we can guess at the selection pressures operating on males and females in mammals, there are few direct measures of selection on particular traits in either sex and our understanding of the comparative pressures operating on the two sexes is largely based on circumstantial evidence. Several field studies of mammals have begun to investigate the factors affecting reproductive success or survival in one or both sexes and some have established correlations between components of reproductive success and variation in morphology or behaviour (e.g. Boonstra & Krebs, 1979; Clutton-Brock *et al.*, 1982, 1988; LeBoeuf & Reiter, 1988; Packer *et al.*, 1988; Cheney *et al.*, 1988; Altmann, Hausfater & Altmann, 1988). However, there have so far been few attempts to convert these figures into direct measurement of selection differentials or gradients (Lande & Arnold, 1983; Gibson, 1987) and no study of a wild mammal has yet compared selection gradients for the same trait between the two sexes.

Polygyny and secondary sexual characters

Presumably as a result of the greater intensity of selection on traits used in competition for mates, the degree of sexual dimorphism increases across mammalian species, with the extent of polygyny among males. For example,

Energetic consequences of polygyny and sexual dimorphism

The pronounced sexual dimorphism found in many polygynous mammals has important energetic consequences. In species where juvenile males are born heavier than females and grow faster during the first months of life (see above), they typically require more food than females and frequently suck longer or more frequently from their mothers (Clutton-Brock, Albon & Guinness, 1981; Trillmich, 1986; Lee & Moss, 1986). Studies of fur seals using radioactive labelling techniques to measure milk uptake confirm that male pups take more milk than females (D. Costa, personal communication). These sex differences in the energy costs of raising male and female offspring have often been interpreted as evidence of active parental discrimination between the sexes. However, except in humans, there is little evidence of active parental discrimination between sons and daughters. In several sexually dimorphic species, males attempt to suck more frequently than females and it is this difference rather than any difference in the behaviour of their mothers that is responsible for their higher suckling rates (Lee & Moss, 1986; T. H. Clutton-Brock, 1991). Similarly, in rhesus macaques, the higher costs of daughters to subordinate mothers are apparently caused by their more frequent attempts to gain access to the mother's nipple arising from the higher rates of aggression that juvenile females receive from other group members (Gomendio, 1989).

The reproductive activities of adult males in polygynous species also have important consequences. In many seasonal breeders, males lose weight rapidly during the breeding season, with the result that they enter the succeeding winter in poor condition. For example, red deer stags lose up to 20% of body weight during the October rut and enter the winter with considerably lower fat reserves than hinds (Mitchell, McCowan & Nicholson, 1976). In aseasonal species, too, males commonly lose condition during periods of active breeding and alternate between breeding and periods of recuperation (Jarman, 1979; Cords, 1986). For example, mature African buffalo bulls in some populations alternate every few weeks between membership of female herds, where they feed less than cows and lose body condition steadily, and foraging alone or in small groups where they regain condition (Prins, 1987; Prins & Iason, 1989). In aseasonal species where males feed little when they are reproductively active, the periodicity of breeding activity is even shorter. In Uganda kob, for example, males defend territories on the lek for around 3 days at a time, subsequently joining all-male herds which graze in other parts of the range before returning to the lek for another period of reproductive activity, usually on the same territory (Buechner & Schloeth, 1962; Leuthold, 1966).

The larger size of mature males can also have an important impact on their choice of foods and feeding sites. In several arboreal primates, males spend less time feeding on the terminal twigs of trees and more time on the ground and, in some species, eat a higher proportion of fruit and a lower proportion of flowers and leaf shoots (Clutton-Brock, 1977). In grazing ungulates, males are often partly or totally segregated from females during the non-breeding season and are commonly found feeding in habitats where food is more abundant but of lower nutritional quality than in areas used heavily by females (e.g. Staines, Crisp & Parish, 1982). This is probably because their energetic requirements increase as around Body Weight$^{0.75}$ whereas the intake of food per bite and intake and, consequently, the rate of food acquisition per unit time increase at a lower function of body weight, possibly as Body Weight$^{0.33}$, the scaling factor for the breadth of the incisor arcade (Clutton-Brock & Harvey, 1983; Illius & Gordon, 1987). Where the standing crop of herbage is very low, males may be unable to satisfy their daily energy requirements in areas where females can still feed economically and may consequently move to feed on less preferred swards where biomass is higher but forage quality is lower (Clutton-Brock & Harvey, 1983; Illius & Gordon, 1987). This suggests that where males and females use the same swards and patches cannot be economically defended by either sex, females may reduce sward height below the level which males can tolerate, gradually excluding them from mutually preferred habitat. On the Isle of Rhum, a two-fold increase in female numbers was associated with a reduction in the use by males of areas of short grassland strongly preferred by females, while females made increased use of areas previously preferred by males (Clutton-Brock, Iason & Guinness, 1987).

Polygyny and differential mortality

In polygynous species, the reproductive activities of males combined with their secondary sexual characters often cause increased mortality when resources are short. In some ungulates, for example, the poor body condition of adult males at the beginning of the winter is associated with a higher risk of winter starvation, especially where high population density is associated with harsh weather (Klein, 1968; Clutton-Brock et al., 1982) and a similar association between food shortage and differential mortality is found in other groups of mammals (Widdowson, 1976) though it is not universal. In addition, breeding males are often more likely than females to be killed by predators, either when they are defending mating territories or when they are regaining condition away from female groups (Schaller, 1972; Prins & Iason, 1988). Especially during periods of rapid population decline, sex differences in mortality can be large in sexually dimorphic species. For example, when

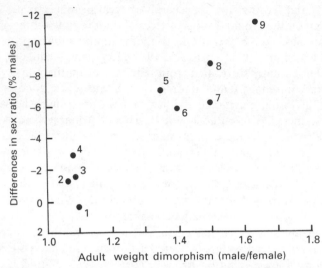

Figure 4. Sex differences in juvenile mortality in the first year of life in different ungulates plotted on the degree of adult body weight dimorphism. (From Clutton-Brock *et al.*, 1985.) Points show the changes in the sex ratio (% males). 1. Zebra, 2. roe deer, 3. sable antelope, 4. feral horse, 5. black-tailed deer, 6. red deer, 7. wapiti, 8. Soay sheep, 9. reindeer.

an introduced population of reindeer on St Matthew Island declined from around 1400 to 22 during the course of a single winter (Klein, 1968) only one of the survivors was a male.

Juvenile mortality also tends to be higher in males than females in sexually dimorphic, polygynous species (Widdowson, 1976; Clutton-Brock, *et al.*, 1985). In this case, it is important to distinguish between mortality of juveniles prior to dispersal and mortality of adolescents during the dispersal phase. Mortality is usually high in the dispersing sex, irrespective of the degree of sexual dimorphism, but sex differences in mortality also occur before dispersal and, across species, sex differential juvenile mortality increases with the degree of sexual dimorphism, especially where food availability is low or conditions harsh (see Figure 4). Though higher rates of mortality in males were initially attributed to the fact that male mammals are heterogametic and may consequently suffer from the effects of deleterious recessive genes carried on their X chromosome, this explanation is unsatisfactory since a positive relationship between sexual dimorphism in adulthood and sex differences in juvenile mortality occurs in birds where females are the heterogametic sex (Clutton-Brock *et al.*, 1985).

Another interpretation of sex differences in mortality is that where the costs of raising successful sons exceed those of raising successful daughters, mothers prematurely terminate investment in sons if they cannot afford to rear them (Trivers & Willard, 1973; McClure, 1981). However, with the exception of humans, there is again no firm evidence of active parental discrimination against offspring of one sex (T. H. Clutton-Brock, 1991), while several studies have shown that male juveniles subjected to food deprivation *in the absence of their parents* suffer higher rates of mortality than females (Widdowson, 1976). At the moment it seems likely that higher mortality in male juveniles in polygynous species is caused by their higher energetic requirements. If so, it is probably a consequence of sexual selection favouring faster growth rates and/or higher metabolic rates in males rather than the outcome of adaptive parental behaviour.

Sex differences in mortality associated with polygyny can have important repercussions for population dynamics. In many polygynous mammals, increased juvenile and adult mortality in males combine to produce an overrepresentation of females in populations close to carrying capacity (Clutton-Brock *et al.*, 1982). This, in turn, can have an important influence on population distribution and on the maximum yield that populations can sustain (Clutton-Brock & Albon, 1989).

Polygyny and the genetic structure of populations

Polygyny also has important consequences for the genetic structure of populations. Male-biased dispersal is a feature of the great majority of mammals in which males are polygynous (Greenwood, 1980; Dobson, 1982). Explanations differ but the persistent aggression directed at adolescent males by dominant males in many polygynous species, and the potentially higher benefits of dispersal to polygynous males compared with females probably both contribute to this trend (Clutton-Brock & Harvey, 1976; Greenwood, 1980; Moore & Ali, 1984; Shields, 1987). There is some evidence that while male-biased dispersal is commonly associated with the defence of female groups by polygynous males, female-biased dispersal is frequently associated with the defence of resources by males, possibly because the benefits of philopatry are enhanced (Greenwood, 1980).

Polygyny is also likely to have important consequences for effective population size (Ne) (Wright, 1931, 1978). Protracted defence of the same female groups by particular males, female-biased sex ratios among breeding adults and high variance in progeny production will all tend to reduce Ne though their effects may be partly offset by male dispersal and the constriction of male breeding lifespans (see above). No data sets for wild mammals yet permit precise calculation of Ne but preliminary analyses suggest that it commonly lies between 10 and 200 in social species and that both biased breeding sex ratios and high variance in male mating success can have a substantial influence on Ne (Chepko-Sade *et al.*, 1987). Since these effects are likely to intensify at high population density in species where adult sex ratios are commonly female-biased because males are the less viable sex (see above), Ne may well prove not to be linearly related to density, falling both at very high and very low densities.

The relatively small effective population sizes typical of many social mammals have several important implications for the genetic structure of populations (Chepko-Sade *et al.*, 1987). They indicate that mild inbreeding within partially isolated local demes may be a common feature of social mammals and that the opportunity for genetic drift may be greater than in other, less sedentary animals (see Shields, 1982). This may help to explain why local sub-populations of mammals commonly show contrasting gene frequencies (e.g. Chesser *et al.*, 1982a, b; Lidicker & Patton, 1987; Bowen & Koford, 1987) and why levels of structural allele heterozygosity are commonly lower than in other taxa (see Nevo, 1978; Chepko-Sade *et al.*, 1987). In addition, the subdivision of populations into small, partially isolated demes favours Wright's shifting balance process in evolution (Wright, 1931, 1932, 1978). Here, the rapid fixation of adaptive gene combinations within local populations, followed by the growth of these sub-populations at the expense of other demes and an increase in production of genetic migrants, can lead to a substantial increase in the rate of evolution (Wade, 1976; Slatkin & Wade, 1978).

Polygyny and sex ratio variation

It is also clear that mating systems can have important consequences for the allocation of parental resources to male and female offspring. The greater energetic requirements of young males in sexually dimorphic species (see above) can have important effects on the costs of rearing sons and daughters to the mother. For example, in red deer, mothers that have reared sons are more likely to die the following winter or, if they survive, are less likely to breed again than mothers that have reared daughters (Clutton-Brock, Albon & Guinness, 1985; T. H. Clutton-Brock, 1991). These fitness costs vary with the social rank and body size of mothers and are more pronounced in small, socially subordinate females than in large, dominant mothers that have priority of access to preferred feeding sites (Gomendio *et al.*, 1990).

The increased costs of rearing sons affect the relative fitness of the offspring of different mothers. In red deer, males born to subordinate mothers show higher mortality than their sisters, whereas the male and female offspring of dominant females show no difference in reproductive success (Clutton-Brock, Albon & Guinness, 1986). Moreover, if males born to subordinate mothers do survive, they tend to show relatively low growth and have low reproductive success in adulthood (Clutton-Brock, Albon & Guinness, 1984, 1986) while the difference in breeding success between females born to low- and high-ranking mothers is less pronounced. As a result, when the lifetime breeding success of male and female offspring is plotted on their mother's rank, the fitness of sons rises more rapidly than that of daughters (see Figure 5a). This effect is clearest when examined within cohorts but remains when data from several cohorts are combined (Figure 5b). Given that a mother's phenotype affects her milk production and thus the early growth of her progeny and that, in many sexually dimorphic species, food availability affects the growth of males more than that of females, these results are unsurprising.

These differences have an important implication. Where maternal phenotype affects the fitness of sons more than of daughters, the sons of superior mothers will, on average, show higher fitness than their daughters whereas the daughters of inferior mothers will show higher fitness than their sons. As Figures 5a and b show, precisely this effect is found in red deer. Where this is the case, mothers will increase the representation of their genotype in succeeding generations if they bias the sex ratio of their progeny towards offspring of the fitter sex (Trivers & Willard, 1973; Frank, 1987). This difference will be accentuated by any tendency for the relative costs of males to be higher to inferior mothers (Gomendio et al., 1990). Thus, in red deer, high-ranking mothers might be expected to produce an excess of sons and low-ranking ones an excess of daughters. As predicted, the sex ratio at birth of offspring produced by different females over their lifetime increases with their social rank, ranging from around 35% male among the most subordinate mothers to around 70% male among the most dominant ones (see Figure 6).

One further line of evidence supports a connection between sex ratio variation and breeding systems. In cercopithecine primates where females form large groups, including most baboons and macaques, a female's status within the troop usually depends on supportive coalitions with her matrilineal kin group (Kawai, 1958; Cheney, 1977; Hausfater, Altmann & Altmann, 1982) and members of high-ranking matrilines typically show higher reproductive success than members of low-ranking ones (Harcourt, 1987). Though relatively little is known of the factors affecting male rank in these species, the available evidence suggests that the rank and fitness of males may be less strongly influenced by maternal rank since they usually disperse from their natal troops at adolescence and their reproductive success is influenced

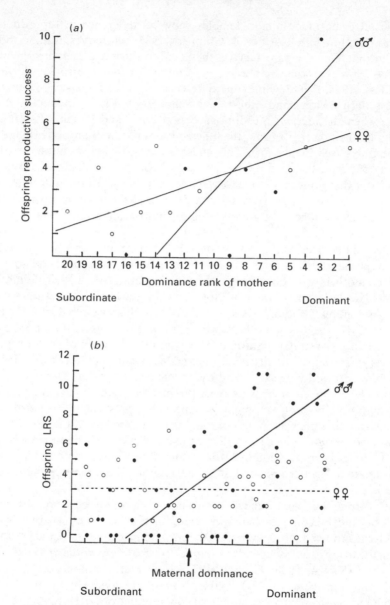

Figure 5. Lifetime reproductive success of male and female offspring born to female red deer of different dominance rank (*a*) for a cohort of seventeen calves born in 1972 (*b*) combining calves born between 1969 and 1974. (From Clutton-Brock *et al.*, 1984.)

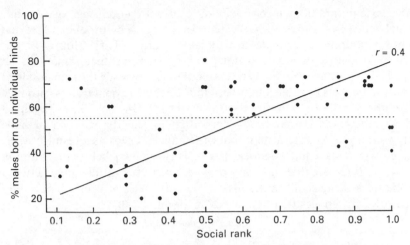

Figure 6. Sex ratio (at birth) of calves born to different red deer hinds throughout their lifespan (from Clutton-Brock *et al.*, 1986).

by the relationships that they develop with unrelated males and females (Strum, 1982; Silk, 1983; Harcourt & Stewart, 1987; Altmann *et al.*, 1988). In three separate populations of baboons and macaques, a consistent (and highly significant) tendency has been found for females belonging to dominant matrilines to produce more *female* offspring than females belonging to subordinate matrilines (baboons: Altmann, 1980; Altmann *et al.*, 1988; rhesus macaques: Simpson & Simpson, 1982, 1985; bonnet macaques: Silk, 1983).

Evidence of systematic variation in the birth sex ratio is now too common for all examples to be dismissed as statistical aberrations (Clutton-Brock & Iason, 1986). A considerable number of recent studies of wild mammals provide convincing evidence that the sex ratio (% males) of offspring at or soon after birth varies in relation to maternal phenotype or nutrition (Clutton-Brock & Iason, 1986). For example, the experimental provisioning of wild common opossums led to a highly significant increase in the sex ratio of pouch young measured shortly after birth compared with control animals (Austad & Sunquist, 1986). Similarly, the experimental reduction of food supplies to pregnant hamsters led to a reduction in the sex ratio at birth from 49·6 to 40·7 % (Labov *et al.*, 1986). These results are intriguing, for they contrast with the persistent failure of agricultural scientists to manipulate the birth sex ratio of domestic mammals and the virtual absence of evidence for genetic variation in the sex ratio in laboratory species (Beatty, 1970; Maynard Smith, 1978; Williams, 1979).

However, as in the case of differential juvenile mortality, it is not yet clear to what extent variations in birth sex ratios are a consequence of adaptive parental strategies and to what extent they are a by-product of sexual selection favouring faster male growth rates *in utero* (T. H. Clutton-Brock, unpublished data). In a proportion of cases parents maintained on an adequate diet produce (birth) sex ratios close to parity while those maintained on inadequate diets or subject to other kinds of environmental stress produce smaller litters including a lower proportion of sons. One possible explanation of these differences is that food deprivation affects the survival of male embryos to a greater extent than that of female embryos as a result of their faster growth rates (Clutton-Brock, 1991). This is a less likely explanation in cases where litter size does not vary or where birth sex ratios range between mothers from being significantly biased towards males to being significantly biased towards females (Clutton-Brock & Iason, 1986).

Conclusions

Differences in male mating systems thus have ramifying consequences for many other aspects of mammalian biology, partly through their direct effects on the genetic structure of populations and partly through their influence on the selection pressures operating on the two sexes. Many mammalian sex differences have probably arisen as a consequence of stronger selection in males for traits that confer success in direct or contest competition. Since it is now clear that many of these traits have important energetic costs and can affect the survival of males, either as juveniles or as adults, it is unsafe to assume that all sex differences increase the fitness of the two sexes. We have so far hardly begun to investigate the consequences of variation in the form or degree of polygyny for the evolution of sex differences. As Harcourt's study of testis size shows, different forms of polygyny can have contrasting consequences for the evolution of male characters. In the future, investigation of the consequences of different forms of polygyny and of differences in the mating system of females may help to shed light on the evolution of many other differences between the sexes.

Here, too, as Robert's work in other areas has shown so clearly, it is important to understand the mechanisms underlying differences in behaviour or reproductive performance. In particular, an understanding of the causes of differences in the costs of raising sons and daughters, of the reasons for differential survival of male and female juveniles and of the mechanisms responsible for variation in the sex ratio at birth could indicate whether these differences are a result of adaptive parental strategies or whether they are by-products of sexual selection for traits that ultimately improve male mating success. In many cases it is largely due to Robert's direct influence or to research that he has guided or stimulated that we are beginning to understand these differences.

References

Albon, S. D. & Clutton-Brock, T. H. (1988). Climate and the population dynamics of red deer in Scotland. In *Ecological Changes in the Uplands*, ed. M. B. Usher and D. B. A. Thompson, pp. 93–107. Oxford: Blackwell Scientific Publications.

Alexander, R. D., Hoogland, J. L., Howard, R. D., Noonan, K. M. & Sherman, P. W. (1979). Sexual dimorphism and breeding systems in pinnipeds, ungulates, primates and humans. In *Evolutionary Biology and Human Social Behavior: An anthropological perspective*, ed. N. A. Chagnon and W. Irons. N. Schituate, Mass.: Duxbury Press.

Altmann, J. (1980). *Baboon Mothers and Infants*. Cambridge, Mass.: Harvard University Press.

Altmann, J., Hausfater, G. & Altmann, S. A. (1988). Determinants of reproductive success in savannah baboons. In *Reproductive Success*, ed. T. H. Clutton-Brock. Chicago: University of Chicago Press.

Armitage, K. B. & Downhower, J. F. (1974). Demography of yellow-bellied marmot populations. *Ecology*, **55**, 1233–45.

Arnold, S. J. (1986). Limits on stabilising, disruptive and correlational selection set by the opportunity for selection. *American Naturalist*, **128**, 143–6.

Austad, S. N. & Sunquist, M. E. (1986). Sex ratio manipulation in the common opossum. *Nature*, **324**, 58–60.

Beatty, R. A. (1970). Genetic basis for the determination of sex. *Philosophical Transactions of the Royal Society of London B*, **259**, 3–13.

Boonstra, R. & Krebs, C. J. (1979). Viability of large and small sized adults in fluctuating vole populations. *Ecology*, **60**, 567–73.

Borgerhoff Mulder, M. (1988). Reproductive success in three kipsigis cohorts. In *Reproductive Success*, ed. T. H. Clutton-Brock. Chicago: University of Chicago Press.

Bowen, B. S. & Koford, R. R. (1987). Dispersal, population size and genetic structure of *Microtus californicus* in empirical findings and computer simulation. In *Mammalian Dispersal Patterns*, ed. D. Chepko-Sade & Z. T. Halpin, pp. 180–92. Chicago: University of Chicago Press.

Bradbury, J. W. (1981). The evolution of leks. In *Natural Selection and Social Behavior: Recent Research and New Theory*, ed. R. D. Alexander and D. Tinkle, pp. 138–69. New York: Chiron Press.

Brown, J. L. (1987). *Helping and Communal Breeding in Birds*. Princeton, NJ: Princeton University Press.

Buechner, H. K. & Schloeth, R. (1965). Ceremonial mating behaviour in Uganda kob (*Adenota kob thomasi* Neumann). *Zeitschrift für Tierpsychologie*, **22**, 209–25.

Cheney, D. L., Seyfarth, R. M., Adelman, S. J. & Lee, P. C. (1988). Reproductive success of vervet monkeys. In *Reproductive Success*, ed. T. H. Clutton-Brock. Chicago: University of Chicago Press.

Cheney, D. L. (1977). The acquisition of rank and the development of reciprocal alliances among free-ranging immature baboons. *Behavioral Ecology and Sociobiology*, **2**, 303–18.

Chepko-Sade, B. D., Shields, W. M. *et al.* (1988). The effects of dispersal and social

247

structure on effective population size. In *Mammalian Dispersal Patterns*, ed. B. D. Chepko-Sade and Z. I. Halpin, pp. 287–321. Chicago: University of Chicago Press.

Chesser, R. K., Smith, M. H., Johns, P. E., Marlowe, M. N., Straney, D. O. & Baccus, R. (1982a). Spatial, temporal and age-dependent heterozygosity of beta-hemoglobin in white-tailed deer. *Journal of Wildlife Management*, **46**, 983–90.

Chesser, R. K., Reuterwall, C. & Ryman, N. (1982b). Genetic differentiation of Scandinavian moose *Alces alces* populations over short geographical distances. *Oikos*, **39**, 125–30.

Clutton-Brock, T. H. (1974). Primate social organization and ecology. *Nature*, **250**, 539–42.

Clutton-Brock, T. H. (1977). Some aspects of intraspecific variation in feeding and ranging behaviour in primates. In *Primate Ecology*, ed. T. H. Clutton-Brock. London: Academic Press.

Clutton-Brock, T. H. (1983). Selection in relation to sex. In *Evolution From Molecules to Men*, ed. B. J. Bendall, pp. 457–82. Cambridge: Cambridge University Press.

Clutton-Brock, T. H. (1988). Reproductive success. In *Reproductive Success*, ed. T. H. Clutton-Brock, Chicago: University of Chicago Press.

Clutton-Brock, T. H. (1991). *The Evolution of Parental Care*. Princeton: Princeton University Press.

Clutton-Brock, T. H. & Albon, S. D. (1989). *Red Deer in the Highlands*. Oxford: Blackwell Scientific Publications.

Clutton-Brock, T. H., Albon, S. D. & Guinness, F. E. (1981). Parental investment in male and female offspring in polygynous mammals. *Nature*, **289**, 487–9.

Clutton-Brock, T. H., Albon, S. D. & Guinness, F. E. (1984). Maternal dominance, breeding success, birth sex ratios in red deer. *Nature*, **308**, 358–60.

Clutton-Brock, T. H., Albon, S. D. & Guinness, F. E. (1985). Parental investment and sex differences in juvenile mortality in birds and mammals. *Nature*, **313**, 131–3.

Clutton-Brock, T. H., Albon, S. D. & Guinness, F. E. (1986). Great expectations: dominance, breeding success and offspring sex ratios in red deer. *Animal Behaviour*, **34**, 460–71.

Clutton-Brock, T. H., Albon, S. D. & Guinness, F. E. (1988). Reproductive success in red deer. In *Reproductive Success*, ed. T. H. Clutton-Brock. Chicago: University of Chicago Press.

Clutton-Brock, T. H., Albon, S. D. & Harvey, P. H. (1980). Antlers, body size and breeding group size in the Cervidae. *Nature*, **285**, 565–7.

Clutton-Brock, T. H., Guinness, F. E. & Albon, S. D. (1982). *Red Deer: the Behaviour and Ecology of Two Sexes*. Chicago: University of Chicago Press.

Clutton-Brock, T. H. & Harvey, P. H. (1976). Evolutionary rules and primate societies. In *Growing Points in Ethology*, ed. P. P. G. Bateson & R. A. Hinde. Cambridge: Cambridge University Press.

Clutton-Brock, T. H. & Harvey, P. H. (1983). The functional significance of variation in body size in mammals. In *Advances in the Study of Mammalian Behavior*, ed. J. F. Eisenberg and D. G. Kleinman. *Special Publication* 7, pp. 632–63. American Society of Mammalogists.

Clutton-Brock, T. H. & Harvey, P. H. (1984). Comparative approaches to investigating adaptation. In *Behavioural Ecology*, ed. J. R. Krebs and N. B. Davies, pp. 7–29. Oxford: Blackwells.

Clutton-Brock, T. H., Harvey, P. H. & Rudder, B. (1977). Sexual dimorphism, socionomic sex ratio and body weight in primates. *Nature*, **269**, 797–800.

Clutton-Brock, T. H., & Iason, G. (1986). Sex ratio variation in mammals. *Quarterly Review of Biology*, **61**, 339–74.

Clutton-Brock, T. H., Iason, G. R. & Guinness, F. E. (1987). Sexual segregation and density-related changes in habitat use in male and female red deer. *Journal of Zoology*, **211**, 275–89.

Clutton-Brock, T. H., Major, M. & Guinness, F. E. (1985). Population regulation in male and female red deer. *Journal of Animal Ecology*, **54**, 831–46.

Cords, M. (1986). Forest guenons and patas monkeys: Male male competition and one male groups. In *Primate Societies*, ed. B. B. Smuts, D. L. Cheney, R. M. Seyfarth, R. W. Wrangham & T. T. Struhsaker, pp. 98–111. Chicago: University of Chicago Press.

de Waal, F. (1982). *Chimpanzee Politics*. London: Allen & Unwin.

Dobson, F. S. (1982). Competition for mates and predominant juvenile male dispersal in mammals. *Animal Behaviour*, **30**, 1183–92.

Douglas Hamilton, I. (1972). On the ecology and behaviour of the African elephant. DPhil thesis, University of Oxford.

Dunbar, R. I. M. (1983). *Reproductive Strategies of Gelada Baboons*. Princeton, NJ: Princeton University Press.

Dunbar, R. I. M. (1988). *Primate Social Systems*. Beckenham, Kent: Croom Helm.

Endler, J. A. (1986). *Natural Selection in the Wild*. Princeton, NJ: Princeton University Press.

Fossey, D. (1983). *Gorillas in the Mist*. Boston: Houghton Mifflin.

Frank, S. A. (1987). Individual and population sex allocation patterns. *Theoretical Population Biology*, **3**, 147–74.

Franklin, W. L. (1983). Contrasting socioecologies of South America's wild camelids: the vicuna and guanaco. In *Advances in the Study of Mammalian Behavior*, ed. J. F. Eisenberg and D. G. Kleiman. *Special Publication 7*, pp. 573–629. American Society of Mammalogists.

Geist, V. (1971). *Mountain Sheep*. Chicago: University of Chicago Press.

Gibson, R. M. (1987). Bivariate versus multivariate analyses of sexual selection in red deer. *Animal Behaviour*, **35**, 292–3.

Glucksman, A. (1974). Sexual dimorphism in mammals. *Biological Reviews*, **49**, 423–75.

Goldizen, A. W. (1987). Tamarins and marmosets: communal care of offspring. In *Primate Societies*, ed. B. B. Smuts *et al.*, pp. 34–43. Chicago: University of Chicago Press.

Gomendio, M. (1989). Suckling behaviour and fertility in rhesus macaques (*Macaca mulatta*). *Journal of Zoology*, **217**, 449–67.

Gomendio, M., Simpson, M. J., Clutton-Brock, T. H., Albon, S. D. & Guinness, F. E. (1990). Contrasting costs of sons and daughters and the evolution of mammalian sex ratios. *Nature*, **343**, 261–3.

Goodall, J. (1968). The behaviour of free living chimpanzees in the Gombe Stream Reserve. *Animal Behaviour Monographs*, **3**, 165–311.

Gosling, L. M. (1986a). The evolution of the mating strategies in male antelope. In *Ecological Aspects of Social Evolution*, ed. D. I. Rubenstein and R. W. Wrangham, pp. 244–81. Princeton, NJ: Princeton University Press.

Gosling, L. M. (1986b). Selective abortion of entire litters in the coypu: adaptive control of offspring reduction in relation to quality and sex. *American Naturalist*, **127**, 772–95.

Grafen, A. (1988). On the uses of data on lifetime reproductive success. In

Reproductive Success, ed. T. H. Clutton-Brock. Chicago: University of Chicago Press.

Greenwood, P. J. (1980). Mating systems, philopatry, and dispersal in birds and mammals. *Animal Behaviour*, **28**, 1140–62.

Harcourt, A. H. (1979a). Social relationships between adult male and female mountain gorillas in the wild. *Animal Behaviour*, **27**, 325–42.

Harcourt, A. H. (1979b). Social relationships among adult female mountain gorillas. *Animal Behaviour*, **27**, 251–61.

Harcourt, A. H. (1987). Dominance and fertility among female primates. *Journal of Zoology*, **213**, 471–87.

Harcourt, A. H., Harvey, P. H., Larsen, S. G. & Short, R. V. (1981). Testis weight, body weight and breeding system in primates. *Nature*, **293**, 55–7.

Harcourt, A. H. & Stewart, K. J. (1987). The influence of help in contests on dominance rank in primates: hints from gorillas. *Animal Behaviour*, **35**, 182–90.

Harvey, P. H., Kavanagh, M. & Clutton-Brock, T. H. (1978). Sexual dimorphism in primate teeth. *Journal of Zoology*, **186**, 475–85.

Hausfater, G., Altmann, J. & Altmann, S. (1982). Long-term consistency of dominance relations among female baboons (*Papio cynocephalus*). *Science*, **217**, 752–5.

Hinde, R. A. (1955a, b). A comparative study of courtship of certain finches. *Ibis*, **97**, 706–45 & **98**, 1–23.

Hinde, R. A. (1956). The biological significance of territories of birds. *Ibis*, **98**, 340–69.

Hinde, R. A. (1958). The comparative studies of species-specific behaviour. In *Evolution and Behavior*, ed. A. Roe & G. G. Simpson. Yale.

Hinde, R. A. (1959). Behaviour and speciation in birds and lower vertebrates. *Biological Reviews*, **34**, 85–128.

Hinde, R. A. (1975a). The concept of function. In *Function and Evolution*, ed. G. Baerends, C. Beer and A. Manning. Oxford: Oxford University Press.

Hinde, R. A. (1975b). The comparative study of non-verbal communication. In *The Body as a Means of Expression*, ed. J. Benthall & T. Polhemus. Allen Lane, Penguin.

Hinde, R. A. (ed.) (1983). *Primate Social Relationships*. Oxford: Blackwell Scientific Publications.

Hrdy, S. B. (1977). *The Langurs of Abu*. Cambridge, Mass.: Harvard University Press.

Huck, U. W., Labov, J. B. & Lisk, R. D. (1987). Food restricting first generation juvenile female hamsters (*Mesocricetus auratus*) affects sex ratio and growth of third generation offspring. *Biology of Reproduction*, **37**, 612–17.

Illius, A. W. & Gordon, I. J. (1987). The allometry of food intake in grazing ruminants. *Journal of Animal Ecology*, **56**, 989–99.

Jarman, M. V. (1979). Impala social behaviour. Territory, hierarchy mating and the use of space. *Advances in Ethology*. Berlin: Paul Parey.

Kawai, M. (1958). On the system of social ranks in a natural group of Japanese monkeys. *Primates*, **1**, 11–48.

Kawata, M. (1985). Mating system and reproductive success in a spring population of red-backed vole, *Clethrionomys rufocanus bedfordiae*. *Oikos*, **45**, 181–90.

Kear, J. (1962). Food selection in finches with special reference to inter-specific differences. *Proceedings of the Zoological Society* (*London*), **138**, 163–204.

Kendrick, K. M. & Baldwin, B. A. (1987). Cells in temporal cortex of conscious sheep can respond preferentially to the sight of faces. *Science*, **236**, 448–50.

Kleiman, D. G. (1977). Monogamy in mammals. *Quarterly Review of Biology*, **52**, 39–69.

Klein, D. R. (1968). The introduction, increase and crash of reindeer on St Matthew Island. *Journal of Wildlife Management*, **32**, 350–67.

Kummer, H. (1978). On the value of social relationships to non-human primates: a heuristic scheme. *Social Science Information*, **17**, 687–705.

Labov, J. B., Huck, U. W., Vaswani, P. & Lisk, R. D. (1986). Sex ratio manipulation and decreased growth of male offspring of prenatally undernourished golden hamsters. *Behavioral Ecology and Sociobiology*, **18**, 241–9.

Lande, R. & Arnold, S. J. (1983). The measurement of selection on correlated characters. *Evolution*, **37**, 120–6.

van Lawick, H. & van Lawick-Goodall, J. (1970). *Innocent Killers*. London: Collins.

LeBoeuf, B. & Reiter, J. (1988). Lifetime reproductive success in Northern elephant seals. In *Reproductive Success*, ed. T. H. Clutton-Brock. Chicago: University of Chicago Press.

Lee, P. C. (1981). Ecological and social inferences on development in vervet monkeys (*Cercopithecus aethiops*). PhD thesis, Cambridge University.

Lee, P. C. & Moss, C. J. (1986). Early maternal investment in male and female African elephant calves. *Behavioral Ecology and Sociobiology*, **18**, 353–61.

Leuthold, W. (1966). Variations in territorial behaviour of Uganda kob *Adenota kob thomasi* (Neumann 1896). *Behaviour*, **27**, 214–57.

Lidicker, W. Z. & Patton, J. L. (1987). Patterns of dispersal and genetic structure in populations of small rodents. In *Mammalian Dispersal Patterns*, ed. D. Chepko-Sade and S. T. Halpin, pp. 144–62. Chicago: University of Chicago Press.

MacKinnon, J. R. (1974). The ecology and behaviour of wild orangutans (*Pongo pygmaeus*). *Animal Behaviour*, **22**, 3–74.

Maynard Smith, J. (1978). *The Evolution of Sex*, Cambridge: Cambridge University Press.

McClure, P. A. (1981). Sex biased litter reduction in food-restricted wood rats (*Neotama floridana*). *Science*, **211**, 1058–60.

Mitchell, B., McCowan, D. & Nicholson, I. A. (1976). Annual cycles of body weight and condition in Scottish red deer. *Journal of Zoology*, **180**, 107–27.

Moehlman, P. D. (1983). Socio-ecology of silver backed and golden jackals (*Canis mesomelas, C. aureus*). In *Recent Advances in the Study of Mammalian Behavior*, ed. J. F. Eisenberg and D. G. Kleiman. *Special Publication 7*. American Society of Mammalogists.

Moore, J. & Ali, R. (1984). Are dispersal and inbreeding avoidance related? *Animal Behaviour*, **32**, 94–112.

Nero, E. (1978). Genetic variations in natural populations: patterns and theory. *Theoretical Population Biology*, **13**, 121–77.

Newton, I. (1967). The adaptive radiation and feeding ecology of some British finches. *Ibis*, **109**, 33–98.

Packer, C. (1979a). Inter-troop transfer and inbreeding avoidance in *Papio anubis*. *Animal Behaviour*, **27**, 1–36.

Packer, C. (1979b). Male dominance and reproductive activity in *Papio anubis*. *Animal Behaviour*, **27**, 37–45.

Packer, C., Herbst, L., Pusey, A. E., Bygott, J. D., Hanby, J. P., Cairns, S. J. &

—10—
What can we say about social structure?

Thelma E. Rowell

Individuals

It is impossible to work with primates for long without coming to see them as individuals who also recognise you as an individual. While early field studies described the behaviour of age/sex classes, and shorter studies may still have to, it is commonplace that table one in a study of primates is a cast of characters, which the reader is expected to remember throughout, as one would in a novel. This is an enormously significant departure from a zoological tradition in which an animal is a specimen of its species, expected to be representative of others of the same age and reproductive condition in all significant ways.

Recognising individuality is not the same as recognising variation in a population. Most branches of biology now use parametric statistical methods to handle variation in anatomy, physiology, or behaviour within a sample, as well as unintentional variation in handling and recording by the biologist. The assumption behind such statistical treatment is precisely that there is a normal form, a Platonic ideal from which the variation is something of an accidental nuisance. This is in fact just the opposite of recognising individuality. Since primates never come in large enough numbers to be able to validate an assumption of a normal distribution, the people who study them were forced to recognise individuality, and in so doing found themselves at the head of a major new direction in studies of animal behaviour. Later, individual differences have been accepted in other taxa, and individuality has been recognised as being worthy of study in its own right (Slater, 1981).

An individual has a history, a series of experiences that cannot be the same as that of any other animal, as well as a genome that is unlikely to be identical to any other. None the less, biology is not an endless series of biographies, because individuals have *similar* histories and *similar* genomes, so that some generalisation does seem to be legitimate. Generalisations lead to concepts and constructs which may be perceived as real entities by both study animals and observers, but this reality of abstraction is at a different level from the reality of the individual, and must always be referred back to it for evaluation. Among people, this tendency to generalise leads to construction of stereotypes of race or gender or age; when confronted with a generalising statement about, for example, what Europeans do, or what middle-aged women do, the sophisticated learn to check it against the known behaviour of a real person who fits the category. Such caution should also be applied to similar stereotypes about what animals do – and equally towards generalisations about what they *should* do.

Models of infragroup structure

The earliest studies of animal social behaviour were in the zoological tradition that animals were specimens of a species. They would interact predictably, exchanging limited stereotyped signals that could be used in identifying a species as reliably as anatomical characters (e.g. Lorenz, 1935).[1] Interactions between two animals were usually considered, occasionally a third was involved. Larger groupings could be seen as aggregations, as at roosts or nesting colonies, or schools of fish (Shaw, 1960), in which all individuals behaved similarly. When, later, animals were studied which lived in groups that were clearly more than simple aggregations, group structure was described first in terms of size and age/sex composition. Since animals of different age, sex, or reproductive state have different requirements, the structure of a group in this limited sense would certainly affect the sum of behaviour seen in the group. Groups were also seen as having a dominance hierarchy (e.g. Schelderup-Ebbe, 1931) which was sometimes linked to a spatial model of group structure, with the highest ranking animals in the middle (Washburn & DeVore 1961; Itani *et al.*, 1963). Such spatial arrangements were later found not to be fixed, but to be linked with short-term costs and benefits such as access to a major food resource or protection from predators (Rhine & Westland, 1981).

Kummer's model

Kummer (1968) made an enormous advance beyond this level of description with his study of the social *organisation* of Hamadryas baboons. He showed that a baboon group could be seen as a nested hierarchy of interacting units,

[1] I quote this paper because it exemplifies the feeling of continuity implicit in Festschriften. It was published in 1935 (the year of my birth) in honour of von Uexkull's 70th birthday.

the smallest being a family unit of an adult male, one or two adult females and their younger offspring. The organisation also had a time dimension: the family unit could, by the nature of the individuals forming it, only be temporary. Kummer described how such units might be formed by young males and even younger females and how a unit might mature and age. At the time it was first published this social system was, as Kummer admitted, a construct which went beyond the observations on which it was based: observations of different animals over a relatively short period were interpreted as sequences. Further field observations, which eventually extended over 17 years, amplified the original picture and interpolated yet another level in the hierarchy of organisation, but the first interpretations proved remarkably robust (Kummer, 1984). Kummer and his colleagues went on to search for rules which baboons use to determine the pattern of interaction among themselves (Kummer, Goetz & Angst, 1974; Kummer, 1975; Bachmann & Kummer, 1980). Such rules form a social system within which the baboons work, and lead to the organisation described earlier. Since rules are discovered by generalising from observations, the individuality of the original actors is discounted when they are formulated: with rules for social behaviour we must return to the classic typological approach of zoology. In his 1978 review of non-reproductive relationships, written for non-zoologists, Kummer emphasised that baboons cannot be seen as merely reacting to each others' sign stimuli and latest move, as in a game of ping-pong. On the contrary, (and the cognitive language is Kummer's own) interactions are purposive, undertaken with the intention of building long-term relationships, in a process which actually requires the *restriction* of response to sign-stimuli from the other animal. The baboon monitors, selects, and alters the behaviour of others as best it can to further its own career goals. Its proximate goals of course change as it moves through life stages, from infancy to old age, and its success in achieving them is limited by the fact that it is in turn being manipulated by others for their own advantage and the fact that it is trying to gain the best from several relationships at the same time. This is a picture of animals with an awareness of both past and future, and finds a place for both the individual and the rule of conduct in a model of a social system. The model as developed does not intend, and is not intended, to explain social behaviour beyond the papionines; it is a model of a model for other taxa working to different rules. A model which stresses the individual was appropriate for a zoologist who was writing early in the 'sociobiological revolution', and specifically in response to Hinde's hierarchical view of social organisation which had been outlined a few years earlier (Hinde, 1975).

Hinde's model

The base of Hinde's hierarchy is also the individual, interacting to form relationships. An important starting point was a serious attempt by Stevenson-Hinde and co-workers to legitimise, by description and repeatable measurements, what all monkey-watchers had long known and privately enjoyed but had taken to be unacceptably subjective: that individual monkeys have personalities which remain consistent over time and across situations (Stevenson-Hinde & Zunz, 1978; Stevenson-Hinde 1983).

In principal the differences between individuals which we call personality could be described in terms of differences in the way that muscles are used to make movements, because that is the only basis of the observer's assessment. Indeed, such a description should be carried out as a technical exercise from time to time, but it would be inappropriate and vastly cumbersome where the level of interest is actually at the next highest level, the interaction between two individuals. A qualitative description provides more suitable scale, or graininess at that level. Hinde (1975) extended this concept, proposing a series of levels of analysis for social behaviour, each with appropriate questions that could not be properly addressed at the level above or below it. Each level concerns properties emergent from the level below it. Thus, the quality of interactions, as well as their frequency, is used to deduce relationships between individuals which may continue and change over lifetime time-scales. Relationships also have emergent properties such as reciprocity or complementarity, or stability, which can be quantified and scaled so that objective comparisons between them are possible. All animals have multiple relationships, and the compromise between these relationships leads to the structure of the group. Groups in turn interact, and in the case of human beings we have a higher level, or series of levels, of institutions to consider. This model has interesting close parallels with a hierarchical view of levels of analysis in ecology developed a little later by Allen and co-workers (Allen & Starr, 1982).

Hinde's model, with its acceptance of the observed subtleties and nuances of social behaviour and its ability to deal with lifetimes, has proved valuable, especially in long-term observations of unmanipulated animals, up to the level of relationships and their interactions or 'compromises'. It is, however, increasingly vague at higher levels of the hierarchical model. The lower levels can be derived each from the preceding one by 'reducing the magnification' of the analysis and lengthening its time-scale, a process which reveals emergent properties at the higher level (Allen & Starr, 1982). I do not think, however, that Hinde convincingly demonstrates that the emergent properties of groups can be derived from the interaction of relationships in the same way. This is, perhaps significantly, the level at which field studies must diverge from captive studies, because it is effectively impossible to study the interaction between groups in captivity (but see Menzel, 1986, for an exception). I shall return to this point later.

Strum and Latour's model

In both human and animal studies, there has been a tendency to reify social structure, to see it as a pre-existing system into which individuals fit themselves. Strum & Latour (1987) question this 'ostensive' model of society. They prefer to view social beings as building and modifying relationships as they go along. Society has no structure – rather, it is *performed* by its members; there is no external system within which individuals work, but only a multitude of personal strategies and interpersonal negotiations. Social structure is abstracted and imposed by the observer of the society. They argue that this 'performative' view better explains the observed variety of baboon social behaviour, which is hard to fit into a more rigid, 'ostensive' structure. I think they would regard Hinde's 'compromises between relationships' as being evidence for the performative view of society rather than a level of social structure.

On the other hand Strum and Latour rather beg the question of how negotiations between individuals can take place without some universal set of rules of communication. The rules themselves have a hierarchical order: at the lowest level there are signals, both motor patterns and structures, which may or may not be learned early in life, but of which all participants must have a common understanding. At the next level the message inherent in these signals is modified by the identities of the message sender and recipient, and it is important to remember that response to signals is not automatic, they may be rejected or ignored. Above that, as Kummer and his colleagues showed (loc. cit.), there are rules for interactions, so that sequences of signal exchanges are far from random. There is need for careful semantic distinction here: while Strum and Latour reject a reified social structure, I think they would not fail to recognise the existence of the rules of communication which have absorbed Kummer and his colleagues. It is easy to confuse the two concepts when considering animal societies.

Strum and Latour also make a distinction which I think is an important contribution to understanding the higher levels of Hinde's hierarchical model. They use a contrast between monkey and human societies to explain a difference in meaning between two terms which are commonly used interchangeably. Monkeys have *complex* societies in that they must make a continual compromise between their many relationships simultaneously; they have no way to separate issues and deal with them one at a time. Their

259

capacity for simultaneous transactions sets a limit to what they can achieve in the way of social arrangements. (To be complex is to 'simultaneously embrace many objects'.) In contrast, people have *complicated* societies. By use of symbols and material resources they can separate social problems into a series of simpler tasks, and this allows each individual to handle a greater elaboration of social arrangements. (To be complicated, literally 'folded together', is to be made of a succession of simple steps.) Thus, in this terminology, human societies have become increasingly complicated but *less* complex as the number of interactants for each individual has increased in growing populations. The step from complexity to complication in Strum and Latour's scheme is the step from groups to institutions in Hinde's hierarchy.[2]

Complexity versus complication as used by Strum and Latour also provide a way of looking at the concept of roles, which Hinde (1978) found to be of extremely limited usefulness in describing non-human social structure. Performing a role means behaving in a way that is defined by others, usually a subset of all individuals known to the actor; sometimes the role is also partly defined by place and circumstances. An actor may be capable of several roles, but only rarely can they be performed simultaneously. An individual successively performing different roles is an example of the complication to which Strum and Latour refer. The conditions for it, usually spatial and temporal separation of partners and circumstances, are only rarely and to a limited extent available to non-humans. Role-playing is characteristic of complicated societies, not complex ones.

The three models of sociality developed by Kummer, Hinde, and Strum and Latour are all derived from experience with primates. Primate studies have made a disproportionate contribution to theories of animal social behaviour. I believe their success has been due largely to an expectation of sophistication in the behaviour of monkeys, because they are our nearest relatives, which overrode the counter-expectation of simple and mechanistic systems of behaviour in all non-human creatures. (Both these sets of expectations have philosophical or religious rather than biological origins.) There was little expectation of sophistication in early Western studies of primates: Carpenter (1964), following Allee (1938) expected and reported little more than simple agonistic hierarchies in free-living primates, and Maslow (1937), from a comparative psychological perspective in the

---

[2] The use of the similar terms complex and complicated for distinguishable attributes of social organisation is useful in that it draws attention to the need for a careful distinction. It may be confusing, however, in that the two words have been used interchangeably and with excessive frequency in describing primate social behaviour, usually with only a vague, hand-waving meaning. To encourage the use of these important concepts, I would suggest using a different term for at least one of them, perhaps elaborate for complicated. I have retained their usage here to stress that the idea is that of Strum and Latour.

laboratory, had similarly limited expectations of social structure. On the other hand, Japanese workers from the beginning expected and found kin recognition among their monkey groups as well as hierarchies (e.g. Itani, 1958), and thus established a lead in appreciating the sophistication of primate social behaviour (Asquith, 1986).

How far can ideas of social behaviour derived from primates be extended to other group-living mammals and beyond? Sociobiological theories have led to recent emphasis on long-term studies of recognised individuals in taxa previously treated only on the 'specimen' basis, and fairly sophisticated social relationships have now been described among rodents (e.g. Sherman, 1980), ungulates (e.g. Berger, 1986) and carnivores (e.g. Rasa, 1983), not to mention many birds.

Group social behaviour

To observe the social behaviour of hyenas is a humbling experience to an experienced monkey watcher: the intensity of sociality among them requires techniques which far outstrip the observation methods developed to record behaviour in primate groups. The models of social behaviour just discussed are built from pairwise interactions. Kummer *et al.* (1974) discussed tripartite interactions, but were able to describe them largely in terms of their constituent pairs, and others have followed the same method. Monkeys also communicate largely with the highly interceptible modalities of vision and hearing. In contrast, a group of hyenas will, for minutes at a time, exchange not only visual and auditory signals but also touch, taste and smell signals, and do so with the group as a whole (Zabel *et al.*, 1988, Krusko, Weldele & Glickman 1988). Although it may be possible to break such an interaction down into pairwise interactions for analysis it would clearly be highly artificial to do so; the reality is that the group is interacting, not that a series of pairs are interacting in quick succession.

I have seen apparently similar behaviour in a flock of rams (*Ovis aries*), which will form a tight huddle, heads down to the centre, tails wagging, pushing and rubbing on each other. Huddles are formed following fights, and may help to re-establish group order. A group of wolves in their greeting or pre-hunting ceremony, howling together, also with heads together and tails waving, might be another and perhaps more familiar example. It is an important characteristic of these group interactions that they are internal to the group. They are not to be confused with situations in which all members of a group are reacting to an external referent (as when mobbing a predator), even though behaviour at such times can be highly synchronised and mutually supportive. Both hyenas and sheep also interact in pairs, of course, recognising and developing long-term relationships with other individuals, but their group behaviour is clearly extremely important, and pair behaviour can merge into group behaviour very easily.

I know of no comparable whole-group interactions among primates[3], and I do not see any easy way to fit such behaviour into the hierarchical models of social structure derived from observations of primates. Here are groups of highly social animals having social exchanges which apparently transcend the relationships of individuals.

Following Hinde's model, we might regard these group interactions as illustrating an emergent property of groups; they are bafflingly difficult to describe adequately, and so one feels they should be higher in the hierarchy of behavioural organisation than the more accessible pairwise relationships. Taking Strum and Latour's model as a guide may, however, lead to the opposite conclusion: group social behaviour is undoubtedly highly *complex* in their sense; it would thus be even more limiting to the elaboration and stability which can be achieved through complication. Perhaps by confining themselves to sequential pairwise interactions, even if very rapidly succeeding each other so as to be almost simultaneous, monkeys can achieve the rudiments of complication in their social structure, and thus increased levels of elaboration and stability when compared with other group-living mammals.

This extension is attractive but uncomfortably pat both with the admiration of the individual acting independently in society, which suffuses western culture, and with '*echelle des entres*' thinking that places anything human at the acme and other primates close behind. In those schemes it 'wouldn't do' for hyenas and sheep to reach levels of social behaviour not achieved by primates, would it? But in any case, studies of group social behaviour are only beginning, and perhaps simpler explanations will emerge.

Groups

It is perfectly possible for populations of animals which rarely meet each other to develop an elaborate social structure – Charles-Dominique (1977) provides examples of lorisoid social systems which work this way – but such systems are difficult to study, and the gregarious group is the next largest unit after individual relationships which has generally been considered. The functions of groups and their evolution have been definitively discussed by Wrangham (1980, 1982, 1983). There is abundant evidence from many species that animals in groups spend more time eating and less time vigilant than do solitary animals and yet the group as a whole maintains better watch

[3] P. Dolhinow suggests to me that the greatly intensified social exchange in a hanuman langur group following social disturbance, during which clusters of animals simultaneously interact, is comparable to the group behaviour of non-primates.

(Berger, 1978; Bertram, 1980; Jarman, 1987). This probably means that being in a group protects from predators, though direct evidence is hard to come by. Groups are supposed to be superior to individuals at finding food in some habitats, and group size can certainly be limited by the availability of food. Groups may provide educational opportunities. On the other hand groups can attract predators, must be internally competitive, and must facilitate transmission of diseases. Since animals do in fact live in groups, the balance must come out in favour of doing so. Wrangham (1980) suggests that, since reproduction of female mammals is usually limited by food or other resources, their interaction with their environment has adaptive priority: females will arrange themselves in their habitat in groups of a size to optimise their resource use. Males' reproduction is limited by their access to receptive females, so they will 'map onto' the female distribution. If there is a resource that males can defend from other males, they may be able to influence the females, but only in so far as they do not interfere with the females' exploitation of their habitat. The variety of mammalian grouping patterns is thus 'explained' by their different use of resources.

Terborgh (1986) sees resource distribution, more specifically the size of patches of available food (for New World monkeys expressed as the diameter of the crowns of fruit trees), as determining group size not only as a present interaction but in an evolutionary sense. Species-typical group size then determines social structure. This extreme view requires that species inhabit ecosystems which are remarkably invariant over space and evolutionary time. The concept of a species-typical group size is difficult to accept. Apart from the difficulty of imagining by what means selection would act to generate species-typical group size, we know that some well-studied species have been found living in a wide range of group sizes even within one study area (e.g. vervets: Wolfheim, 1983, Table 97). Macaques can respond to changing environment by drastically changing group size, witness the enormous troops of provisioned *Macaca fuscata* (ibid, Table 127). Similarly, many canids can live as monogamous pairs or in packs according to the available prey (Zabel, 1986), and the 'solitary' rhinoceros lived in small herds when there were enough rhino to make herds (Owen-Smith, 1975). Terborgh uses the number of males in a group as being synonymous with social structure. This simplification risks tautology, and also ignores the very different organisation of, for example, 'multimale' groups of talapoins (Rowell, 1973) and cynocephalus baboons (Smuts, 1985) On the other hand, on a shorter-than-evolutionary time-scale, food availability and predation will determine group size and composition through birth and survival rates and this in turn will obviously determine the number and type of personal relationships available to its members and hence the compromises which will be reached between them (Berman, 1984).

Evolutionary discussions of groups are entertaining but ultimately unsatisfactory in that they cannot be tested. There is no way that the order of adaptations that have led to modern social systems can be discovered, and it may be impossible to unravel the interlocking effects of different aspects of the environment (past or present) on a particular group, since anything which changes in that environment, by experiment or by chance, will affect several aspects of it.

Explanations of groups such as those referred to here have not had recourse to the lower levels of the hierarchy discussed earlier; in describing what groups do, the internal social relationships of groups do not seem to be particularly relevant. Instead, the interesting questions seem to be about how groups interact with their environment, and with other groups, and not about the mechanisms through which the groups themselves are maintained.

In several ways, groups seem to transcend the individuals which compose them. A baboon group of roughly the same size using roughly the same area in roughly the same way may be revisited over many decades, far longer than the lifespan of any of its members. The identity of the group is in its traditions. Kawai (1965) showed how traditions continue and how they can be changed in macaque groups. Perpetuating traditions is not confined to primates: sheep are also well known for their traditions, and they may well be the rule rather than the exception among herd animals. Thus a hill farm in northern Britain is always sold with its ewe flock, and stock is recruited from ewe lambs born on the farm, brought up by their mothers to find the local resources in a severe environment. Newly introduced ewes, lacking the local traditions, would suffer heavy mortality in winter.

Monkeys in a group moving through a forest give the impression that they all know where they are going, that the whole route is anticipated by all members. They certainly move with assurance towards new foraging sites well out of sight of the present position, as the observer is able to appreciate only after much experience following them. Sometimes the group pauses for a while and then changes direction in a way the observer had not predicted; was this a change of plan, or was the pause also anticipated? A monkey who was left behind can catch up without difficulty even though the group is out of sight and sound; occasionally I have seen a monkey take a short cut and then doze until the group came along several hours later. Decision making was described by Kummer (1968), and Rowell (1966) as a process in which route suggestions are made and then selected among by more influential members of the group. Norton (1986) tried to identify leaders among his baboons, but the most complete and analytical study of this question is that of Sigg & Stolba (1981) and Sigg (1986), of hamadryas baboons groups. They were able to show that decisions made at the start of the day allowed baboons which had not been in sight of each other during foraging to meet at a particular waterhole later in the day. This was not achieved by a follow-my-leader mechanism. Within the day-route, local foraging patterns by family groups of hamadryas are determined by the senior female of the family (Sigg, 1980). The detailed route of a subgroup can be described in terms of following a more experienced leader, just as the oldest ewe present usually leads a subgroup of sheep. The baboons' day-route constrains the decisions of the subgroup leaders, and perhaps similar interactions decide the movements of the sheep. Group home ranges and day ranges constrain the foraging patterns of individuals, that is, their interaction with the space in which they live.

Populations?

Groups interact with other groups, most frequently by avoidance or animosity, and again place is a frequent component or determinant of the interaction. Territoriality is an extreme form of place-determined group interaction. It draws the attention of the observer away from intragroup interactions and towards intergroup interactions, and to the social structure of a whole population.

A territorial encounter is much to do with group identification, of 'us' versus 'them'. In a border dispute between blue monkeys (*Cercopithecus mitis*), threats and rushes towards the ranks of the other group are alternated with excited grooming within the group. Threats are exchanged by adult and juvenile females, only rarely by the males, but the adult male of the group is often at the centre of the threatening cluster, and is assiduously groomed. When a troop split, the us/them dichotomy was set up in a week or two (Cords & Rowell, 1986). Encounters along the new border, between females which had only recently been fellow troop members, seemed particularly fierce, as if the new distinction between 'us' and 'them' needed reinforcing. In this case we know that group members were well acquainted with the members of the neighbouring group, and this is probably also true of adjacent groups whose history is not known. Resident male blue monkeys certainly distinguish their resident neighbour and tolerate his presence, when an intruder would be chased. In fact two resident males may cooperate in 'hunting' an intruding male until he flees beyond the territories of both their groups.

While a female blue monkey's acquaintance is probably limited to her own group and the adjacent groups, because females rarely leave their natal groups, males range much more widely. Sub-adult males leave their group and may travel with each other or with an adult male for a while. The adult males form loose and perhaps intermittent associations which need more study. Adult males move through the territories of many female groups, and must be acquainted with group members and other males over a wide area.

Each mating season our study group of blue monkeys in the Kakamega forest is visited by males we recognise from previous years and also by males that are new to us, but it would be unwise to assume that 'strange' males are also unfamiliar to the older females of the group or to the other males. It seems that the female groups are linked throughout a wide area by the more mobile males. We are limited, by practicality, to trying to understand a small corner of an open system whose extent we cannot determine. One possibility is that there is a closed group of perhaps a dozen subgroups, within which the males circulate but which they rarely leave; another that the system is really open, and knows no barriers other than distance and no limits other than the extent of suitable habitat. This last closely corresponds, I think, to the Japanese workers' concept of a species-wide social system, or specia of Imanishi (described by Asquith, 1986). A combination of experience and anecdotes of several species of African monkeys (baboons, patas, colobus, deBrazzas, blue monkeys and redtails) suggests to me that adult males might have something like a Poisson distribution of travel lengths, with most males mostly making short moves within a study area, some moving longer distances within an area, while occasional males are encountered far from others of the species, apparently moving between suitable habitats.

Habitat suitable for many larger mammals occurs in patches between which travel is difficult or impossible for them; this is becoming increasingly true as human populations take exclusive control of ever greater areas. Such habitat-constrained populations are often quite small, of the order of tens or hundreds of individuals. Even migratory birds such as geese or cranes which fly thousands of miles between seasonal parts of their total range are divided up into populations with different routes, which rarely intermingle. Interactions between members of these place-defined populations will be possible but rare (in the brief time-scale of research, not necessarily in ecological or evolutionary time). Does interaction within them add up to something so organised as to be recognisable as a population-wide element of social structure? The answer will depend on the ability of individuals to recognise others and remember them between infrequent encounters, and the longevity which can allow a network of acquaintance to build up. For the elephant, fabled both for its good memory and its longevity, Moss & Poole (1983) have suggested that such a population-wide system is indeed a reality.

Conclusions

So, what can we say about social structure? There seems to be general agreement on some hierarchical, nesting system of sociality, although whether the hierarchy is of organisation or simply of description is still under discussion. On the whole we can say increasingly little about animal social systems as we move up the hierarchy, to the point of being increasingly doubtful about whether the higher levels exist or not. We have become fairly sophisticated about the lower levels of the hierarchy, largely thanks to Hinde's leadership, and we now accept a degree of complexity and continuity in relationships which would have been unthinkable 30 years ago. (It is ironic that this increasing understanding has provided ammunition to a movement against animal behavioural research which is surely biting the hand that fed it.) Hinde has pointed out that each level of social organisation has emergent properties not deducible from a component of the lower level. This is indeed a general property of hierarchical organisation (Allen & Starr, 1982). I perceive a gap between the level of individual relationships and that of the group, with interest in the two levels coming from different backgrounds and directed towards very different goals. The gap parallels the divergence, characteristic of present-day studies in animal behaviour, between those interested in the mechanisms of behaviour and those interested in its evolution, even though these are ultimately inseparable aspects of the same subject. Perhaps the near impossibility of studying the behaviour of groups in captivity (because their edges are artificial) is the root cause, so that the real divergence is to a large extent a practical one between people who work in the field and those who work with captive animals.

Social structure above the group, beyond territoriality, is merely adumbrated. Hinde indicated human institutions as the next level in his hierarchy, but that is not the only way to go, and it may be a unique human dimension of complication. Sociality at and above the group level among animals is concerned with and determined by place. This may be the simplest of uses of instruments or symbols which Strum and Latour suggested are necessary for complication, as opposed to complexity, of social structure. Because of the extent of supra-group sociality in time and space, our understanding of it can only expand slowly. It may be that we are now underestimating social structure at this level as much as we used to underestimate the lower levels of the hierarchy before.

References

Allee, W. C. (1938). *The Social Life of Animals*. New York: Norton.

Allen, T. F. H. & Starr, T. B. (1982). *Hierarchy: Perspectives for Ecological Complexity*. Chicago: University of Chicago Press.

Asquith, P. J. (1986). Anthropomorphism and the Japanese and Western traditions in primatology. In *Primate Ontogeny, Cognition, and Social Behaviour*, ed. J. P. Else and P. C. Lee, pp. 61–72. Cambridge: Cambridge University Press.

Bachmann, C. & Kummer, H. (1980). Male assessment of female choice in hamadryas baboons. *Behavioural Ecology and Sociobiology*, **6**, 315–21.

Berger, J. (1978). Group size, foraging, and anti predator ploys: an analysis of bighorn sheep decisions. *Behavioural Ecology and Sociobiology*, **4**, 91–9.

Thelma E. Rowell

Berger, J. (1986). *Wild Horses of the Great Basin*. Chicago: University of Chicago Press.

Berman, C. A. (1984). Variation in mother–infant relationships: traditional and non-traditional factors. In *Female Primates: Studies by Women Primatologists*, ed. M. Small. New York: Alan R. Liss.

Bertram, B. C. R. (1980). Vigilance and group size in ostriches. *Animal Behaviour*, **28**, 278–86.

Carpenter, C. R. (1952). Social behaviour of non-human primates. Reprinted in Carpenter (1964) below.

Carpenter, C. R. (1964). *Naturalistic Behaviour of Non-human Primates*. Pennsylvania: Pennsylvania State University Press.

Charles-Dominique, P. (1977). *Ecology and Behaviour of Nocturnal Primates*. New York: Columbia.

Cords, M. & Rowell, T. E. (1986). Group fission in Blue monkeys of the Kakamega Forest, Kenya. *Folia Primatologica*, **46**, 70–82.

Hall, K. R. L. and DeVore, I. (1965). Baboon Social Behaviour. In *Primate Behaviour*, ed. I. DeVore. New York: Holt, Rhinehart and Winston.

Hinde, R. A. (1974). Interactions, Relationships, and Social Structure in Non-human Primates. *Symposium of the 5th Congress of the International Primatological Society*, pp. 13–24.

Hinde, R. A. (1978). Dominance and role – two concepts with dual meanings. *Journal of Sociological and Biological Structure*, **1**, 27–38.

Itani, J. (1958). On the acquisition and propagation of a new food habit in the natural group of the Japanese monkey in Takasakiyama. *Primates*, **1**, 84–98.

Itani, J., Tokuda, K., Furuya, Y., Kano, K. & Shin, Y. (1963). The social construction of natural troops of Japanese monkeys in Takasakiyama. *Primates*, **4**, 1–42.

Jarman, P. J. (1987). Group size and activity in Eastern grey kangaroos. *Animal Behaviour*, **35**, 1044–50.

Kawai, M. (1965). Newly acquired pre-cultural behaviour of the natural troop of Japanese monkeys on Koshima islet. *Primates*, **6**, 1–30.

Krusko, N. A., Weldele, M. L. & Glickman, S. E. (1988). Meeting ceremonies in a colony of juvenile spotted hyenas. Paper presented at the Montana meetings of the animal behaviour society.

Kummer, H. (1968). Social organisation of Hamadryas baboons. A field study *Biblioteca Primatologica*, **6**, 1–18. Basel: Karger.

Kummer, H. (1975). Rules of dyad and group formation among captive gelada baboons (*Theropithecus gelada*). In *Proceedings of the Symposium of the 5th Congress of the International Primatological Society*, Nagoya (1974), ed. S. Kondo, M. Kawai, A. Ehura and S. Kawamura, pp. 129–59. Tokyo: Japan Science Press.

Kummer, H. (1978). On the value of social relationships to non-human primates: a heuristic scheme. *Social Science Information*, **17**, 687–705.

Kummer, H. (1984). From laboratory to desert and back: a social system of hamadryas baboons. *Animal Behaviour*, **32**, 965–71.

Kummer, H., Goetz, W. & Angst, W. (1974) Triadic differentiation: An inhibitory process protecting pair bonds in baboons. *Behaviour*, **49**, 62–87.

Lorenz, K. (1935). Der Kumpan in der Umwelt des Vogels. *Journal für Ornithologie*, **83**, 137–213.

Maslow, A. H. (1937). The role of dominance in social and sexual behaviour of infra-human primates. IV. The determination of a hierarchy in pairs and in a group. *Journal of Genetic Psychology*, **49**, 161–98.

Menzel, C. R. (1986). An experimental study of territory maintenance in captive titi monkeys (*Callicebus moloch*). In *Primate Ecology and Conservation*, ed. J. P. Else and P. C. Lee, pp. 133–44. Cambridge: Cambridge University Press.

Moss, C. J. & Poole, J. H. (1983). Relationships and social structure of the African elephant. In *Primate Social Relationships: An Integrated Approach*, ed. R. A. Hinde, pp. 314–24. Oxford: Blackwell.

Norton, G.W. (1986). Leadership: decision-making processes of group movements in yellow baboons. In *Primate Ecology and Conservation*, ed. J. P. Else and P. C. Lee, pp. 145–56. Cambridge: Cambridge University Press.

Owen-Smith, R. N. (1975). The social ethology of the white rhinoceros, *Ceratotherium simum* (Burchell 1817). *Zeitschrift für Tierpsychologie*, **38**, 337–84.

Rasa, O. A. E (1983). A case of invalid care in wild dwarf mongooses. *Zeitschrift für Tierpsychologie*, **62**, 235–40.

Rhine, R. J. & Westlund, B. J. (1981). Adult male positioning in baboon progression: order and chaos revisited. *Folia Primatologica*, **35**, 77–116.

Rowell, T. E. (1966). Forest living baboons in Uganda. *Journal of Zoology* (*London*), **149**, 344–64.

Rowell, T. E. (1973). Social organisation of wild talapoin monkeys. *American Journal of Physiological Anthropology*, **38**, 93–598.

Schelderup-Ebbe, T. (1931). Die Despotie in sozialen Leben der Vogel. *Forsch. Voelkerpsychol. soziologie*, **10**, 77–140.

Shaw, E. (1960). The development of schooling behaviour in fishes. *Physiological Zoology*, **33**, 79–86.

Sherman, P. (1980). The limits of ground squirrel nepotism. In *Sociobiology: Beyond Nature–Nurture*, ed. G. W. Barlow and J. Silverberg, pp. 505–44. Colorado: Westview Press.

Sigg, H. (1980). Differentiation of female positions in hamadryas one-male units. *Zeitschrift für Tierpsychologie*, **53**, 265–302.

Sigg, H. (1986). Ranging patterns in hamadryas baboons: evidence for a mental map. In *Primate Ontogeny, Cognition, and Social Behaviour*, ed. J. P. Else and P. C. Lee, pp. 87–92. Cambridge: Cambridge University Press.

Sigg, H. & Stolba, A. (1981). Home range and daily march in a hamadryas baboon troop. *Folia Primatologica*, **36**, 40–75.

Slater, P. J. B. (1981). Individual differences in animal behaviour. *Perspectives in Ethology*, **4**, 35–50.

Smuts, B. B. (1985). *Sex and Friendship in Baboons*. New York: Aldine.

Stevenson-Hinde, J. (1983). Individual characteristics: a statement of the problem, consistency over time, predictability across situations. In *Primate Social Relationships, an Integrative Approach*, ed. R. A. Hinde, pp. 28–34. Oxford: Blackwell.

Stevenson-Hinde, J. & Zunz, M. (1978). Subjective assessment of individual rhesus monkeys. *Primates*, **19**, 473–82.

Strum, S. B. & Latour, B. (1987). Redefining the social link: from baboons to humans. *Social Science Information*, **26**, 783–802.

Terborgh, J. (1986). The social system of New World primates: an adaptionist view. In *Primate Ecology and Conservation*, ed. J. P. Else and P. C. Lee, pp. 199–212. Cambridge: Cambridge University Press.

Wolfheim, J. H. (1983). *Primates of the World*. Seattle: University of Washington Press.

Wrangham, R. W. (1980). An ecological model for female-bonded primate groups. *Behaviour*, **75**, 262–300.

Wrangham, R. W. (1982). Mutualism, kinship and social evolution. In *Current Problems in Sociobiology*, ed. King's College Sociobiology Group, pp. 269–89. Cambridge: Cambridge University Press.

Wrangham, R. W. (1983). Ultimate factors in determining social structure. In *Primate Social Relationships; an Integrated Approach*, ed. R. A. Hinde, pp. 255–61 and 325–33. Oxford: Blackwells.

Zabel, C. J. (1986). The reproductive behaviour of the red fox (*Vulpes vulpes*): a longitudinal study of an island population. PhD thesis, University of California, Santa Cruz.

Zabel, C. J., Glickman, S. E., Frank, L. G., Woodmansee, K. B. & Keppel, G. (1988). Coalition formation in a colony of prepubertal spotted hyenas. In *Coalitions and Competition in Animals*, ed. S. Harcourt and F. W. de Waal, Oxford: Oxford University Press (in press).

—11—

On declaring commitment to a partner

M. J. A. Simpson

Introduction

This essay has grown out of a constellation of ideas which Robert Hinde articulated in the 1970s (Hinde & Stevenson-Hinde, 1976, p. 462 and pp. 464–7; Hinde, 1979). Central among these ideas is the question of the value of a relationship (Kummer, 1978) to the participants involved in it. I present it in the spirit of a tradition, which Robert Hinde has done so much to foster, of looking to see where ideas from animal and human studies illuminate each other.

When the success of the relationship depends on the identities of the partners involved, and when each participant has some choice of partners, then for each participant, the other partner could be said to have a certain value, relative to the other partners that the participant in question might have. Hinde & Stevenson-Hinde (1976) argued that such a view would explain many anomalies in the literature of non-primate communication, especially the distribution of social grooming in primate groups. These and other activities could be means by which individuals express social approval (p. 464).

As a starting point, I take the view that a primate's act of choosing to groom a particular partner can sometimes be the groomer's way of declaring its view of the value of that partner. I argue that we would expect to find situations where 'views of value' should be translated into promises or declarations of future commitment to a relationship with that partner. Situations where it should pay an individual to declare the extent of its commitment to its partner are those in which commitment as such has some value to the partnership, in addition to the values of the skill and prowess that the individual can bring to a partnership. In such situations I shall argue

271

that an individual declares commitment to a particular partner in order to make itself more attractive as a potential partner, and thus to increase the range of partners interested in reciprocating its choice, thereby increasing its own choice.

Phrases like 'declaring the value of a partner' and 'declaring commitment to a partner' have mentalistic overtones. I shall nevertheless first try to develop my argument in the utilitarian terms of 'how does this course of action best pay an individual', and I shall try to define commitment in operational terms. Then I shall look for evidence of primate grooming as a 'commitment-declaring' activity, and also try to indicate when we may expect to find comparable activities in other species. Finally, I shall explore how our mentalistic language with its words like 'commitment', 'loyalty', 'trust' and 'love' deals with commitment declaring in our own species. But first of all, I shall briefly review current views of the role of primate grooming.

The question of how primate grooming can be 'regarded, like alliances, as functioning to maintain and reinforce relationships' (Harcourt, 1988) is still an open one. Dunbar (1988) raises the question of why grooming, which can be given with little cost (and often paid back in kind) should weigh as much as help given in an alliance, which may be given at considerable risk? Surely the possibility of cheating would devalue grooming, and the only possible true test of a partner's performance in an alliance situation can be just that performance? (See also Bond's [1989 a, b] arguments about cheating.) Dunbar's (1988) discussion of grooming 'as the main process used in servicing relationships' (p. 223) and 'building and reinforcement of the trust and familiarity between animals that makes it possible for them to form reliable coalitions' (p. 254) includes suggestions for mechanisms by which trust can be promoted. (Dunbar does not define 'trust'. Nor do I, except to suggest that trust enables one individual to accept the commitment of another as valid. Below the meaning of commitment is discussed further.) One suggestion is that individuals come to trust those in whose presence they relax. The evidence that physical contact and grooming can be relaxing (Mason, 1965; Terry, 1970) and pleasurable (Falk, 1958) is good, but the functional question remains of why the recipients of grooming ('groomees' for short) should be prepared to let themselves be relaxed and pleasured, and why they should let the experience count for anything in other contexts. In short, the question of generalisation of trust outside the grooming context seems to be begged, obvious as the trust of a groomee abandoning its body to the partner seems to be. The suggestion that grooming sessions provide the necessary familiarity to allow prediction of an ally's future behaviour (Dunbar, 1988, p. 254) also raises questions about what dimensions of grooming performance are relevant predictors of contribution in a coalition to the groomee. Why should eager and single-minded devotion shown in grooming be shown in a coalition?

The way towards the argument to be developed in this essay is pointed by Dunbar's (1988) observation that time 'has to be invested in grooming' and the frequent observation (Harcourt, 1988, 1990) that an individual behaves as if it knows not only that it has been chosen by a particular partner, but also the other allies and enemies of its partner. The value of being chosen will often depend on who has been passed over (e.g. is the chosen one groomed more than the dominant male?), and on the potential of the groomer in other contexts. When time is limited and when there is a number of alternative partners, grooming attention could become a token of potential attention in other contexts (is the chosen one being groomed by the dominant male?). (For people who own more than one dog or cat, the apparent value to their pets of such attention is often underlined by the jealous reaction of the one who gets less).

Development of the principle

When should one individual declare to another how much it values that other?

First, their partnership should indeed be valuable to the individual, in the sense that its joint tasks yield more per unit effort to the individual than would carrying out the same tasks alone (as in 'mutualistic' relationships (Wrangham, 1982), exemplified below).

Secondly, there should be some choice of partners. If only one partner is available, or if all are equally promising, then the individual should simply team up with the only or nearest available one. If there is some choice, then better endowed individuals will find they have more choice, because more will be interested in choosing them.

In some groups it may be clear to every group member that there is some best possible combination of partnerships for the individuals concerned. For example, there could be a group of four individuals, whose fighting power decreases in order from Individual 1 to Individual 4, but all teams of two are more powerful than is any of the individuals alone. In this example I follow Wrangham (1980). Thus if Individual 1 is a primate who first comes upon a stand of mushrooms and if the individuals act singly, Individual 1 can defend and take all the mushrooms. However, it could pay Individual 2 to team up with Individual 3, for the pair of them could then take the mushrooms over from Individual 1. The partnership will pay both Individuals 2 and 3 so long as Individual 2 does not 'defect' and corner all the mushrooms once Individual 1 is out of the way. If (as in Wrangham's 1980 argument) the food source is sufficiently clumped to make it profitable to fight for, and if it is sufficiently divisible to allow both individuals access once it has been won, then Individual 3 can gain something from the partnership. Less divisible resources bring the possibility that one partner will defect by taking all. However, Individual 2's defection would pay him in the long run only if it were unlikely to have to call on Individual 3 again, or if Individual 3 were forgetful and/or forgiving (Axelrod & Hamilton, 1981; Axelrod, 1984). In this chapter, which refers to relatively stable groups of individuals which can recognise each other, I will not consider these possibilities further. Less divisible prizes, like oestrous females, bring special problems of reciprocation, which may be solved by some combination of chance and convention (such as 'prior possession' shown in Kummer, Gotz & Angst, 1974). For example, in anubis baboons, the individual who solicited help from his partner in wresting an oestrous female from a third male in possession usually became the one who eventually took over the female (Packer, 1977). 'Reciprocation' in such a partnership would occur if each of the two partners was first to come across oestrous females in possession of other males approximately equally often.

Once Individuals 2 and 3 are paired up, Individuals 1 and 4 could team up and together prove nearly as powerful as the team of Individuals 2 and 3. If extraneous 'chance' factors can also determine which team wins on any one occasion, the weaker team could at least sometimes beat the stronger one. For example, if 2 and 3 happen to be feeding on a slope still slippery with morning dew, and 1 and 4 come upon them from higher ground, they could surprise them with a charge from above. Unless the stronger team wins every time, it should pay members of the weaker team to stay together, so that each member has some as opposed to no chance of getting part of the spoils.

As stated so far, the argument need give no reason to expect a team member to declare the value of its partner to anyone. Everyone's potential as a team-mate is evident to everyone else because relevant strengths and skills are adequately assessed, for example, from physique and fighting ability. It may pay everyone to declare or advertise their power and skill, perhaps honestly (cf. Zahavi, 1975, 1977a, b), but not necessarily extravagantly. (The extent to which it will in the long term pay an individual to exaggerate its prowess in display is debatable, and it has been argued that it should not exaggerate unduly (Bond 1989a, b, cf. Dawkins & Krebs, 1978). In a stable group it should become evident whose performance fails to live up to its display.) Individuals may of course discover each other's potential in other contexts, for example as they play together. Moreover, in grooming sessions an individual could also keep up to date on the physical state of current and potential partners and rivals. The declaration and assessment of prowess should be distinguished from the declaration and assessment of commitment, to be discussed below.

Can an individual always be sure of another's potential as a partner? And how much does potential, as it might be assessed on some ideally refereed field of play, count for success in 'real-life' situations? And if testing real situations are infrequent, past successes may be out-of-date history. How far back should such history count? For how long, once a partnership begins to lose more than the occasional fight, should a team member go on finding unlucky circumstances to blame, rather than the performance of its partner? If chance plays a relatively major role in determining outcomes, perhaps skill and strength count for less than we might expect? Moreover, how should individuals choose among several partners of approximately equal skill and strength?

In circumstances when the foregoing questions arise, it is possible that the promptness, appropriateness and persistence of the partner's response and contribution to the team's effort, especially its persistence in the face of inadequate moment-by-moment feedback about success, become as valuable as more easily assessed qualities like skill and strength. Thus, other things being equal, when an individual comes upon a stand of mushrooms, a weak partner who comes quickly to defend and share the stand is more valuable than a potentially strong one who is slower. For until the members of the other teams get together, the first team to take possession wins all, in a situation where teams are stronger than individuals.

In situations where the readiness of one individual to come to the aid of a particular other counts for much it will pay every individual both to declare his commitment to its partner, and given a choice of partners, to choose the one promising most commitment. If committed joint action is much needed, but only on rare occasions, such declarations may count for much.

Commitment is only proved by prompt help to a particular partner in the face of risk, and such readiness depends partly on the partner's close attention to the individual potentially in need. But in more leisurely situations, commitment to a partner should be declared by directing attention selectively to that partner: using some activity to one partner that can only be directed to one partner at a time, but might as equally easily have been directed to others. Among non-human primates, grooming is one possible activity of this kind. This is not to deny the many other possible functions of grooming (e.g. Hutchins & Barash, 1976; Hart & Hart, 1988; B. L. Hart, unpublished data), and the many other reasons social individuals have for attending to each other (Chance, 1970).

Summary of the principle

Some of an individual's social behaviour could be directed to declare commitment to a partner in a partnership where success in certain joint activities may depend to some degree on commitment, as well as sheer skill and power (prowess). Commitment to a partner is expressed by attention to it in the form of prompt help, especially in risky activities (like fighting) whose outcome cannot be predicted from the partnership's prowess alone, and by directing other social activities, like grooming, to the partner, at the expense of others. Such a commitment-declaring function of social behaviour would be of adaptive value to an individual in the following conditions:

1. There are tasks which, when done cooperatively yield more per individual than when done singly;
2. The individuals live in a relatively stable group in which individuals recognise each other, and remember their partners' behaviour in leisurely social situations and performance in cooperative tasks;
3. Partners differ in value; and
4. An important proportion of one individual's value to another lies in its commitment to that other, as well as in its strength and skill (prowess) as shown in cooperative tasks, and sometimes shown off in play and display;
5. There is competition for partners;
6. The size of partnership is limited compared with the number of available partners.

In social groups in which the above conditions obtain, an individual's commitment to a particular partner should reflect the value of that partner to it.

In so far as commitment is valuable to a partner, an individual should attempt to win and keep its partner by declaring its commitment to that partner promising the best combination of commitment and prowess. (From this last point follow interesting problems of optimisation which will not be pursued. For example, how will a particular individual compare a potential partner who promises much commitment and shows little prowess with one promising less commitment and more prowess? Additional problems of optimisation arise when the same partnership cooperates in different kinds of task. For example, commitment may count for relatively little in a valuable honey-hunting chimpanzee partner – sheer knowledge of hive sites and agility and brute strength for reaching and breaking hives open quickly being at a premium, while in a valuable baboon-hunting partner, commitment in the form of readiness to stand firm against angry male baboons may count for much.)

How general is the principle?

Limits to its application

The value of the partner will not be declared when the rewards from the cooperative activity are sufficiently large and/or frequent, or when all partners are potentially equally adequate, or when there are no alternative partners to choose among. Choice may also be irrelevant in so far as companions are equivalent flock or herd members. For diluting exposure to a predator, or minimising heat loss, any companions are better than none, often the more the better (Hamilton, 1971). In flying in a loose 'V' a flock of pelicans could increase its chance of detecting a thermal, because the part of the skein encountering the thermal will kink upwards. By closing up like a purse net around a shoal of fish, all pelican partners may be equally important in preventing the shoal from breaking through their ring. Sometimes any 'leader' might do, as in some forms of mobbing.

Sometimes the process of value declaration, as suggested by the principle, is relevant only for a short time. The value of a potential partner may be paramount only in making initial choices, especially when once-and-for-the-whole-breeding-season choices must be made quickly on the basis of what is immediately apparent (see also discussion by Rowley, 1983). Thus the longer she takes over choosing, the fewer free territories remain for an unattached female bird patrolling early in the breeding season. As she chooses, a female bird might do well to note a territory-owning male's commitment to his territory, as well as his condition. Indeed the vigour with which a male initially attacks an intruding female, as well as the amount of time its resources leave him free to sing in it, could be important information for her.

Once in an established relationship, as in the case of a territory-owning pair, but perhaps in many other cooperative relationships, choice may become progressively less important to the extent that experience of each other improves the value of the partnership as it improves their ability to cooperate. Moreover, in the case of some territorial animals, experience of the best feeding places and escape routes in the shared territory could progressively enhance its value to the established members. As such relationships become established, we may find that occasions when each declares its partner's values become rarer: the two come to 'take each other for granted' to the extent that their knowledge of each other has made each the best partner for the other.

In partners who are potential rivals, familiarity through prolonged intimacy can have other consequences. For example, by regularly grooming a partner, the groomer could keep accurately up-to-date with its physical condition, including the relatively rapid changes in physique of a male primate moving into its prime, and the less rapid wasting of muscle accompanying ill-health and/or dotage. Thus partners who know each other well suffer the risk that they will be discarded and also treated as rivals in the event of deterioration, which may be quickly and accurately discerned. At the same time, accurate knowledge of its partner's physique may enable an individual to embark on a conflict at a time when it can be fairly sure of

277

winning quickly and decisively. This is one of the explanations Kummer *et al.* (1978, p. 37) offered for 'the puzzling tendency' of hamadryas males to risk fighting for a desired object (a female or a can that slowly released corn) more especially with a partner with whom they are previously on grooming terms.

Cases from primate grooming which may be consistent with the principle

Although no studies have been designed to test the principle, results from some fit it, and are presented to show the perspectives it offers. Alone, of course, 'post hoc' fits are not very strong evidence, even when they explain more than alternative models.

How an individual distributes his grooming among partners will be different according to whether other partners are available. Thus Stammbach & Kummer (1982) argued that grooming in groups of female hamadryas baboons was used as if to maintain and defend a valuable relationship, in contrast to grooming in dyads, when it seemed to be used more for improving poor relationships.

A study by Bachmann & Kummer (1980) suggests that a hamadryas male can assess the value of another male to one of his unit group females. In an experimental situation, 'rival' males were less likely to 'encroach' upon a female in possession of an 'owner' male, if that female had been following her 'owner' more readily and therefore needing less herding by him. Also consistent with the view that the rival males were able to assess the value of the relationship between the female and the 'owner' to the female is the finding that fights between 'rivals' and 'owners' are less likely to end with the 'rival' in possession of the female if the female often 'clasps' the 'owner' between bouts of fighting. Gelada baboons show a similar phenomenon (Dunbar & Dunbar, 1975). During pauses in a fight between two male gelada baboons for a female, the female may groom one of the males, and the male groomed most often is more likely to win her.

In all studies of partner-directed activities in which there is limited space near the partner, such as primate grooming, competition for access can complicate interpretation. Thus greater competition for access to higher-ranking partners may limit the access of lower-ranking ones (Seyfarth, 1980). The Seyfarth model also proposes that, in so far as competition does not prevent it, an individual should groom higher-ranking partners more. This is consistent with the view that she should declare their greater value by grooming them more. For this reason, dominant individuals grooming those ranking below them should groom the ones ranking closer to them more, on the grounds that individuals higher up the hierarchy are potentially more powerful allies, or rivals when not allies. The Seyfarth model is not always confirmed (e.g. Fairbanks, 1980; Silk, 1982; de Waal & Luttrell, 1988). Close attention to proximate mechanisms and thus to other possible consequences of grooming (de Waal 1986, 1989) suggest several other hypotheses (not necessarily exclusive) that should also be considered in every case (as should Silk's (1982) 'reciprocal altruism', 'protection' and 'extortion' hypotheses (not discussed further in this chapter), and Smuts's (1985) 'reciprocity hypothesis', considered later). Thus the tension-reducing effect of grooming (e.g. Mason, 1965; Terry, 1970; de Waal, 1982, p. 177; Boccia, 1987; Schino *et al.*, 1988) may sometimes have conciliatory consequences (de Waal, 1986), and in some species other kinds of contact may be involved, such as embracing and kissing in chimpanzees (de Waal & Roosmalen, 1979). In terms of this chapter's principle, conciliation directed by a dominant individual to a subordinate one who has been disciplined and now shows, by suitable submissive behaviour, that it recognises the other's dominant position, should be shown to the degree that the dominant one values the other's partnership (see also de Waal, 1982). (Grooming is often only one among several behaviour patterns with possible conciliatory functions [see de Waal & Yoshihara, 1983; Cords, 1988].)

The 'similarity principle' (de Waal & Luttrell, 1986) was invoked to explain the initial grooming preferences in rhesus females which establish bonds with females whom they most resemble in genetic and social background, age, hierarchical position and social class. The authors suggest that such 'similarity' may be an efficient criterion for an individual to use in her first 'screening' in her search for coalition partners, because the more the two females resemble each other, the more common interests they are likely to have. In terms of the principle put forward in this chapter, a partner's 'similarity' to the chooser is an important aspect of her potential value to the chooser, to be declared by the chooser's grooming.

That individuals should compete to groom dominant individuals (e.g. Seyfarth, 1980) complicates the interpretation of grooming frequency and duration scores when grooming occurs in social groups in which not all potential partners are present all the time, and/or when the effects of competition are not allowed for. For this reason, Simpson's (1973) study can only be taken as suggestive. Among 11 adult male chimpanzees, the alpha male (Mike) proved to be an exceptionally generous groomer to the other high-ranking males. Pairs involving this alpha male were thus exceptions to the rule that, in a pair, the lower-ranking one grooms his higher-ranking partner for longer than vice versa. Thus this alpha male generally groomed his partners longer than they groomed him (Simpson, 1973). Shortly after this study Mike lost his position. It is arguable, in terms of the principle presented

usually be reliable indications of kinship, so that individuals which have groomed one more will both be preferred partners, and closer kin. In this simple form, such a mechanism could then be a preadaptation of grooming as a way of declaring value of any kind.

Given such a mechanism, individuals could respond to partners' potential value, irrespective of relatedness, for example when expressing a choice between two equally closely related partners, or between a moderately related partner which is not strongly committed to a cooperative relationship and an unrelated partner which is very committed. In such situations, grooming would be declaring the partner's value as well as providing an intrinsically useful service.

Comparative studies

The commitment principle predicts how certain social activities occur together, given opportunities for some kinds of cooperation. Moreover, under certain conditions where there is a choice of partners for cooperative activity, particular social activities may come to function to declare commitment to a partner. Such an activity should be one that can be directed at one partner at the expense of another, and able to be performed reasonably successfully with most partners. Most primates in a grooming group are sufficiently skilled to perform adequately as grooming partners, just as in a cocktail party most people can make adequate small talk. As Tiger and Fox's phrase 'grooming talk' (1969) suggests, some people may nevertheless use small talk to declare and improve their allegiances. Among mammals, other activities involving touch, including sexual ones, as well as clearly directed looking or calling, are possible candidates. For example, in porcupines (Sever & Mendelssohn, 1988) as well as human beings, copulations more frequent than necessary for conception could reinforce the bond between a mated pair, and it would be easy to elaborate the human case in terms of the principle presented here (see also Morris, 1967). The porcupine case must wait for more evidence about the social systems within which pairs live: the principle would predict that frequent copulation would go with mate choice remaining open and relatively easy. Crook (1980) cites Wrangham's (1976) observation that some young male gelada baboons, when in their all-male groups and before they leave to join harem groups, masturbate each other, and he presents Wrangham's suggestion that mutual sexual activity in creating relationships between males could also amount to a form of collaborative support in obtaining and defending harems in competition against rival males. Dunbar & Dunbar (1975) describe how members of the all-male group may support an individual male in his attempts to take over harem groups from incumbent males, for example by calling as he fights. The principle predicts that his sexual partner(s) in the all-male group would give more support in his take-over attempts.

Among birds, directed courtship displays, 'gifts' of nest material, and courtship feeding could all indicate commitment to the partner, and I would predict that such activities would be more frequent and/or elaborate in one partner when opportunities for, and possible gains from, infidelity in the other are greater. Thus an elaborate nest, like that made by a pair of hamerkops (Wilson & Wilson, 1984; Wilson, Wilson & Durkin, 1987), which can take them 30 hours to build, contain on average 8000 items, and which may, when finished 'bear the weight of a heavy man standing on top' (Brown, Urban & Newman, 1982), could in part be an expression of their commitment to each other.

Human applications: general comments

The perspective on commitment developed so far could be seen as taking a somewhat utilitarian view: partners in risky endeavours who are more committed to each other can do better for themselves out of the partnership. An interesting tension arises when this view is applied to the human case. Thus an operational definition of commitment, declared as special attention to a particular partner, and proven as coming quickly to help in the face of uncertainty about an outcome, suggests that a committed partner is trustworthy in the Oxford English Dictionary sense of inspiring confidence and loyal in the sense that it adheres faithfully to its promise of help. But when commitment becomes an important issue in determining the success of a partnership, this view goes beyond a particular utilitarian approach of calculating the partner's assets, in terms of its strength, skill, etc. For, as I have argued, commitment becomes relevant at the point where asset calculations reach their limits, as when partners are effectively equivalent in terms of 'objectively' measurable prowess, perhaps because all partners are approximately equally well endowed, perhaps also because of the unpredictable nature of circumstances that truly put the partnership to a test. Within a reflective and articulate partnership, tension can arise about the relative value given by each partner to the other one's prowess and commitment. For prowess can be calculated on the basis of past performance, while commitment is promised at the point where calculation reaches its limit. Perhaps it is for this reason that to consider commitment in utilitarian terms can feel like questioning a partner's commitment.

The view that 'if one gives love to another, one simultaneously increases the amount one has for oneself' (Hinde, 1979, p. 243, in discussing Foa & Foa's (1974) view of exchange) can be mapped onto my argument. For the individual promising commitment to a loved partner, if it succeeds in inspiring more commitment from that partner, brings about an overall increase in commitment in the relationship. In so far as promises – not necessarily explicit – of commitment that can be honoured are generated by both sides, much more has been added to the partnership than a mere exchange of words or gestures.

In theory individuals in a partnership should be as interested in what they get out of it as what they bring to it. Process of reciprocation and exchange are often involved in the transactions between partners, and have been much discussed (e.g. Chadwick-Jones, 1976, 1987), and can (i) help ensure that gains from the partnership were approximately matched, and perhaps (ii) help each partner monitor the value of the partnership, in terms of what it yields. Thus (i), if one is gaining less than the other in a reasonably well-matched partnership, the other may be taking unfair advantage, and one should look elsewhere, and (ii), in its simple form, Axelrod & Hamilton's (1981) TIT FOR TAT model of reciprocal altruism requires that if the protagonists are to meet again, each should never be the first to defect, but do what the other did on the preceding move.

Mutualism, cooperation, altruism and reciprocity

The commitment principle is concerned with partnerships, characterised as mutualistic or cooperative, in the sense that each partner gains more for itself by cooperating than it would have done by acting alone. When only one partner can benefit in the short run, as when they jointly win some indivisible resource, from which only one partner at a time can benefit (like the oestrous females won by the anubis baboons described by Packer, 1977), the other partner is 'altruistic' in the sense of being 'unselfish' or 'acting with regard for others'. But on a longer time-scale, so long as the 'altruistic' one also gains oestrous females more often from the partnership than alone, he is also acting for himself. Moreover, the balance of 'altruistic' acts exchanged need not be strict, nor need the exchange be strictly reciprocal, especially when the partners take complementary roles, as they do prototypically as mated pairs producing offspring.

The words 'exchange', 'reciprocity' and 'altruism' often occur together, the first two sometimes seem to be used interchangeably, and as Janus (1989) has pointed out, reciprocal trading of benefits is often described as 'reciprocal altruism' (Trivers, 1971). (Note that 'altruism' likely to be 'reciprocated' is not strict altruism, as Trivers argued (1971) (see also Wrangham, 1982). The term 'altruistic' is often used loosely in the context of reciprocal altruism to imply that an act so described does not benefit the actor in the short term [e.g. Silk, 1982, p. 165].) However, it should be recognised that altruism is a common but not necessary feature of reciprocity, and vice versa (Janus, 1989). While 'exchange' and 'reciprocity' will be shown in many kinds of cooperative partnerships, they need not be, as when two individuals pull together to bring a stiff fruit-bearing branch within reach and then each takes the closest fruit. Reciprocity, as defined by the two minimal requisites that (i) people should help those who have helped them, and (ii) people should not injure those who have helped them (Gouldner, 1960) has been seen as a defining characteristic of friendship (Youniss, 1986; discussion by Janus, 1989), and as especially important in the development of childrens' relationships. In 6 to 7-year-old children, Youniss (1986) describes reciprocity as a 'literal practice' (including turn-taking and retaliation) that determines friendship and develops into a refined principle, understood through rights and obligations. Here reciprocity is seen as a propensity which underlies the development of human friendships, and many adult social institutions.

In real-life friendships, even among non-human primates, 'literal' reciprocity is unlikely to be found, and the TIT FOR TAT model will often require sophistication. For example, if the first baboon to ask for help gets the oestrous female (Packer, 1977), and if it is a matter of chance who comes upon the next oestrous female first, getting the female first even two or three times running perhaps should not be counted as 'defecting', as opposed to doing so six or more times running. Here a distinction must be made between a temporary run of bad luck and persistent 'cheating'.

What is 'reciprocated' can be so complex as to make it a matter of debate as to whether reciprocity is at issue. For example, can the loyalty of a faithful individual to the temporarily faithless partner be seen as something 'given' to the faithless one, on the latter's return, if it returns? Should the loyal partner then expect something, even loyalty, in return? Moreover, apparently simple reciprocal relationships are not necessarily friendly. Thus among people, too literal demands on reciprocity by one partner can indicate a deteriorating relationship (discussion in Janus, 1989) in which the two must keep even with each other, and in which there is all too little 'give and take'. It should also be borne in mind that sometimes gifts need not express any intention of initiating a reciprocal exchange. Thus the generosity of presentation on the part of the giver may aggressively aim to put the donor in his debt, and giving may be motivated only be a desire to impress (cf. discussion of the evolution of reciprocal sharing by Moore (1984)).

Human applications: possible scenarios

Cooperation between two partners only: social approval and gratitude

In this chapter, I have emphasised that what is likely to cement partnerships is social approval that reflects commitment to the other for its potential value in the future, and where gestures of approval may be promises of what will be committed to that other in the future. Such gestures could be seen as more like cheques – of little value as pieces of paper, but promises which are as good as the bank balance behind them – and less like cash used to pay off a past debt. Social approval can also be shown in the form of gratitude, although I do not believe that gratitude alone is enough to ensure the perpetuation of the kinds of committed relationships I have been considering. Interestingly, Homans (1961, p. 63; more formally stated in 1974, p. 54) found gratitude to be a problem for his model in which a more competent office worker helps a less competent one in the office in exchange for the gratitude of the less competent one. Homans thought that, with time, satiation effects could cause the competent worker to find the other's gratitude becoming less valuable to him, so that the latter would have to increase his efforts at ingratiation. The problem arises if gratitude or 'social approval' is only something exchanged for time given up to help in the office, there could be a progressive deterioration in the rate of exchange between social approval and working time given up. Moreover, the cost of being increasingly ingratiating might hurt the less competent worker's pride increasingly, to the point where he would rather struggle alone.

Partnership maintained without the need for declarations of commitment

This example is intended to show that some kinds of partnership can persist without the need for declarations of commitment. An exchange of service between two people may persist if (i) the service given by someone is more expensive to the partner than to himself, and (ii) the service returned is more expensive to self than to the partner (Homans, 1961, 1974). For example, an English and a German research worker work in the same laboratory, and need to write scientific articles in German and English, respectively. Both can write well in their own languages and both translate reasonably well, but neither writes well in his non-native language. In this situation, both should gain if each translates the others' articles. Thereby each avoids the time-consuming struggle of working a foreign language article up to a stylistically acceptable level, and each ends up with a well-written article.

If one of the participants in the transaction were someone contacted anonymously through some agency, and if he were paid in money rather than kind, the principle that both would gain would still hold, for the translator would gain more per hour by translating and earning money thereby than, say, growing his own food, just as the English scientist gains more per hour by doing science than by struggling with the niceties of German.

Whether the relationship existing for the purpose of the 'exchanges' considered above is face-to-face, or anonymous, the satisfaction of the scientists with their translations will be sufficient to ensure its survival, and no additional declarations of commitment should be necessary. In the view of our (naïve) scientists, money is involved only as a convenient way of putting goods and services that may be exchanged on a common agreed scale of value, independent of the identities of the participants in the exchange. In other words, when I pay for a service I trust that I will gain more by paying and using the time I save to do something else, than if I had struggled with the job myself, and the person providing the service hopes thereby to gain more than he would have done by doing something else. Money, of course, can also be 'made' competitively, and our perspective may offer something to understanding partnerships interested in this (below).

Partnership in which commitment is needed

In this example, declarations of commitment, even if they are only implicit, may be necessary. In a larger laboratory, there could be two or three English speakers who understand German, and two or three German speakers who understand English. Proficiency in translating would vary from scientist to scientist, and consequently there would be some advantage to being choosy. Assuming that each scientist wants to get the very best partner, it will nevertheless be difficult to judge who is best (for example because in practice each gets different translating tasks, and perhaps differences in translating prowess are small anyway). Then a partner's commitment to the partnership may come to count for much: a prompt mediocre translation which an editor can always correct being more valuable than one done well but maybe next week. If someone believes that commitment is critical, he will make extra efforts to show how he values his partner: declaring this by inviting him home to dinner, standing him drinks at the bar, and so on. And the partner may reciprocate, on the grounds that such a committed partner must be valuable. While it may look as if their 'exchange' now includes a variety of extra-laboratory activities, these are the declarations of commitment which ensure that the partnership, whose job is the exchange of skills, continues. Here we should note that in real life, with experience of each others' writing styles, etc., partners will become more valuable with time, so that alternative partners will become less attractive, and accordingly the need to declare commitment will decrease. Tiger & Fox's chapter heading 'Men court Men' (1969), rewritten as 'People court People', could be used to paraphrase the present model's application to the early stages in a variety of kinds of human pairing, including marriages.

Cooperation, risk and rivalry

In some cooperative ventures the testing times are widely spaced in time, and much can hang on the performance of one or both partners. In war, sport, crime, business and some marriages, there may be rare and unpredictable crucial moments when success, and even the survival of the participants, can hang on their nerve and skill, often in the face of great uncertainty. As well as being skilled, strong and brave, a valuable partner should value the other's life and the relationship as his own, and not defect at some critical moment.

The partners should also advertise their assets as conspicuously and honestly as possible (cf. Zahavi 1975, 1977a, b). Much individual 'display', especially when it occurs in large groups, as in chimpanzees, may be a way of focusing attention on one's qualities (Reynolds & Luscombe, 1969). In human life, for example, business 'meetings' should be travelled to in a conspicuous and 'expensive' manner (e.g. by Concorde) and conducted lavishly to show off one's power and wealth to the best advantage, and also to show that all this is being devoted to the prospective partner and not to someone else. If the meeting also provides settings, like poker games or hunting trips, in which relevant qualities (e.g. of nerve, patience, cunning) of all partners can be shown off and assessed, so much the better. Tiger & Fox's (1969) observation of white American men who reserve their expensive bottles of whisky for when they meet in groups to go hunting, keeping the cheaper brands for everyday use at home, may be explained not simply as something men do in groups, but as one way of affirming the special value of their hunting partners, who may also be prospective business partners. While one's assets can be calculated against scales generally 'agreed' in the culture or group in question (e.g. in terms of make of car driven, brand of whisky drunk), one's commitment is almost by definition not calculable, but perhaps can be contrasted as the proportion of what one has that one is willing to risk for the partnership. While such commitment is not truly tested until the partnership faces its real tasks, it can be expressed meanwhile in terms of how attention is apportioned between the potential partner and others.

Choices for one partner may often prove to be to the detriment of someone who was, or might otherwise have been, a partner, as when coalition partners change (e.g. de Waal, 1982), and when coalitions or partnerships compete against each other. In human life it often seems that the availability of a rival group or team can intensify the pleasure of comradeship within each team. Perhaps 'football hooligans' are teams of fans who are doing their best to create such a rival group. Fighting such a group could provide each member with opportunities to show his commitment and value to his team by displaying and proving his nerve and prowess in action.

Conclusion

This chapter has considered the principle that in animal and human life commitment can be a valuable quality in a partner, and that declaring commitment, by attending selectively to that partner in some special way in times of leisure, can be a way of strengthening a partnership. Stated thus, the principle may seem banal. But it becomes interesting when we ask about the conditions in which it could apply. These limits are indicated by the list of questions that should produce 'yes' answers for an individual before it decides whether to declare its commitment to a partner. Does it value a relationship or partnership because of the identity of that partner? Is the choice of possible partners to some degree open? Does the value of a partner in the relationship depend partly on the commitment it promises, to be put to the test in its readiness to join in endeavours which are 'risky' in the sense that their outcomes cannot with certainty be calculated in advance from the situation and the partners' prowess?

It remains to be seen whether the principle can be spelt out for more rigorous testing. It will be particularly difficult to assess the amount of commitment a partner shows during a cooperative task. This is because tasks in which commitment counts are risky because it is difficult to assess how each partner contributes to their joint successes or failures. Meanwhile, I believe that following out the kinds of thought experiments presented here can be suggestive. The point is not whether they fit, for of course I chose examples specially to show the principle off. But do the fits seem creakily contrived, or do they invite the reader to try fitting other examples (such as involving courtship and marriage contracts, or jealousy among humans and animals, or the attachments that form between gamblers and the appurtenances of their risky 'partnerships'), or to formulate living scenarios that can be looked for in the world, or devised and tested in the laboratory? Second, as a human primate, how do you feel about applying the principle to yourself? That, of course, is a test for you as well as the principle. I feel glad that the pleasures of forming cooperative relationships may be sufficiently explained by a design that is built around the potential value of a cooperative relationship to myself. I feel free to temper any concern I might harbour about whether I can be truly 'altruistic', in the sense of acting only for another, with my suspicion that after all I may be designed by Natural Selection to enjoy doing things which show and prove my commitment to others (but cf. Asch's passionate 1959 discussion, which also provides a perspective on social psychologists' thinking on the subject through the previous half century). My feelings are mixed when I reflect that cooperative tasks can become even more pleasurable when there are others to compete against: we love to hate our enemies. Doing without enemies in our shrinking 'global village' is going to make awesome demands on our understanding of love, cooperation and competition (Hinde, 1989). I am grateful to Robert Hinde for doing so much to put us to this task.

Acknowledgements

While writing this essay I was supported by the MRC. This chapter has gained much from Patrick Bateson's editing, and I owe much to John Chadwick-Jones, Magdalena Janus and Hans Kummer for discussions of some of the topics of this essay, and to all the people with whom I have worked, for my experience of commitment and cooperation.

References

Asch, S. E. (1959). A perspective on social psychology. In *Psychology: A Study of a Science. Study 1. Conceptual and Systematic, Vol. 3. Formulations of the Person in the Social Context*, ed. S. Koch, pp. 363–83. New York: McGraw-Hill.

Axelrod, R. (1984). *The Evolution of Cooperation*. New York: Basic Books.

Axelrod, R. & Hamilton, W. D. (1981). The evolution of cooperation. *Science*, **211**, 1390–6.

Bachmann, C. & Kummer, H. (1980). Male assessment of female choice in hamadryas baboons. *Behavioral Ecology and Sociobiology*, **6**, 315–21.

Boccia, M. L. (1987). The physiology of grooming: a test of the tension-reduction hypothesis. *American Journal of Primatology*, **12**, 330.

Bond, A. B. (1989a). Toward a resolution of the paradox of aggressive displays: I. Optimal deceit in the communication of fighting ability. *Ethology*, **81**, 29–46.

Bond, A. B (1989b). Toward a resolution of the paradox of aggressive displays: II. Behavioral efference and the communication of intentions. *Ethology*, **81**, 235–49.

Brown, L. H. Urban, E. K. & Newman, K. (1982). *The Birds of Africa, Vol. 1*. London: Academic Press.

Bygott, J. D. (1974). *Agonistic Behaviour and Dominance in Wild Chimpanzees*. PhD thesis, University of Cambridge.

Bygott, J. D. (1979). Agonistic behavior, dominance, and social structure in wild chimpanzees of the Gombe National Park. In *The Great Apes, Perspectives on Human Evolution, Vol. V*, pp. 405–27. Menlo Park, Calif.: Benjamin/Cummins.

Chadwick-Jones, J. K. (1976). *Social Exchange Theory*. London: Academic Press.

Chadwick-Jones, J. K. (1987). Social psychology and primatology: proximate explanations. *Ethology*, **74**, 164–9.

Chance, M. R. A. (1970). *Social Groups of Monkeys, Apes and Men*. London: Jonathan Cape.

Chapais, B. (1985). An experimental analysis of a mother–daughter rank reversal in Japanese Macaques (*Macaca fuscata*). *Primates*, **26**, 407–23.

Cords, M. (1988). Resolution of aggressive conflicts by immature long-tailed macaques (*Macaca fascicularis*). *Animal Behaviour*, **36**, 1124–35.

Crook, J. H. (1980). *The Evolution of Human Consciousness*. Oxford: Clarendon Press.

Dawkins, R. & Krebs, J. R. (1978). Animal Signals: Information or Manipulation? In *Behavioural Ecology: an Evolutionary Approach*, ed. J. R. Krebs and N. B. Davies, pp. 292–309. Oxford: Blackwell.

de Waal, F. (1982). *Chimpanzee Politics: Power and Sex among Apes.* London: Jonathan Cape.

de Waal, F. B. M. (1986). The integration of dominance and social bonding in primates. *Quarterly Review of Biology*, **61**, 459–79.

de Waal, F. B. M. (1989). *Peacemaking among Primates.* Cambridge, Mass.: Harvard University Press.

de Waal, F. B. M. & Luttrell, L. M. (1986). The similarity principle underlying social bonding among female rhesus monkeys. *Folia Primatologica*, **46**, 215–34.

de Waal, F. B. M. & Luttrell, L. M. (1988). Mechanisms of social reciprocity in three primate species: symmetrical relationship characteristics or cognition? *Ethology and Sociobiology*, **9**, 101–18.

de Waal, F. B. M. & van Roosmalen, A. (1979). Recognition and consolation among chimpanzees. *Behavioral Ecology and Sociobiology*, **5**, 55–66.

de Waal, F. B. M. & Yoshihara, D. (1983). Reconciliation and redirected affection in rhesus monkeys. *Behaviour*, **85**, 224–41.

Dunbar, R. I. M. (1988). *Primate Social Systems.* London: Croom Helm.

Dunbar, R. I. M. & Dunbar, P. (1975). Social dynamics of gelada baboons. *Contributions to Primatology, Vol. 6.* Basel: Karger.

Fairbanks, L. A. (1980). Testing a model of rank-related attractiveness. *Animal Behaviour*, **28**, 853–9.

Falk, J. L. (1958). The grooming behavior of the chimpanzee as a reinforcer. *Journal of the Experimental Analysis of Behaviour*, **1**, 83–5.

Foa, U. G. & Foa, E. B. (1974). *Societal Structures of the Mind.* Springfield, Ill.: Thomas.

Gouldner, A. V. (1960). The norm of reciprocity: a preliminary statement. *American Sociology Review*, **25**, 161–78.

Hamilton, W. D. (1971). Geometry for the selfish herd. *Journal of Theoretical Biology*, **31**, 295–311.

Harcourt, A. H. (1988). Social expertise and the evolution of intellect in monkeys, apes and humans. In *Machiavellian Intelligence*, ed. R. W. Byrne and A. Whiten, pp. 132–51. Oxford: Clarendon Press.

Harcourt, A. H. (1990). Social influences on competitive ability: alliances and their consequences. In *Comparative Socioecology of Animals and Man*, ed. R. Foley & V. Standen, pp. 223–42. Oxford: Blackwell.

Hart, L. A. & Hart, B. L. (1988). Autogrooming and social grooming in impala. *Annals of the New York Academy of Sciences*, **525**, 399–402.

Hinde, R. A. (1979). *Towards Understanding Relationships.* London: Academic Press.

Hinde, R. A. (1989). Patriotism: is kin selection both necessary and sufficient? *Politics and the Life Sciences*, **8**, 55–61.

Hinde, R. A. & Stevenson-Hinde, J. (1976). Towards understanding relationships: dynamic stability. In *Growing Points in Ethology*, ed. P. P. G. Bateson and R. A. Hinde, pp. 451–79. Cambridge: Cambridge University Press.

Homans, G. C. (1961) Social Behaviour: its Elementary Forms. In *International Library of Sociology and Social Reconstruction*, ed. W. J. H. Sprott. London: Routledge & Kegan-Paul.

Homans, G. C. (1974). *Social Behaviour: its Elementary Forms*, revised edition. New York: Harcourt Brace.

Hutchins, M. & Barash, D. P. (1976). Grooming in primates: implications for its utilitarian function. *Primates*, **17**, 145–50.

Janus, M. C. (1989). Social development and behavioural reciprocity in young rhesus monkeys with their siblings and non-siblings. PhD thesis, University of Cambridge.

Kummer, H. (1978). On the value of social relationships to nonhuman primates: a heuristic scheme. *Social Science Information*, **17**, 687–705.

Kummer, H. (1979). In *Human Ethology: Claims and Limits of a New Discipline*, ed. M. von Cranach, K. Foppa, W. Lepenies and D. Ploog. Cambridge: Cambridge University Press.

Kummer, H., Abegglen, J. J., Bachmann, Ch., Falett, J. & Sigg, H. (1978). Grooming relationship and object competition among hamadryas baboons. In *Recent Advances in Primatology*, *Vol. I. Behaviour*, ed. D. J. Chivers & J. Herbert, pp. 31–8. London: Academic Press.

Kummer, H., Gotz, W. & Angst, W. (1974). Triadic differentiation: an inhibitory process protecting pair bonds in baboons. *Behaviour*, **49**, 62–87.

Mason, W. A. (1965). Determinants of social behavior in young chimpanzees. In *Behavior of Nonhuman Primates: Modern Research Trends, Vol. II*, ed. A. M. Schrier, H. F. Harlow and F. Stollnitz, pp. 335–64. New York: Academic Press.

Moores, J. (1984). The evolution of reciprocal sharing. *Ethology and Sociobiology*, **5**, 5–14.

Morris, D. (1967). *The Naked Ape*. London: Jonathan Cape.

Packer, C. (1977). Reciprocal altruism in *Papio anubis*. *Nature*, **265**, 441–3.

Reynolds, V. & Luscombe, G. (1969). Chimpanzee rank order and the function of displays. In *The Second Conference of the International Primatological Society*, *Behaviour, Vol. 1,* ed. C. R. Carpenter. Basel: Karger.

Riss, D. & Goodall, J. (1977). The recent rise to the alpha-rank in a population of free-living chimpanzees. *Folia Primatologica*, **27**, 134–51.

Rowley, I. (1983). Re-mating in birds. In *Mate Choice*, ed. P. Bateson, pp. 331–60. Cambridge: Cambridge University Press.

Schino, G., Scucchi, S., Maestripieri D. & Turillazzi, P. G. (1988). Allogrooming as a tension-reduction mechanism: a behavioral approach. *American Journal of Primatology*, **16**, 43–50.

Sever, Z. & Mendelssohn, H. (1988). Copulation as a possible mechanism to maintain monogamy in porcupines, *Hystrix indica*. *Animal Behaviour*, **36**, 1541–2.

Seyfarth, R. M. (1980). The distribution of grooming and related behaviour among adult female vervet monkeys. *Animal Behaviour*, **28**, 798–813.

Seyfarth, R. M. & Cheney, D. L. (1984). Grooming, alliances and reciprocal altruism in vervet monkeys. *Nature*, **308**, 541–3.

Silk, J. B. (1982). Altruism among female *Macaca radiata*: explanation and analysis of patterns of grooming and coalition formation. *Behaviour*, **79**, 162–88.

Simpson, M. J. A. (1973). The social grooming of male chimpanzees: a study of eleven free-living males in the Gombe Stream National Park, Tanzania. In *Comparative Ecology and Behaviour of Primates*, ed. R. P. Michael and J. H. Crook, pp. 411–505. London: Academic Press.

Smuts, B. B. (1985). *Sex and Friendship in Baboons*. New York: Aldine.

Stammbach, E. (1988). Group responses to specially skilled individuals in a *Macaca fascicularis* group. *Behaviour*, **107**, 241–66.

Stammbach, E. & Kummer, H. (1982). Individual contributions to a dyadic interaction: an analysis of baboon grooming. *Animal Behaviour*, **30**, 964–71.

Terry, R. L. (1970). Primate grooming as a tension reduction mechanism. *Journal of Psychology*, **76**, 129–36.

Tiger, L. & Fox, R. (1969). *Men in Groups*. Bristol: Nelson, Western Printing Services.

Trivers, R. L. (1971). The evolution of reciprocal altruism. *Quarterly Review of Biology*, **46**, 35–57.

Wilson, R. T. & Wilson, M. P. (1984). The breeding biology of the Hamerkop *Scopus umbretta* in central Mali. In *Proceedings of the 5th Pan-African Ornithological Congress*, pp. 855–65.

Wilson, R. T., Wilson, M. P. & Durkin, J. W. (1987). Aspects of the reproductive ecology of the Hamerkop *Scopus umbretta* in central Mali. *Ibis*, **29**, 382–8.

Wrangham, R. W. (1976). Research Report to Science Research Council London.

Wrangham, R. W. (1980). An ecological model of female-bonded primate groups. *Behaviour*, **75**, 262–300.

Wrangham, R. W. (1982). Mutualism, kinship and social evolution. In *Current Problems in Sociobiology*, ed. King's College Sociobiology Group, pp. 269–89. Cambridge: Cambridge University Press.

Youniss, J. (1986). Development in reciprocity through friendship. In *Altruism and Aggression, Biological and Social Origins*, ed. C. Zahn-Waxler, E. Mark Cummings and R. Iannotti, pp. 88–106. Cambridge: Cambridge University Press.

Zahavi, A. (1975). Mate selection – a selection for a handicap. *Journal of Theoretical Biology*, **53**, 205–14.

Zahavi, A. (1977 a). The cost of honesty (further remarks on the handicap principle). *Journal of Theoretical Biology*, **67**, 603–5.

Zahavi, A. (1977 b). Reliability in communication systems and the evolution of altruism. In *Evolutionary Ecology*, ed. B. Stonehouse and C. M. Perrins, pp. 253–9. London: Macmillan.

Commentary

— 3 —

All three of the papers on social organisation in mammals concern problems close to my own interests, and all three focus on issues in which studies of non-humans help in the understanding of our own species.

Tim Clutton-Brock was a student in Jane Goodall's camp when I first visited it. At least, he was there sometimes, but most of the time he lived on his own, in a valley down the lake, near his Colobus monkeys. I much valued the days I spent with him watching the Colobus from paths he had cut in the forest, and the discussions we had when he returned to Cambridge. But he is not quite right in saying that the evolution of sex differences is tangential to my main interests, for it is a crucial issue in the understanding of human behaviour. Men and women behave very differently in close relationships, as Peplau (1983) and others have beautifully documented. The forerunners of some of these differences can be seen even in preschool children. Experiential factors account in large measure for the development of these differences, and the details differ enormously between cultures. However, the *direction* of the differences is virtually pan-cultural. The most reasonable explanation of this, and one which integrates otherwise diverse facts about behavioural differences between men and women, is an evolutionary one (Alexander & Noonan, 1979; Hinde, 1984). Clutton-Brock's synthesis of mammalian data on how the mating system affects the selection pressures operating on the two sexes suggests many exciting leads that could be followed up in our own species.

In a co-adapted complex the investigator always has the problem of where to start. Lorenz (1966) tended towards the view that in animals the nature of social structure was a consequence of the nature of the individuals, whereas in humans there are important influences from the culture on the individuals. In my own work (Hinde, 1987) I have stressed how, in humans, the socio-cultural structure both affects and is affected by the nature of individuals, and it is necessary to consider the cause–effect relations that operate both ways between them. In his chapter in this volume, Clutton-Brock is concerned not with immediate causation but with selection pressures. Taking the mating system as his starting point, he asks how it 'affects' the selection pressures on the two sexes and thus their morphological, physiological and behavioural characteristics. Mating systems are certainly environmentally influenced, but the nature and behaviour of individuals must influence the impact of selection in any particular environment. Thus in both animals and humans it is necessary to come to terms with dialectic relations between social structure and the nature and behaviour of individuals, whether one is considering immediate causation or selection pressures. Clutton-Brock's work constitutes a major contribution to this enterprise.

Thelma Rowell's chapter takes me back, not quite to the days when we sat through the night waiting to watch hamsters give birth, but at least to the times when we set up the Madingley monkey colony together and, later, when we watched gorillas, baboons and elephants in Uganda. On many occasions I have valued her as a critic – I recently came across a long, long letter with pages of constructive comments, on an early book on social behaviour. Here she stresses first an issue that has already come up in several other contexts in this book, the importance of coming to terms with individual differences: I learned much more from her on this score when we were watching monkeys. I am also grateful to her (and to Judy Dunn, see below) for raising the issue of levels of social complexity – individuals, interactions, relationships and groups. I am wholly in sympathy with the main thrust of what she has written here. Since the 1971 paper that she cites, I (e.g. 1987) have elaborated the earlier scheme in four ways that affect her argument somewhat by:

1. Stressing the dialectical relations between levels. Thus the nature of an interaction is affected both by the nature of the individuals involved and by the nature of the relationship in which it is embedded, the nature of a relationship is affected by its component interactions and by the group in which it is embedded, and so on.
2. Pointing out that the several levels of social complexity are to be regarded not as entities but as processes in continuous creation by the agency of the dialectic relations between levels.
3. Regarding institutions not simply as an additional level beyond groups, but as part of the socio-cultural structure – the system of values, beliefs, institutions, etc. in the society in question. The socio-cultural structure itself influences and is influenced by the several levels of social complexity.

4. Arguing that roles and culture could each be seen from two points of view – that of the external observer, who sees their consequences in behaviour, and that of the participant individual, for whom they are causative.

Such issues lead to more resemblances between my approach and that of Strum & Latour (1987) than would be apparent from the 1974 paper. Nevertheless, I would still emphasise that at times it is important to distinguish between the levels, because new properties appear at each one.

I agree with Thelma Rowell that group behaviour poses special problems and that we do not yet know how to cope with them. In the long run, it is important not to become mystical about them. The cases she describes must surely be made up of:

1. Individuals responding to individuals;
2. Individuals responding to signals emitted by groups of individuals simultaneously; and/or
3. Groups of individuals responding to the signals of groups.

Michael Simpson, with whose work on Siamese fighting fish, chimpanzees and monkeys I have had the good fortune to be in contact for over thirty years, takes on the challenging task of relating the human concepts of commitment, trust and cooperation to animal data. In my view his review is highly successful in demonstrating that certain aspects of animal behaviour, such as much of the social grooming of non-human primates, can best be understood as declaring commitment to the cooperative or mutualistic task of a partnership. Indeed, his review has implications for the sparse but increasing work on these topics in our own species – as, for instance, that of Mary Lund (1985). She studied students living together in their last year at university, who would have to decide whether they would stay together or follow their separate careers. Interestingly, the best predictors of whether the pair would actually stay together turned out to be not how much they said they loved each other, nor how much they felt they were getting out of the relationship, but how committed they felt and the costs they felt they were incurring on behalf of the relationship. I am grateful to Michael Simpson that this volume contains a chapter which explores in such an imaginative fashion both how insights into our own behaviour can facilitate our understanding of animals, and how advances in the understanding of animals can pose questions which augment our understanding of ourselves.

References

Alexander, R. D. & Noonan, K. M. (1979). Concealment of ovulation, parental care and human social evolution. In *Evolutionary Biology and Human Social Behaviour*, ed. N. A. Chagnon and W. Irons. Massachusetts: Duxbury.

Hinde, R. A. (1984). Why do the sexes behave differently in close relationships? *Journal of Social and Personal Relationships*, **1**, 471–501.

Hinde, R. A. (1987). *Individuals, Relationships and Culture*. Cambridge: Cambridge University Press.

Lorenz, K. (1966). *On Aggression*. London: Methuen.

Lund, M. (1985). The development of investment and commitment scales for predicting continuity of personal relationships. *Journal of Social and Personal Relationships*, **2**, 3–23.

Peplau, L. A. (1983). Roles and gender. In *Close Relationships*, ed. H. H. Kelley *et al.* New York: Erlbaum.

Strum, S. B. & Latour, B. (1987). Redefining the social link: from baboons to humans. *Social Science Information*, **26**, 783–802.

R.A.H.

V
Human behaviour

—12—

Ethological light on psychoanalytical problems

John Bowlby

Any attempt to understand the emotional life of human beings entails the study of intimate and committed human relationships. This may seem obvious. From time immemorial they have been the bread and butter of novelists and playwrights; and it is the field in which those ministers of religion who take their pastoral duties seriously labour. Medical practitioners also have recognised, sometimes rather unwillingly, the part played by disturbed relationships, and by separations and bereavements, in the ailments of their patients. Yet, although of the greatest consequence for human happiness, the field has for long remained intractable to scientific study.

For most of this century the only discipline committed to the systematic study of emotions and relationships has been psychoanalysis, with its many variants and schools of thought. Initiated by Freud at the turn of the century it was at that time but one of several comparable and competing attempts that had one thing in common: all of them were rooted in medicine. That meant that the early formulations of psychoanalytic and related theory were strongly influenced by the physiology of the day, which was then making striking advances. Thus it followed that the first theorising was cast in terms of the individual organism, its energies and drives, with only marginal reference to relationships. Yet, by contrast, the principal feature of the innovative technique for treating patients that Freud had introduced is to focus attention on the relationships patients make with their therapists. From the start, therefore, there was a yawning gulf between the phenomena with which the therapist was confronted and the theory that had been advanced to account for them.

Of the many later attempts that Freud made to reformulate his theory, the line of thought that has proved most productive is, not surprisingly, one concerned with relationships. This formulation takes as its starting point the observation, made repeatedly during the treatment of patients with emotional and relationship problems, that in the relationship with their therapists patients tend to create, without realising it, most of the very same problems that have been troubling them in their other intimate relationships. When this propensity is examined, with the aim of helping the patient escape from slavery to it, much circumstantial evidence emerges to suggest that the troublesome patterns were initially laid down during childhood in relationships with parents.

As is well known, the particular patterns that Freud first held to be the influential prototypes for later intimate relationships, especially the ones that give trouble, are those labelled Oedipal. In that formulation, of course, the emphasis is on the sexual component of relationships; and that was the component Freud always emphasised, largely because so many of his patients were having major problems in their sexual relationships. Nevertheless, at the end of a long life wrestling with problems of emotions and relationships, Freud came to realize that the earliest relationship in every person's life is the relationship with his or her mother. It was that relationship, he came to believe, that was really the prototype of later love-relations, and that it was so irrespective of the person's sex (Freud, 1931).

During the past fifty years the notion that the form taken by a child's relationship with his or her mother during the early years (and to a lesser degree the relationship with the father) has a far-reaching influence on personality development and mental health, through its effect on the capacity for making committed relationships, has gradually become recognised throughout the psychotherapeutic world as one of the two or three most fruitful among the bewildering array of overlapping and competing theories that have gathered around Freud's initial formulations. Whilst psycho-analysis and its variants have from the first offered critics a thousand easy targets, credit is nonetheless due to the therapists for having had the courage to address serious and difficult problems that are of great consequence for human happiness and which have long been shunned by others. Furthermore, the constant effort exerted by many of them to place the discipline on a better scientific footing is at long last paying off. To that outcome Robert Hinde has made a very significant contribution.

I first met Robert Hinde in the spring of 1954. Having trained in psychoanalysis before the War and working in a child guidance clinic, I was struck by the high incidence of severely disrupted relationships with mother-figures in the early histories of children and adolescents who had been referred to the clinic on account of repeated and apparently incorrigible stealing. This led me, for research purposes, to focus on the consequences of periods of separation of child from mother-figure during the first five years of life, in particular separations in which a child is put in a strange place with strange people. First-hand observations of young children admitted to residential nursery or hospital and not visited by parents revealed the intense and prolonged distress they suffer. Moreover, visits home showed that the child's relationship with the mother is seriously disturbed for weeks or longer after reunion. These observations lent considerable support to the hypothesis that the experience of separation and loss of mother-figure in the early years could have adverse effects on development, at least in some cases.

That raised a question. If the disruption of a child's relationship with mother-figure in the early years creates much distress and anxiety, what is so special about the relationship that has been disrupted? During the early 1950s the answer to that question was regarded as obvious: interest in mother stems from the food she provides, namely the cupboard love theory of mother-love. Were that to be true, however, a child would be expected to take a shift from one feeding figure to another in his stride, which was certainly not the case. Since at that time Lorenz's work on imprinting was becoming known in England, a theory of bond formation independent of food reinforcement appeared as a plausible alternative.

Early in 1954, at a meeting in London of a Study Group on the Psychobiological Development of the Child convened by the World Health Organization, Lorenz told me of a visit he had just made to Cambridge. During a discussion there Robert Hinde had introduced him to a new idea, that of a consummatory situation. I was at once struck by its relevance to my problem and decided to investigate. Shortly afterwards, Robert Hinde and I were to find ourselves on the same platform at a meeting of what later was to become the Royal College of Psychiatrists: the topic was 'The Biological Background of Human Behaviour'. The organisers had hoped to have Lorenz and Tinbergen and had settled on us as their second strings. Among those present and taking part in the discussion I recall J. B. S. Haldane.

That meeting was of the greatest consequence for me. Ethology was an exciting new world, but a strange one. I badly needed a guide and Robert Hinde was willing to be one. Looking back I realise the many blunders I made and the patience with which he steered me into better ways. All the papers I wrote in the following years, in which I strove to represent the merits of an ethological approach to my clinical colleagues, were vetted by him, vettings that, to my dismay and subsequent gratitude, usually called for extensive rewriting. Of special value early on was his critique of the concept of drive (Hinde, 1956) and, later, the typed drafts of major parts of the first edition of his *Animal Behaviour* (1966) which he lent me in 1965 when I was starting work on my volume on *Attachment* (Bowlby, 1969). Whatever merits my own volume has owe a tremendous debt to his.

Among other great contributions Robert Hinde has made to the clinical field are the systematic observations he and his colleagues, notably Thelma Rowell and Yvette Spencer-Booth, made on the development of mother–infant relations in rhesus monkeys and on the effects on them of brief separations. During the 1950s the view that separation from and loss of mother-figure during the early years could have long-lasting consequences on human children met with derision and incredulity in many quarters. Debate was often heated. Harlow's work quelled the heat and initiated serious discussion; but it had manifest limitations. Hardly any human child suffers the extreme degrees of maternal deprivation and imprisonment to which Harlow's monkeys were subjected, and some of the measures he used of subsequent effects were far from subtle. It was therefore of particular value that the observations made at Cambridge included, first, a normative study of how infant–mother relationships develop during the infant's early years (Hinde & Spencer-Booth, 1967) and, later, studies using sensitive measures of the effects on subsequent behaviour of periods of separation of one or two weeks in the middle of the first year (Hinde & Spencer-Booth, 1971). The resemblance of the responses of rhesus infants to those of human infants and toddlers proved sufficiently great to confirm that rhesus monkeys provide a suitable animal model for studying the problem, and that the findings from the rhesus experiments could be used as leads for the further study of human subjects (Hinde, 1974). Moreover, some of the methods of observation and of analysis of data elaborated in the rhesus studies could clearly be adapted for use with humans.

My reason for dwelling on these events of the 1950s and 1960s is, of course, because of the rich harvest that is now being garnered from these early sowings. Twenty years ago the many clinicians who regarded the childhood years as being especially influential in determining the course of personality development had singularly little reliable information about those years to go upon; and the vacuum was filled by speculation, most of it, unfortunately, appallingly wide of the mark. The scene today is transformed.

Attachment theory and research

The affectional bond that almost always develops between a child and his or her mother-figure is nowadays conceived as being the consequence of certain preprogrammed patterns of behaviour in the child which quickly become focused on whoever is caring for him or her, most frequently the natural mother. The effect of their action is to bring the child and mother-figure close together and to maintain them there, hence the inclusive term 'attachment behaviour'.

Although most frequently in action during childhood, attachment behaviour is believed to be characteristic of human beings from the cradle to the grave. It includes crying and calling, which elicit care, following, touching and clinging, and also strong protest whenever a child is left alone or with strangers. As a child grows older the frequency and intensity with which attachment behaviour is exhibited diminish. Nevertheless, all these forms of behaviour persist into adult life and are especially evident whenever a person is frightened, distressed or sick.

The particular patterns of attachment behaviour shown by an individual turn partly on age, sex and current circumstances and partly on particular experiences had with attachment figures earlier in life. The variations in patterns, and in the caregiving practices that determine their development, have been the subject of an intensive research effort during the past decade because of the mounting evidence that they are of great relevance for understanding the origins of individual differences in personality development and mental health.

Before describing these variations, however, it is useful to list the basic features of attachment theory as they contrast with the previously most widely held theory, that postulating a 'dependency need'.

1. Attachment behaviour is conceived as any form of behaviour that results in a person attaining or retaining proximity to some other preferred individual. So long as the attachment figure remains accessible and responsive the behaviour may consist of little more than checking by eye or ear on the whereabouts of the figure and exchanging occasional glances and greetings. In certain circumstances, however, following or clinging to the attachment figure may occur and also calling or crying, which are likely to elicit his or her caregiving.

2. As a class of behaviour with its own dynamic, attachment behaviour is conceived as distinct from feeding behaviour and sexual behaviour and of at least an equal significance in human life.

3. During the course of healthy development attachment behaviour leads to the development of affectional bonds or attachments, initially between child and parent and later between adult and adult. The forms of behaviour and the bonds to which they lead are present and active throughout the life cycle (and by no means confined to childhood as other theories assume).

4. Attachment behaviour, like other forms of instinctive behaviour, is mediated by behavioural systems which early in development become goal-corrected. Homeostatic systems of this type are so structured that, by means of feedback, continuous account is taken of any discrepancies there may be between initial instruction and current performance so that behaviour becomes modified accordingly. In planning and guiding goal-corrected behaviour use is made of

representational models both of the self's capabilities and of the relevant features of the environment. The goal of attachment behaviour is to maintain certain degrees of proximity to, or of communication with, the discriminated attachment figure(s).

5. Whereas an attachment bond endures, the various forms of attachment behaviour that contribute to it are active only when required. Thus the systems mediating attachment behaviour are activated only by certain conditions, for example, strangeness, fatigue, anything frightening, and unavailability or unresponsiveness of the attachment figure, and are terminated only by certain other conditions, for example a familiar environment and the ready availability and responsiveness of an attachment figure. When attachment behaviour is strongly aroused, however, termination may require touching, or clinging, or the actively reassuring behaviour of the attachment figure.

6. Many of the most intense emotions arise during the formation, the maintenance, the disruption and the renewal of attachment relationships. The formation of a bond is described as falling in love, maintaining a bond as loving someone, and losing a partner as grieving over someone. Similarly, threat of loss arouses anxiety and actual loss gives rise to sorrow; while each of these situations is likely to arouse anger. The unchallenged maintenance of a bond is experienced as a source of security and the renewal of a bond as a source of joy. Because such emotions are usually a reflection of the state of a person's affectional bonds, the psychology and psychopathology of emotion is found to be in large part the psychology and psychopathology of affectional bonds.

7. Attachment behaviour has become a characteristic of many species during the course of their evolution because it contributes to the individual's survival by keeping him or her in touch with one or more caregivers, thereby reducing the risk of harm, for example from cold, hunger or drowning and, in the human's environment of evolutionary adaptedness, especially from predators. ('Dependency' theory not only neglects function but regards the behaviour as regrettable and to be outgrown as soon as possible.)

8. Behaviour complementary to attachment behaviour and serving a complementary function, that of protecting the attached individual, is caregiving. This is commonly shown by a parent, or other adult, towards a child or adolescent, but is also shown by one adult towards another, especially in times of ill health, stress or old age.

9. In view of attachment behaviour being potentially active throughout life and also of its having the vital biological function proposed, it is

held a grave error to suppose that, when active in an adult, attachment behaviour is indicative either of pathology or of regression to immature behaviour. (The latter view has been characteristic of almost all other versions of psychoanalytic theory.)

10. Disturbed patterns of attachment behaviour can be present at any age due to development having followed a deviant pathway. One of the commonest forms of disturbance is the over-ready elicitation of attachment behaviour, resulting in anxious attachment. Another is a partial or complete deactivation of attachment behaviour.

11. Principal determinants of the pathway along which an individual's attachment behaviour develops, and of the pattern in which it becomes organised, are experiences with attachment figures during the years of immaturity – infancy, childhood and adolescence.

12. On the way in which an individual's attachment behaviour becomes organised within his or her personality turns the pattern of affectional bonds made during later life.

In considering further the attachment control system postulated as present within the child, it is evident that for it to operate efficiently, it requires to have at its disposal as much information as possible about self and attachment figure, not only in regard to their respective locations and capabilities but in regard also to how each is likely to respond to the other as environmental and other conditions change. Observations lead to the conclusion that towards the end of the first year of life a child is acquiring a considerable knowledge of the immediate world and that during subsequent years this knowledge is best regarded as becoming organised in the form of internal working models, including models of self and mother. The function of these models is to simulate happenings in the real world, thereby enabling the individual to plan behaviour with all the advantages of insight and foresight. Although our knowledge of the rate at which these models develop during the earliest years is still scanty, there is good evidence that by the fifth birthday most children are using a sophisticated working model of mother or mother-substitute which includes knowledge of her interests, moods and intentions, all of which can then be taken into account (Light, 1979). With such a complementary model, the child is already engaging in a complex intersubjective relationship with the mother who, of course, has her own working models both of her child and of herself. Because these models are in constant use, day in and day out, their influence on thought, feeling and behaviour becomes routine and largely outside awareness.

Long before a child reaches five, however, the patterns of interactions with the mother are known to range vastly in diversity, from smooth running and happy to being filled with friction and distress of every kind and degree, and also are apt to persist. For practical reasons, therefore, the more we know

307

about how they originate the better. It is here that recent research by developmental psychologists has made such huge strides.

Patterns of attachment and their determinants

Three principal patterns of attachment present during the early years are now reliably identified, together with the family conditions that promote them. One of these patterns is judged by clinicians to be consistent with the child developing healthily and two to be predictive of disturbed development. Which pattern any one individual develops during these years is found to be profoundly influenced by the way his parents (or other parent-type figures) treat him. The evidence for this conclusion is now weighty and derives from a number of prospective research studies of socio-emotional development during the first five years. This research tradition was first set in train by Mary Ainsworth during the 1960s (Ainsworth *et al.*, 1978; Ainsworth, 1985) and has since been exploited and expanded, notably in the USA by Mary Main (Main & Weston, 1981; Main & Stadtman, 1981; Main, Kaplan & Cassidy, 1985), Alan Sroufe (1983, 1985) and Everett Waters (Waters, Vaughn & Egeland, 1980; Waters & Deane, 1985), and in Germany by Klaus & Karin Grossmann (Grossmann, Grossmann & Schwan, 1986).

The pattern of attachment believed consistent with healthy development is that of secure attachment, in which the individual is confident that a parent (or parent figure) will be available, responsive and helpful in adverse or frightening situations. With this assurance, the child feels bold in explorations of the world and also competent in dealing with it. This pattern is found to be promoted by a parent, in the early years especially by the mother, being readily available, sensitive to her child's signals and lovingly responsive when protection and/or comfort and/or assistance is sought.

A second pattern is that of anxious resistant attachment in which the child is uncertain whether a parent will be available or responsive or helpful when called upon. Because of this uncertainty the child is always prone to separation anxiety, tends to be clinging, and is anxious about exploring the world. This pattern is promoted by a parent being available and helpful on some occasions but not on others and, clinical evidence shows, by separations and, later, especially by threats of abandonment used as a means of control.

A third pattern is that of anxious avoidant attachment in which the children have no confidence that, when seeking care, they will be responded to helpfully and, on the contrary, expect to be rebuffed. Such individuals attempt to live their lives without the love and support of others. This pattern is the result of their mothers constantly rebuffing them when approached for comfort or protection. The most extreme cases result from repeated rejection and ill-treatment, or prolonged institutionalisation. Clinical evidence suggests that, if it persists, this pattern leads to a variety of personality disorders of very different degrees of severity, from compulsively self-sufficient individuals to persistently delinquent ones.

Much evidence suggests that, at least in families where caregiving arrangements remain stable, the pattern of attachment between child and mother, once established, tends to persist. For example, in two different samples (Californian and German) the patterns of attachment to mother at 12 months were found, with but few exceptions, still to be present at 6 years (Main *et al.*, 1985; Wärtner, 1986). Furthermore, prospective studies in Minneapolis (Sroufe, 1983) have shown that the pattern of attachment characteristic of the pair, as assessed when the child is aged 12 months, is highly predictive also of behaviour outside the home in a nursery group, $3\frac{1}{2}$ years later. Thus children who showed a secure pattern with mother at 12 months are likely to be described by their nursery teachers as cheerful and cooperative, popular with other children, resilient and resourceful. Those who showed an anxious avoidance pattern are likely to be described later as emotionally insulated, hostile or antisocial and as unduly seeking of attention. Those who showed an anxious resistant pattern are also likely to be described as unduly seeking of attention and as either tense, impulsive and easily frustrated or else as passive and helpless. These findings have been replicated in Germany by G. J. Suess, K. E. Grossmann and L. A. Sroufe (unpublished data).

Confirmation of the teacher's descriptions comes from independent observers and laboratory assessments of the same children (Sroufe, 1983; La Fréniere & Sroufe, 1985). An experimental study done in Germany (Lütkenhaus, Grossmann & Grossmann, 1985) shows that at 3 years of age children earlier assessed as securely attached respond to potential failure with increased effort, whereas the insecurely attached do the opposite. In other words, the securely attached children are responding with confidence and hope that they can succeed whilst the insecure are already showing signs of helplessness and defeatism.

In a number of these studies detailed observations have been made of the way the children's mothers treated them. Great variability is seen, with high correlations between a mother's style of interaction and the child's pattern of attachment to her. For example, in one such study (Matas, Arend & Sroufe, 1978), made when the children were $2\frac{1}{2}$ years old, mothers were observed whilst their children were attempting a task that they could not manage without a little help. Mothers of secure toddlers enabled their children to focus on the task, respected their attempts to complete it on their own, and responded with the required help when called upon; communication between them was harmonious. Mothers of insecure infants were less sensitive to the toddlers' state of mind, either not giving support and help when appealed to or else intruding when the children were striving to solve the problem themselves.

In discussing these and similar findings Bretherton (1987) emphasises the easy flow of communication between a mother and her child in the secure partnerships and concludes that this easy communication is possible only when a mother is intuitively alive to the crucial part she plays in providing her child with a secure base, variously encouraging autonomy, providing necessary help or giving comfort according to her child's state of mind.

Mothers of insecure infants deviate from this sensitive pattern of mothering in a great variety of ways. One, common amongst mothers of avoidant infants, is to scoff at her child's bids for comfort and support (Main *et al.*, 1985). Another, well known to clinicians and the effects of which are now being observed by developmentalists (Sroufe *et al.*, 1985; Main & Solomon, 1986), is a mother who fails to respect her child's desire for autonomy and discourages exploration. This is usually a mother who, not having had a secure home base during her childhood, is consciously or unconsciously seeking to invert the relationship by making her child her own attachment figure. In the past this has too often been labelled 'over-indulgence' or 'spoiling', which has led to appalling confusion about what is best for a child.

It is not difficult to understand why patterns of attachment, once developed, tend to persist. One reason is that the way a parent treats a child, whether for better or for worse, tends to continue unchanged; another is that each pattern tends to be self-perpetuating. Thus a secure child is a happier and more rewarding child to care for, and also is less demanding, than an anxious one. An anxious ambivalent child is apt to be whiny and clinging, whilst an anxious avoidant child keeps his distance, is bad-tempered and is prone to bully other children. In each of these cases the child's behaviour is likely to elicit an unfavourable response from the parent so that vicious circles develop.

Although for the reasons given patterns, once formed, are likely to persist, this is by no means necessarily so. Evidence shows that during the first 2 or 3 years pattern of attachment is a property of the relationship[1], for example the pattern of child to mother may differ from the pattern to father, and also that if the parent treats the child differently the pattern will change accordingly. These changes are amongst much evidence reviewed by Sroufe (1985) that stability of pattern, when it occurs, cannot be attributed to inborn characteristics immune to environmental influence. On the contrary, the evidence points unmistakably to the conclusion that a host of personal characteristics, traditionally termed temperamental and hitherto often

---

[1] This is a point that was in danger of being overlooked and to which Robert Hinde drew special attention (Hinde, 1982).

believed to be inborn and unchangeable, are environmentally induced. True, neonates differ from each other in many many ways. Yet the evidence is clear from repeated studies that infants described as difficult during their early days are enabled by sensitive mothering to become happy easy toddlers. Contrarily, placid newborns can be turned into anxious, moody, demanding or awkward toddlers by insensitive or rejecting mothering. Not only did Ainsworth demonstrate this in her original study, but it has been found repeatedly in subsequent ones.

Thus, during the earliest years features of personality believed crucial to mental health remain relatively open to change because they are still responsive to the environment. As a child grows older, however, clinical evidence shows that both the pattern of attachment and the personality features that go with it become increasingly a property of the child and also increasingly resistant to change. This means that he or she tends to impose it, or some derivative of it, upon new relationships, such as those with the teacher and other children in the Minneapolis study. Similarly, experience shows that the child tends also to impose it or some derivative of it on to a foster-mother or a therapist.

This tendency to impose earlier patterns on to new relationships, and in some measure to persist in doing so despite absence of fit, is, it will be remembered, the very problem that has from the start been at the centre of psychoanalytic attention.

By far the most valuable aspects of the new conceptual framework, to which the contribution made by Robert Hinde's understanding of ethology has been indispensable, are the reformulation of old questions in a researchable form and the development of new methods of answering them. The stage, therefore, is now set for a great expansion of productive research. Meanwhile, clinicians are beginning to apply such reliable knowledge as is so far available and are, inevitably, extrapolating in the huge areas where it still is not – as I have sometimes been doing in this exposition.

References

Ainsworth, M. D. S. (1985). I. Patterns of infant–mother attachment: antecedents and effects on development. II. Attachments across the life span. *Bulletin of the New York Academy of Medicine*, **61**, 771–91 and 792–812.

Ainsworth, M. D. S., Blehar, M. C., Waters, E. & Wall, S. (1978). *Patterns of Attachment: Assessed in the Strange Situation and at Home*. Hillsdale, NJ: Erlbaum.

Bowlby, J. (1969). *Attachment and Loss, Vol. 1. Attachment* (second edition, 1982). London: Hogarth Press.

Bretherton, I. (1987). New perspectives on attachment relations: security, communication and internal working models. In *Handbook of Infant Development*, 2nd edition, ed. J. Osofsky, pp. 1061–100. New York: John Wiley.

John Bowlby

Freud, S. (1931). *Female Sexuality*, Standard Edition 21. London: Hogarth Press.
Grossmann, K. E., Grossmann, K. & Schwan, A. (1986). Capturing the wider view
of attachment: a reanalysis of Ainsworth's strange situation. In *Measuring
Emotions in Infants and Children. Vol. 2*, ed. C. E. Izard and P. B. Read, pp. 124–71.
New York: Cambridge University Press.
Hinde, R. A. (1956). Ethological models and the concept of drive. *British Journal of
the Philosophy of Science*, **6**, 321–31.
Hinde, R. A. (1966). *Animal Behaviour: A Synthesis of Ethology and Comparative
Psychology* (second edition, 1970). New York: McGraw-Hill.
Hinde, R. A. (1974). *Biological Bases of Human Social Behaviour*. New York:
McGraw-Hill.
Hinde, R. A. (1982). Attachment: some conceptual and biological issues. In *The
Place of Attachment in Human Behaviour*, ed. C. M. Parkes and J. Stevenson-
Hinde, pp. 60–76. New York: Basic Books.
Hinde, R. A. & Spencer-Booth, Y. (1967). The behaviour of socially living rhesus
monkeys in their first two and a half years. *Animal Behaviour*, **15**, 169–96.
Hinde, R. A. & Spencer-Booth, Y. (1971). Effects of brief separation from mother on
rhesus monkeys. *Science*, **173**, 111–18.
La Fréniere, P. & Sroufe, J. A. (1985). Profiles of peer competence in the pre-school:
with relations between measures, influence of social ecology and relation to the
attachment history. *Developmental Psychology*, **21**, 56–69.
Light, P. (1979). *Development of a Child's Sensitivity to People*. Cambridge:
Cambridge University Press.
Lütkenhaus, P., Grossmann, K. E. & Grossmann, K. (1985). Infant–mother
attachment at twelve months and style of interaction with a stranger at the age of
three years. *Child Development*, **56**, 1538–42.
Main, M., Kaplan, N. & Cassidy, J. (1985). Security in infancy, childhood and
adulthood: a move to the level of representation. In *Growing Points of Attachment
Theory and Research*, ed. I. Bretherton and E. Waters, pp. 66–104. Monograph of
the Society for Research in Child Development, Serial No. 209. Chicago:
University of Chicago Press.
Main, M. & Solomon, J. (1986). Discovery of an insecure disorganized/disoriented
attachment pattern. In *Affective Development in Infancy*, ed. T. B. Brazelton & M.
Yogman, pp. 95–124. Norwood, NJ: Ablex.
Main, M. & Stadtman, J. (1981). Infant response to rejection of physical contact by
the mother: aggression, avoidance and conflict. *Journal of the American Academy
of Child Psychiatry*, **20**, 292–307.
Main, M. & Weston, D. R. (1981). The quality of the toddler's relationship to mother
and to father related to conflict behaviour and the readiness to establish new
relationships. *Child Development*, **52**, 932–40.
Matas, L., Arend, R. A. & Sroufe, L. A. (1978). Continuity of adaptation in the
second year: the relationship between quality of attachment and later competence.
Child Development, **49**, 547–56.
Sroufe, L. A. (1983). Infant–caregiver attachment and patterns of adaptation in pre-
school: the roots of maladaptation and competence. In *Minnesota Symposium in
Child Psychology, Vol. 16*, ed. M. Perlmutter, pp. 41–81. Minneapolis: University
of Minnesota Press.
Sroufe, L. A. (1985). Attachment classification from the perspective of infant–
caregiver relationships and infant temperament. *Child Development*, **56**, 1–14.
Sroufe, L. A., Jacobvitz, D., Mangelsdorf, S., DeAngelo, E. & Ward, M. J. (1985).

Generational boundary dissolution between mothers and their preschool children: a relationship systems approach. *Child Development*, **56**, 317–25.

Wärtner, U. G. (1986). Attachment in infancy and at age six, and children's self-concept: a follow-up of a German longitudinal study. Doctoral dissertation, University of Virginia.

Waters, E. & Deane, K. A. (1985). Defining and assessing individual differences in attachment relationships: Q-methodology and the organization of behaviour in infancy and early childhood. In *Growing Points of Attachment Theory and Research*, ed. I. Bretherton and E. Waters, pp. 41–65. Chicago: University of Chicago Press.

Waters, E., Vaughn, B. E. & Egeland, B. R. (1980). Individual differences in infant–mother attachment relationships at age one: antecedents in neonatal behaviour in an urban economically disadvantaged sample. *Child Development*, **51**, 208–16.

(John Bowlby died on 2nd September, 1990)

—13—

Temperament and attachment: an eclectic approach

Joan Stevenson-Hinde

The futility of a dichotomy between the biological and social aspects of human nature is now generally recognized. (Hinde, 1989, p. 251).

Introduction

'In studies of psychological development, the child must be seen not as an isolated unit, but as a social being, forming part of a network of relationships. Interactions, relationships, social groups, and the sociocultural structure form successive levels of complexity, each level involving properties not relevant to lower levels.' (Hinde & Stevenson-Hinde, 1987, p. 1). Nevertheless, the nature of the interactions depends in part on what each participant brings to a situation. In the field of Child Development, two approaches have made major contributions to identifying and organising features of individuals which predict subsequent behaviour: temperament theory (e.g. Thomas & Chess, 1977; Buss & Plomin, 1984; Kohnstamm, Bates & Rothbart, 1989) and attachment theory (e.g. Bowlby, 1969/82; Ainsworth *et al.*, 1978; Parkes, Stevenson-Hinde, & Marris, 1990).

Unfortunately, the very success of each approach has led to one being pitted against the other. 'One sometimes senses a metaphorical struggle between the temperament and attachment constructs to project their broad explanatory powers and ensnare a piece of the infant's limited behavioral repertoire for their own purposes' (Goldsmith, Bradshaw & Rieser-Danner, 1986, pp. 28–9). While temperament constructs are held to be 'inherent', 'biologically based', or 'constitutional', attachment constructs are held to be relational. One is reminded of the nature/nurture controversy, which led many to conclude that 'such dichotomies are not only false but sterile' (Hinde, 1966/70, p. 426; see also Hebb, 1953; Lehrman, 1953; Beach 1955).

Indeed, such a dichotomy may lead to the false assumption that temperament, being 'constitutional', should take priority over relational constructs. For example, 'How do individual differences in the various

315

dimensions of temperament influence the developing attachment relationship?' (Goldsmith *et al.*, 1986, p. 5) is a more common question than the reverse, 'How does the attachment relationship affect dimensions of temperament?' (but see Sroufe, 1985). Neither question deals with the whole. Taking a systems perspective, in which there is a 'cycle of interaction' among elements of a system (e.g. Minuchin, 1985), such questions of priority fade away.

An eclectic approach

While isolation may be necessary during a theory's infancy, and displays of strength during its adolescence, maturity calls for a broadened view. The fruitfulness of an eclectic approach has been particularly demonstrated by Robert Hinde over the years (e.g. Hinde, 1966/70, 1979, 1987). He himself was influenced by meetings in the 1950s that brought together people with diverse orientations, organised on one side of the Atlantic by a physiological psychologist (Frank Beach) and on the other side by a psychiatrist (John Bowlby). In each case, integration was achieved by focusing on a particular area: sexual behaviour for Beach and the mother/child relationship for Bowlby. The outcome of such integration speaks for itself (e.g. Beach, 1948, 1965; Bowlby, 1969/82, 1973, 1980).

Another area that could benefit from an eclectic approach is the development of fearfulness or 'behavioural inhibition' in infants and young children. This refers particularly to 'the initial reaction to unfamiliar or challenging events' (Kagan, 1989, p. 2). While dimensions of temperament vary among theories of temperament, many include a dimension related to such reactions (reviewed in Rothbart, 1989). Since temperament is not a trait itself, but a 'rubric for a group of related traits' (Goldsmith *et al.*, 1987, p. 506), fearfulness will be used here as an exemplar of temperament.

Although well established as a temperament trait, and indeed 'one that has received the most attention thus far' (Kagan, 1989, p. 2), fearfulness may also be viewed from an attachment perspective as partially an outcome of insecurity of attachment. That is, a secure attachment relationship should dissipate fear and permit exploration, while an insecure relationship should augment fearfulness (Bowlby, 1969/82). Which is primary, the temperament or the attachment? As argued above, this is not a particularly fruitful question. If instead we return to the level of observables, then 'fearfulness' is indexed by fearful behaviour (see Stevenson-Hinde, 1989 for a clarification of terminology) and 'attachment' by attachment behaviour (see Hinde, 1982 for a clarification of terminology). Thus, we shall ask 'How does fearful behaviour develop in relation to attachment behaviour?'

With fearful behaviour, one may specify the contexts in which it occurs; differences in the intensity, quality, and patterning of the behaviour; and differences in outcome, with respect to avoiding or approaching the fear-eliciting stimulus. Similarly, with attachment behaviour, one may specify context, behaviour, and outcome. This allows each to be regarded as a 'behaviour system' (with quotes indicating 'theory language' as opposed to 'data language'). Such a term is a 'software' one, comparable to a computer program that performs a particular job irrespective of whether the computer into which it is fed employs valves, transistors, or integrated circuits' (Hinde, 1982, pp. 63–4; see also Hinde, 1966/70, Chapter 8). Thus 'behaviour system' is used here in an organisational rather than explanatory sense.

With a behaviour systems approach, 'Differences in responsiveness of one individual at different times can be understood on the basis of variations in the balance between different motivational systems' (Baerends, 1976, p. 733). Baerends' studies of incubating herring gulls exemplify this. For example, when given a choice of two egg models on the rim of a nest, an incubating herring gull normally retrieves the larger one first. However, when accompanying behaviour suggests a relatively high tendency to escape (escape system) compared with the tendency to incubate (incubation system), the smaller egg will be retrieved first (Baerends & Kruijt, 1973). While the precision of Baerends' experiments is not yet matched with human subjects, the concept of a behavioural system is nevertheless useful as a way of organising behavioural data. Distinct, but interacting behaviour systems have been postulated for both wary/fearful behaviour and attachment behaviour (e.g. Bowlby, 1969/82; Bretherton & Ainsworth, 1974; Bischof, 1975). For example, when a female stranger approached 2-year-olds, they looked at mother, remained in proximity with mother, and touched mother more than did 3 or 4-year-olds. It was therefore inferred that the stranger activated a fear behaviour system which then activated an attachment behaviour system, and that the activation was less in the older children (Greenberg & Marvin, 1982).

Methodological issues

Within a postulated behaviour system, intercorrelations between responses, or between different aspects of the same response, may be far from perfect. For example, in our present study with $2\frac{1}{2}$-year-olds, fear of stranger was assessed by *latency* to approach a female stranger when asked to come and see what she had in her hand, as well as by *ratings* of fear expressed. These measures were taken from video-tapes of the Ainsworth strange situation (Ainsworth *et al.*, 1978) with mother present (Episode 2), immediately after mother and child had been in the strange room on their own for 3 minutes (Episode 1). (Please note that with this sample of 'normal' $2\frac{1}{2}$-year-olds, 'wariness' is a more appropriate descriptor than 'fear' since the relevant behaviour was usually subtle.) Each rating was based on observational criteria, concerning the occurrence of wary/fearful behaviour patterns, involving facial expression (e.g. eyes wide; 'underbrow look'; ambivalent smile with lips compressed or while biting bottom lip), body posture and movement (e.g. tense or frozen postures; shoulders raised), and avoidant behaviour to stranger (e.g. look, turn or move away; hide). Ratings on a four-point scale were made when the stranger (i) entered the room, (ii) sat down, (iii) invited the child to approach her and see what she had in her hand, and (iv) sat on the floor to play with the child. The correlation between the sum of the four ratings and the latency was $r = 0.44$ ($N = 82$, $p < 0.001$, two-tailed). On the one hand, this is highly significant; on the other hand, it is far from perfect. Similar levels of intercorrelations among indices of fear occur in other studies (e.g. Reznick, 1989).

One reason for modest intercorrelations is measurement error. However, this is unlikely to be the sole reason, since similar correlations between measures of fear in a given context occur even in highly controlled situations with a standard stimulus. For example, chaffinches (*Fringilla coelebs*) and many other song birds emit a predictable and stereotyped 'mobbing' display to a stationary novel object or potential predator (for further description see Marler & Hamilton, 1966, p. 248–9). One component of this display is a discrete alarm call, which sounds like a 'chink' (see sound spectrograms in Marler & Hamilton, 1966, pp. 464–7). This response may be studied in the laboratory, by presenting an isolated chaffinch with a stationary stimulus for varying amounts of time, and with varying interstimulus intervals. The preparation has provided an excellent means of studying behavioural habituation (Hinde, 1970). Of interest here is that the alarm call may be taken as an index of 'fear'. Thus, the stronger the stimulus (e.g. stuffed owl > toy dog), the shorter the latency to the first alarm call, the higher the rate of occurrence over the first 6 minutes of the stimulus presentation, and the higher the rate during the second 6 minutes relative to the first 6 minutes (i.e. the response wanes more slowly with a stronger stimulus). Turning to intercorrelations, the correlation between rate of responding in the first 6 minutes and latency to the first response was $r = -0.59$ ($N = 100$) for an owl stimulus and -0.33 for a toy dog, and the correlation between rate of responding in the first 6 minutes and relative rate in the second 6 minutes was $+0.38$ for an owl and $+0.42$ for a dog. 'The correlations, however, are not very high, and indicate considerable independent individual variation in these response characteristics' (Hinde, 1960, p. 404).

Modest correlations between responding in the first versus the second part of a test could arise from differences in the duration of activation of a fear behaviour system given a constant stimulus. With the other correlations, two different types of measurement are involved: while the ratings are descriptions by 'the movements involved', latency to approach involves 'description by consequence' (Hinde, 1966/70, pp. 10–13). Thus, one child may have a high latency to approach but show little fear, while another may approach right away but show fearful behaviour while doing so.

Similarly, with an attachment behaviour system, alternative behaviour patterns may be employed by different children in the same context or by the same child in different contexts. For example, in contexts where the inferred goal may be gaining and/or maintaining proximity with an attachment figure, a human infant may cry, cling, suck or even smile (e.g. Bowlby, 1969/82; Ainsworth *et al.*, 1978). To the extent that different children have different 'preferred' patterns for a particular context, then intercorrelations between patterns will be low. Similarly, to the extent that a given child has a different pattern for different contexts (e.g. crying on separation but smiling on reunion), then correlations across contexts, or cross-situational consistency, will be low. Nevertheless, each child may be behaving entirely predictably. Thus, for both fearful behaviour and attachment behaviour, alternative behaviour patterns may be used toward a common goal, depending on the individual and the context.

Common features of attachment and fear behaviour systems

What features do an attachment behaviour system and a wary/fearful behaviour system have in common? The remainder of this chapter pursues this question.

Context

Particular stimuli which elicit attachment behaviour may be internal (e.g. illness, fatigue) or external (e.g. separation from the attachment figure). However, the context in which such stimuli occur is crucial (see also Radke-Yarrow, Chapter 16). For example, if a child is at home and used to mother coming and going from one room to another, attachment behaviour may not be activated when she leaves the room. On the other hand, attachment behaviour is likely to be activated if the child is in a strange situation and the mother leaves (see Ainsworth *et al.*, 1978).

Similarly, the occurrence of fearful behaviour depends crucially on context, as well as on aspects of a stimulus which is novel and/or perceived to be potentially harmful. As with attachment behaviour, fearful behaviour is more likely to occur in the context of a strange situation than at home, and with increased distance from mother (e.g. Sroufe, Waters & Matas, 1974; Skarin, 1977).

Outcome

In the sense of having a predictable outcome, both fearful and attachment behaviour may be viewed as 'goal-directed' (Hinde & Stevenson, 1969). A predictable goal of attachment behaviour is gaining and/or maintaining proximity or communication with an attachment figure (e.g. Bowlby, 1969/82, Chapter 12; Ainsworth *et al.*, 1978). In human infants, heart rate may accelerate upon separation from mother and decrease once proximity is regained (Sroufe & Waters, 1977).

The outcome of fearful behaviour is to decrease or avoid proximity to and/or interaction with the feared object, either through a caregiver's intervention or through the child's own behaviour. Avoidance of a fear-eliciting stimulus has been likened to 'cut-off' behaviour, with the outcome of decreasing 'arousal' as indicated by a decrease in heart rate (Sroufe & Waters, 1977). For example, gaze aversion to a stranger occurred when heart rate acceleration was near its peak, and the infant again looked at the stranger when the rate neared basal level. Additionally, one may postulate an approach/avoidance conflict. In the above example of an owl eliciting alarm behaviour in a chaffinch, if a postulated avoidance threshold became lower than an approach threshold, then flight would ensue, with the outcome of decreased arousal (see Hinde, 1954). In fact, this may not be too far off as an explanation of the behaviour of a child who does show some fear of a stranger but does not actually move away. If the stranger were to become too intrusive, then 'flight' would occur instead. (It should be noted that some dimensions of temperament, such as 'activity' and 'intensity of expression' [see e.g. Thomas & Chess, 1977; Goldsmith *et al.*, 1987], do not have an obvious outcome and therefore cannot be viewed as a goal-directed behaviour system. Nevertheless, most of the present headings do apply to all dimensions.)

Function

In evolutionary terms, a common function of both a fear and an attachment system is thought to be protection from harm (Bowlby, 1969/82; Sroufe, 1977; Ainsworth *et al.*, 1978). Fear of the unfamiliar or of being left alone would have been essential for survival in the environment in which we evolved. Interestingly, children's 'irrational fears' such as fear of the dark, fear of water and fear of snakes are more ubiquitous in children than are fears more appropriate to the present day, such as fear of cars or guns (Marks, 1987). Thus, our propensities both to fear certain situations and to maintain proximity with mothers may have been guided by natural selection, with the common function of protection from harm.

320

Development

Early appearance. Behaviour patterns such as sucking, clinging, smiling, or crying, which can all serve as attachment behaviour, are present from birth. Similarly, components of fearful behaviour, such as crying or startle responses, are present from birth. However, in the above sense of a goal-directed behaviour system, both an attachment and a fear behaviour system may properly be inferred only over the last half of the first year of life. For example, the onset of negative responses to a stranger, such as a frown or gaze aversion, occurs during the second half of the first year (e.g. Schaffer, Greenwood & Parry, 1972; Waters, Matas & Sroufe, 1975). Over a similar age range, attachment behaviour becomes more 'organised' (e.g. Bowlby, 1969/82; Ainsworth *et al.*, 1978). Both coincide with a developmental shift in the expression of emotionality (Emde, Gaensbauer & Harmon, 1976).

Changes in expression. Age-appropriate behaviour is observed in relation to both systems. For example, while an infant may cry when mother leaves, an older child may follow mother, or still later ask her where she is going. Similar developmental changes occur with fearful behaviour. Whereas an infant might cry on meeting a stranger, a toddler might withdraw and/or have a fearful expression, and an older child might look down and have a relatively long latency to speak to the stranger. Such changes need not imply instability, but rather they may reflect 'heterotypic continuity' (Kagan, 1971).

Narrowing the range of objects of attachment or fear. An infant's attachment behaviour initially occurs in an undirected manner, then is undiscriminatingly directed to any available person, and finally to preferred figures. Attachment preferences do not emerge until about 4 months of age (Bowlby, 1969/82; Ainsworth *et al.*, 1978).

Similarly, stimuli which elicit fear are initially wide-ranging, and then become narrowed. A particularly good example of 'tuning' a fear response, and of the importance of interactions with others for doing this, is provided by Seyfarth & Cheney's (1986) experiments with vervet monkeys. The adults of this species respond with a different alarm call to each of three types of predators: snakes, mammalian predators, and birds of prey. Young vervets initially respond to a wide range of objects. They may give a response appropriate to a bird of prey to a falling leaf. However, they come to give an alarm call appropriate to each type of predator, and not to falling leaves, through observing adults, especially their mothers. With humans, some infants are particularly prone to the acquisition of learned fears (Bronson & Pankey, 1977).

Changes in objects of attachment or fear.   In addition to the range of appropriate stimuli narrowing during development, the nature of appropriate stimuli changes as well. With attachment behaviour, whereas parental figures are preferred early on, humans turn to peers in adolescence and adulthood. This does not mean that early attachments disappear, just that new ones are preferred. Parents may still be turned to when all else fails, and their loss mourned (Weiss, 1982; Ainsworth, 1990).

Similarly with fearful behaviour, while a strange adult is an appropriate stimulus for eliciting mildly fearful (or wary: see Sroufe, 1977) behaviour in infants, a more potent stimulus in early childhood is an unfamiliar peer(s) (Kagan, Reznick & Snidman, 1987). Still later, a situation which involves being evaluated may produce behaviour indicating 'fear of negative evaluation' (e.g Asendorpf, 1986), something not observed at earlier ages.

Social influences

Fearful behaviour.   Social influences on fearful behaviour may be inferred from studies involving comparisons between boys and girls in terms of what social interactions were associated with the behaviour in question. Take for example shyness, rated from maternal interview questions about initial approach/withdrawal to strange people and places (Garside *et al.*, 1975). Individuals were consistent from 42 to 50 months (Spearman $r = 0.61$, $N = 41$, $p < 0.001$, two-tailed). For girls at 50 months, shyness was significantly *positively* correlated with: mother sensitive to child, mother enjoys child, joint activities with mother and with father, a positive relationship with the sibling, and conversational questions to mother. On the other hand, shyness was *negatively* correlated with: child actively hostile to mother, child passive (i.e. not engaged) with mother, mother/child activity changes (implying that they did not do one thing for long), child reactively hostile to peers in nursery school, and both peers and adults disconfirming the child. For 50-month-old boys, each set of correlations went in the opposite direction (for details see Hinde, Stevenson-Hinde & Tamplin, 1985; Simpson & Stevenson-Hinde, 1985).

Similar associations have been found by Radke-Yarrow and her colleagues in their research on families with and without a history of psychiatric disorder. They found that 'Mothers seemed not to be pleased with shyness in boys. Boys' shyness was associated with less joyfulness in their mothers. Mothers' interactions with shy girls, in contrast, where characterised by tenderness, affection, and sadness' (Radke-Yarrow, Richters & Wilson, 1988, p. 58). They also found that behavioural correlates of shyness differed between boys and girls, with shyness in boys associated with tension and negative mood and shyness in girls 'associated with a more complex set of personal qualities, including tension, sadness, lower levels of anger and social competence, and higher levels of affection and compliance' (p. 58).

During the interviews in our own study, some mothers complained that their sons should have grown out of their shyness, having been in nursery school for a year, while others commented with pleasure that their daughters still preferred being at home with them. Thus, mothers (and fathers) may have different attitudes towards shyness in boys and shyness in girls, with shyness in boys becoming less acceptable as they get older. This agrees with the findings of Kagan *et al.* (1987), that of children selected as being inhibited or uninhibited at 21 months, more boys than girls had changed from inhibited to uninhibited at $5\frac{1}{2}$ years. On the other hand, 'A much smaller group of originally uninhibited children, about 10% and typically girls from working-class families, became more inhibited at later ages. The interviews with these mothers suggested they wanted a more cautious child and encouraged such a profile' (p. 1462).

Attachment behaviour.   Perhaps the most interesting and potentially fruitful measures of interactions involve not intensity, but quality and patterning (see e.g. Ainsworth *et al.*, 1978; Hinde, 1979; Radke-Yarrow *et al.*, 1988). For example, Ainsworth's system of coding reunion behaviour with mother relies not just on the intensity of the attachment behaviour shown, but also on the quality and patterning of responses. Three basic patterns observed on reunion have proved particularly useful in predicting later behaviour. They may be briefly described as:

Secure: Calm, intimate interactions with full gaze and positive affect, indicating that the relationship is 'special';

Insecure–avoidant: Ignoring or minimal responses, gaze aversion, turning away.

Insecure–ambivalent: Immature, whiny, dependent behaviour, often with ambivalence to physical proximity/contact.

In addition, an *Insecure–controlling* pattern has been found in children aged $2\frac{1}{2}$–7 years, in which the child takes control of the reunion. This may be done in a neutral manner, or with elements of caregiving or punitive behaviour. (Detailed descriptions of such patterns may be found in Ainsworth *et al.*, 1978 (for infants); Cassidy & Marvin, 1989 (for 3 to 4-year-olds), and Main & Cassidy, 1988 (for 6-year-olds).)

Such patterns of attachment have been related both to antecedent mother–infant interactions as well as to subsequent behaviour (see also Bowlby, Chapter 12; Rutter, Chapter 14). In addition to the classic work of Ainsworth (summarised in Ainsworth *et al.*, 1978), the Grossmanns' longitudinal studies have related maternal sensitivity – reflected in affectionate holding, appropriate reactions to crying, and frequent responses to vocalisations, often with a tender-warm voice quality – to a secure classification with mother in the strange situation (Grossmann *et al.*, 1985; Grossmann & Grossmann, 1990a). Insecure patterns are viewed as strategies developed by the child in the course of interacting with an attachment figure who does not show the above characteristics of sensitivity. Thus, an Insecure–avoidant pattern upon reunion may reflect a strategy of independence from a rejecting mother (Main & Weston, 1982), while an Insecure–ambivalent pattern may reflect a strategy of emphasised dependence to an unpredictable mother (Egeland & Farber, 1984), and an Insecure–controlling pattern may reflect a child who has had to 'take charge' with a mother who is emotionally unavailable, due to problems of her own, such as depression or lack of resolution of mourning (Ainsworth & Eichberg, 1990; Main & Hesse, 1990; Radke-Yarrow, 1990).

Individual differences

Upon reunion with mother after a brief separation, most infants regain proximity with mother in a positive and relaxed way. However, some infants show insecure patterns of attachment, as described above. Given stable family circumstances, such individual differences in the quality of attachment to mother have been shown to be stable over the first 6 years (reviewed by Bowlby, Chapter 12).

With fearful behaviour, consistent individual differences are also documented, from infancy to childhood (e.g. Rothbart, 1989). For example, in a sample of extreme children, selected at 21 months as being either inhibited or uninhibited, indices of behavioural inhibition were significantly correlated over the years, with $r = 0.67$ ($p < 0.001$) from 21 months to $7\frac{1}{2}$ years (Kagan *et al.*, 1988). Ways in which individual differences may operate as either protective factors or risk factors for later disorders are considered by Bowlby (Chapter 12) and by Rutter (Chapter 14) in this volume.

Interplay between fear of strangers and patterns of attachment

Both temperament and attachment theorists would agree that, other things being equal, insecure children should be most fearful. With our sample of $2\frac{1}{2}$-year-olds, we found a significant negative correlation of $r = -0.32$ ($N = 82$) between fear of stranger and security ratings which ranged from 1 (highly insecure) to 9 (highly secure). One would also expect the above attachment strategies to be associated with the expression of fear. Thus, children emphasising *dependence* would be expected to be observed as most fearful, while those with *avoidant* or *controlling* strategies should hide their fearfulness as much as possible. Finally, the children classed as very secure should be able to express their feelings freely to a sensitively responsive mother (e.g. Grossmann & Grossmann, 1990b), with no 'strategy' required, if they were indeed frightened. In our sample of $2\frac{1}{2}$-year-olds, the *Very secure* children were the least fearful, and the *Insecure–ambivalent* children the most fearful. Within the secure subclassifications (i.e. Very secure, Secure–reserved, Secure–dependent, and Secure–controlling), the most fearful were the children classes as *Secure–dependent* (Stevenson-Hinde & Shouldice, 1990).

Although our own ratings of fearful behaviour assessed quality as well as intensity, to our knowledge fearful behaviour has not been coded for its patterning with respect to context and time. Such coding would have the advantage of implying something about the 'fit' between the behaviour and the context in which it occurs. It might therefore provide more homogeneous measures over different contexts and over time than measures along a single dimension. For example, while low fear may be appropriate in the laboratory situation of meeting an adult female stranger, it may not be appropriate in other situations. Coding for patterns would necessitate careful development of coding systems suitable for particular contexts and particular ages. Yet to jump ahead, one outcome might be classifications generally described as 'shows fearful behaviour that is appropriate to the type and intensity of the fear-eliciting stimulus and appropriate changes in the behaviour over time'; 'over-reacts in terms of the intensity, quality and duration of the fearful behaviour'; or 'under-reacts', avoids, 'cuts off' the fearful stimulus, thereby decreasing the opportunity for exploration of the object'. Predicted parallels with attachment behaviour are obvious, and knowledge of both patterns would say a lot about a child's behavioural style.

Conclusion

I have argued that pitting 'temperament' against 'attachment' has not been particularly fruitful. When a dimension of temperament, namely fearfulness, and attachment are described in terms of behavioural systems, barriers between the two approaches fade away. There is no reason to assert that a 'fear behaviour system' is any more 'biological' or 'constitutional' or primary than an 'attachment behaviour system'. Both share common properties, in terms of the relevance of context, outcome, and function. In addition, both are early appearing, change during development, and are influenced by interactions with others. Finally, both show consistent individual differences from infancy to early childhood, and probably beyond.

The postulation of discrete behavioural systems should not obscure relations between them. Activation of a fear behaviour system may lead to activation of an attachment behaviour system in all infants or young children, many times over. Furthermore, such activation will occur in the context of close relationships, with influences being mutual during the course of development.

Acknowledgements

I should like to acknowledge funding by the Medical Research Council, London and to thank J. Bowlby, R. A. Hinde, R. S. Marvin, and L. A. Sroufe for their helpful comments on the manuscript.

I hope this chapter will speak for, and live up to, the influence of Robert Hinde's work on my own thinking. Although the chapter is explicitly concerned with temperament and attachment approaches, an ethological approach is pervasive. For this, I am grateful to Robert, as well as to Bill Thorpe and others from Madingley, including the editor of this volume.

References

Ainsworth, M. D. S. (1990). Attachment and other affectional bonds across the life cycle. In *Attachment Across the Life Cycle*, ed. C. M. Parkes, J. Stevenson-Hinde and P. Marris. New York: Routledge (in press).

Ainsworth, M. D. S., Blehar, M. C., Water, E. & Wall, S. (1978). *Patterns of Attachment*. Hillsdale, NJ: Erlbaum.

Ainsworth, M. D. S. & Eichberg, C. G (1990). Effects on infant–mother attachment of mother's unresolved loss of an attachment figure or other traumatic experience. In *Attachment across the Life Cycle*, ed. C. M. Parkes, J. Stevenson-Hinde and P. Marris. New York: Routledge (in press).

Asendorpf, J. (1986). Shyness in middle and late childhood. In *Shyness: Perspectives on Research and Treatment*, ed. W. H. Jones, J. M. Cheek and S. R. Briggs, pp. 91–103. New York: Plenum Press.

Baerends, G. P. (1976). The functional organization of behaviour. *Animal Behaviour*, **24**, 726–38.

Baerends, G. P. & Kruijt, J. P. (1973). Stimulus selection. In *Constraints on Learning*, ed. R. A. Hinde and J. Stevenson-Hinde, pp. 23–50. New York: Academic Press.

Beach, F. A. (1948). *Hormones and Behavior*. New York: Hoeber.

Beach, F. A. (1955). The descent of instinct. *Psychological Review*, **62**, 401–10.

Beach, F. A. (ed.) (1965). *Sex and Behavior*. New York: John Wiley.

Bischof, N. (1975). A systems approach toward the functional connections of fear and attachment. *Child Development*, **46**, 801–17.

Bowlby, J. (1969/82). *Attachment and Loss, Vol. 1. Attachment*. London: Hogarth Press.

Bowlby, J. (1973). *Attachment and Loss, Vol. 2. Separation*. New York: Basic Books.

Bowlby, J. (1980). *Attachment and Loss, Vol. 3. Loss, Sadness and Depression*. New York: Basic Books.

Bretherton, I. & Ainsworth, M. D. S. (1974). Responses of one-year-olds to a stranger in a strange situation. In *The Origins of Fear*, ed. M. Lewis and L. A. Rosenblum, pp. 131–64. New York: John Wiley.

Bronson, G. W. & Pankey, W. B. (1977). On the distinction between fear and wariness. *Child Development*, **48**, 1167–83.

Buss, A. H. & Plomin, R. (1984). *Temperament: Early Developing Personality Traits.* Hillsdale, NJ: Erlbaum.

Cassidy, J. & Marvin, R. S. (1989). *Attachment Organization in Preschool Children: Coding Guidelines.* Seattle: MacArthur Working Group on Attachment.

Egeland, B. & Farber, E. A. (1984). Infant–mother attachment: Factors related to its development and changes over time. *Child Development*, **55**, 753–71.

Emde, R. N., Gaensbauer, T. & Harmon, R. (1976). Emotional expression in infancy: A biobehavioral study. *Psychological Issues*, Monogr. 37. New York: International Universities Press.

Garside, R. F., Birch, H., Scott, D., Chambers, S., Kolvin, I., Tweddle, E. G. & Barber, L. M. (1975). Dimensions of temperament in infant school children. *Journal of Child Psychology and Psychiatry*, **16**, 219–31.

Goldsmith, H. H., Bradshaw, D. L. & Rieser-Danner, L. A. (1986). Temperament as a potential developmental influence on attachment. In *Temperament and Social Interaction during Infancy and Childhood: New Directions for Child Development, No. 31*, ed. J. V. Lerner, & R. M. Lerner, pp 5–34. San Francisco: Jossey-Bass.

Goldsmith, H., Buss, A. H., Plomin, R. Rothbart, M K., Thomas, A., Chess, S., Hinde, R. A. & McCall, R. B. (1987). What is temperament? Four approaches. *Child Development*, **58**, 505–29.

Greenberg, M. T. & Marvin, R. S. (1982). Reactions of preschool children to an adult stranger: A behavioral systems approach. *Child Development*, **53**, 481–90.

Grossmann, K. & Grossmann, K. E. (1990a). Newborn behavior, early parenting quality and later toddler–parent relationships in a group of German infants. In *The Cultural Context of Infancy, Vol. II*, ed. J. K. Nugent, B. M. Lester and T. B. Brazelton. Norwood, NJ: Ablex (in press).

Grossmann, K. F. & Grossmann, K. (1990b). Attachment quality as an organizer of emotional and behavioral responses. In *Attachment Across the Life Cycle*, ed. C. M. Parkes, J. Stevenson-Hinde, & P. Marris. New York: Routledge (in press).

Grossmann, K., Grossmann, K. E., Spangler, G., Suess, G. & Unzner, L. (1985). Maternal sensitivity and newborns' orientation responses as related to quality of attachment in northern Germany. In *Growing Points of Attachment Theory and Research*, ed. I. Bretherton & E. Waters. *Monographs of the Society for Research in Child Development*, **50**, (1–2, Serial No. 209).

Hebb, D. O. (1953). Heredity and environment in mammalian behaviour. *British Journal of Animal Behaviour*, **1**, 43–7.

Hinde, R. A. (1954). Changes in responsiveness to a constant stimulus. *British Journal of Animal Behaviour*, **2**, 41–55.

Hinde, R. A. (1960). Factors governing the changes in strength of a partially inborn response, as shown by the mobbing behaviour of the chaffinch (*Fringilla coelebs*): III. The interaction of short-term and long-term incremental and decremental effects. *Proceedings of the Royal Society*, B, **153**, 398–420.

Hinde, R. A. (1966/70). *Animal Behaviour: A Synthesis of Ethology and Comparative Psychology*, 2nd edition. New York: McGraw-Hill.

Hinde, R. A. (1970). Behavioural habituation. In *Short-term Changes in Neural Activity and Behaviour*, ed. G. Horn & R. A. Hinde, pp. 3–40. Cambridge: Cambridge University Press.

Hinde, R. A. (1979). *Towards Understanding Relationships*. London: Academic Press.

Hinde, R. A. (1982). Attachment: Some conceptual and biological issues. In *The Place of Attachment in Human Behavior*, ed. C. M. Parkes and J. Stevenson-Hinde, pp. 60–76. New York: Basic Books.

Hinde, R. A. (1987). *Individuals, Relationships and Culture: Links between Ethology and the Social Sciences.* Cambridge: Cambridge University Press.

Hinde, R. A. (1989). Ethological and relationship approaches. *Annals of Child Development,* **6,** 251–85.

Hinde, R. A. & Stevenson, J. G. (1969). Goals and response control. In *Development and Evolution of Behavior,* ed. L. R. Aronson *et al.,* pp. 216–37. New York: Freeman.

Hinde, R. A. & Stevenson-Hinde, J. (1987). Interpersonal relationships and child development. *Developmental Review,* **7,** 1–21.

Hinde, R. A., Stevenson-Hinde, J. & Tamplin, A. (1985). Characteristics of 3–4 year olds assessed at home and interactions in preschool. *Developmental Psychology,* **21,** 130–40.

Kagan, J. (1971). *Change and Continuity in Infancy.* New York: John Wiley.

Kagan, J (1989). The concept of behavioral inhibition to the unfamiliar. In *Perspectives on Behavioral Inhibition,* ed. J. S. Reznick, pp. 1–23. Chicago: University of Chicago Press.

Kagan, J., Reznick, J S. & Snidman, N. (1987). The physiology and psychology of behavioral inhibition in children. *Child Development,* **58,** 1459–73.

Kagan, J. Reznick, J. S., Snidman, N., Gibbons, J. & Johnson, M. O. (1988). Childhood derivatives of inhibition and lack of inhibition to the unfamiliar. *Child Development,* **59,** 1580–9.

Kohnstamm, G. A., Bates, J. E. & Rothbart, M. K. (ed.) (1989). *Temperament in Childhood.* New York: John Wiley.

Lehrman, D. S. (1953). A critique of Konrad Lorenz's theory of instinctive behaviour. *Quarterley Review of Biology,* **28,** 337–63.

Main, M. & Cassidy, J. (1988). Categories of response to reunion with the parent at age 6: predictable from infant attachment classifications and stable over a 1-month period. *Developmental Psychology,* **24,** 415–26.

Main, M. & Hesse, E. (1990). Lack of resolution of mourning in adulthood and its relationship to infant disorganization: Some speculations regarding causal mechanisms. In *Attachment in the Preschool Years: Theory, Research and Intervention,* ed. M. Greenberg, D. Cichetti and M. Cummings. Chicago: University of Chicago Press (in press).

Main, M. & Weston, D. (1982). Avoidance of the attachment figure in infancy: Descriptions and interpretations. In *The Place of Attachment in Human Behavior,* ed. C. M. Parkes and J. Stevenson-Hinde, pp. 31–59. New York: Basic Books.

Marks, I. M. (1987). *Fears, Phobias and Rituals.* Oxford: Oxford University Press.

Marler, P. & Hamilton, W. J. (1966). *Mechanisms of Animal Behavior.* New York: John Wiley.

Minuchin, P. (1985). Families and individual development: Provocations from the field of family therapy. *Child Development,* **56,** 289–302.

Parkes, C. M., Stevenson-Hinde, J. & Marris, P. (ed.) (1990). *Attachment across the Life Cycle.* New York: Routledge (in press).

Radke-Yarrow, M. (1990). Attachment patterns in children of depressed mothers. In *Attachment across the Life Cycle,* ed. C. M. Parkes, J. Stevenson-Hinde and P. Marris. New York: Routledge (in press).

Radke-Yarrow, M., Richters, J. & Wilson, W. E. (1988). Child development in a network of relationships. In *Relationships within Families: Mutual Influences,* ed. R. A. Hinde and J. Stevenson-Hinde, pp. 48–67. Oxford: Clarendon Press.

Reznick, J. S. (1989). Behavioral inhibition in a normative sample. In *Perspectives on*

Behavioral Inhibition, ed. J. S. Reznick, pp. 25–49. Chicago: University of Chicago Press.

Rothbart, M. K. (1989). Behavioral approach and inhibition. In *Perspectives on Behavioral Inhibition*, ed. J. S. Reznick, pp. 139–57. Chicago: University of Chicago Press.

Schaffer, H., Greenwood, A. & Parry, M. (1972). The onset of wariness. *Child Development*, **43**, 164–75.

Seyfarth, R. & Cheney, D. (1986). Vocal development in vervet monkeys. *Animal Behaviour*, **34**, 1640–58.

Simpson, E. E. & Stevenson-Hinde, J. (1985). Temperamental characteristics of three- to four-year-old boys and girls and child–family interactions. *Journal of Child Psychology and Psychiatry*, **26**, 43–53.

Skarin, K. (1977). Cognitive and contextual determinants of stranger fear in six- and eleven-month-old infants. *Child Development*, **48**, 537–44.

Sroufe, L. A. (1977). Wariness of strangers and the study of infant development. *Child Development*, **48**, 731–46.

Sroufe, L. A. (1985). Attachment classification from the perspective of infant–caregiver relationships and infant temperament. *Child Development*, **56**, 1–14.

Sroufe, L. A. & Waters, E. (1977). Heart rate as a convergent measure in clinical and developmental research. *Merril-Palmer Quarterly*, **23**, 3–25.

Sroufe, L. A., Waters, E. & Matas, L. (1974). Contextual determinants of infant affective response. In *The Origins of Fear*, ed. M. Lewis & L. Rosenblum, pp. 49–72. New York: John Wiley.

Stevenson-Hinde, J. (1989). Behavioral inhibition: Issues of context. In *Perspectives on Behavioral Inhibition*, ed. J. S. Reznick, pp. 125–38. Chicago: University of Chicago Press.

Stevenson-Hinde, J. & Shouldice, A. (1990). Fear and attachment in 2·5-year-olds. *British Journal of Developmental Psychology* (in press).

Thomas, A. & Chess, S. (1977). *Temperament and Development*. New York: Brunner/Mazel.

Waters, E., Matas, L. & Sroufe, L. A (1975). Infants' reactions to an approaching stranger: description, validation, and functional significance of wariness. *Child Development*, **46**, 348–56.

Weiss, R. S. (1982). Attachment in adult life. In *The Place of Attachment in Human Behavior*, ed. C. M. Parkes and J. Stevenson-Hinde, pp. 171–84. New York: Basic Books.

—14—

A fresh look at 'maternal deprivation'

Michael Rutter

Bowlby's (1951) World Health Organization monograph on *Maternal Care and Mental Health* made a major impact when it first appeared and, although it was published nearly 40 years ago, its concepts and policy recommendations continue to excite controversy (Ernst, 1988). This is evident, for example, in the continuing disputes over possible ill-effects associated with maternal employment (Gottfried & Gottfried, 1988) and group day care (Belsky, 1988; McCartney & Galanopoulos, 1988; Terr, 1989), and in the arguments over whether or not parental loss in early childhood predisposes to depression in adult life (Tennant, 1988). It might appear at first sight that there has been little progress because these issues so closely parallel those that led to vigorous debate in the 1950s. However, this impression is mistaken. The accumulation of research findings has led to important shifts in the intellectual battleground; some of the original tenets have come to be generally accepted while others have had to be abandoned. Perhaps, most crucially, the growth of knowledge has raised new issues of considerable theoretical and practical importance. The time seems opportune to re-evaluate the concept of 'maternal deprivation' and to consider where it has led us and what are the directions for future research.

It is particularly appropriate to do so in this volume because Robert Hinde has played such a central role in the clarification of ideas on the topic; because his experimental studies with rhesus monkeys both established the reality of behavioural effects from separation experiences and indicated some of the mechanisms involved (Hinde, 1977; Hinde & McGinnis, 1977); because his thinking on the development of relationships has been so seminal (Hinde, 1979; Hinde & Stevenson-Hinde, 1987a); and because his current research is continuing to focus attention on key issues in human social development (Hinde & Stevenson-Hinde, 1987b). It is significant that, in the

331

first volume of his trilogy on *Attachment*, Bowlby (1969) expressed his strong reliance on Robert Hinde (see also Bowlby, Chapter 12). My own indebtedness is at least as great as I made clear in my 1972 (Rutter, 1972) reassessment of 'maternal deprivation'. This chapter provides a welcome opportunity to acknowledge the huge extent to which my own research and concepts have been influenced by Robert Hinde's concepts and ideas and, more personally, to express gratitude for the innumerable occasions when his wise guidance (always given generously however busy he has been) has been crucial.

1951 Postulates regarding 'maternal deprivation'

The 1951 monograph originally arose out of a WHO request to assess the mental health consequences for 'children who are orphaned or separated from their families for other reasons and need care in foster homes, institutions or other types of group care' (Bowlby, 1951, p. 7). The finding, based on many studies (albeit often of uncertain quality), that such children frequently suffer psychological problems was scarcely surprising. However, the inferences based on this finding gave rise to vigorous dispute. Bowlby's general proposition was that 'the prolonged deprivation of the young child of maternal care may have grave and far-reaching effects on his character and so on the whole of his future life' (Bowlby, 1951, p. 46). The main tenets underlying this conclusion may be summarised as follows: (i) the association represents a causal relationship, attributable to life experiences; (ii) the key factor in 'maternal deprivation' is the lack of a warm, intimate, and continuous relationship with the mother; (iii) such deprivation includes quite brief mother–child separations as well as long-term foster care (Bowlby, Robertson & Rosenbluth, 1952); (iv) the ill-effects stem from deprivation in infancy, rather than from experiences in middle childhood or later; (v) infancy represents a critical period so that good experiences later cannot compensate (good mothering 'is almost useless if delayed after the age of $2\frac{1}{2}$ years': p. 49); (vi) although some children escape damage, the effects tend to be permanent; and (vii) the consequences of deprivation are wide-ranging, encompassing especially psychopathic character development but also cognitive impairment, anxiety and depression.

Although Bowlby's review dealt almost entirely with studies of children experiencing prolonged institutional care or severely disrupted discordant family relationships, the concept of deprivation was extended very broadly by other writers to include the experiences stemming from group day care (WHO Expert Committee on Mental Health, 1951) or from having a mother with a job outside the home (Baers, 1954). It should be added that, of course, Bowlby's (1988) current views differ in several crucial respects from those espoused in 1951 (see Bowlby, Chapter 12). In no respect does this essay constitute a critique of Bowlby's theoretical position; rather, it seeks to outline some of the ways in which a high influential report led to research that has greatly advanced our knowledge on the nature of and influences on social development. Only brief reference is made to research undertaken up to the late 1970s, as it has been reviewed previously (Rutter, 1981a). Instead, the main focus is on issues and findings that are of current importance and which seem likely to guide future research and practice.

However, it is necessary to start with the features that first gave rise to controversy. Five may be singled out. First, critics argued that the observed effects might well be a consequence of genetic factors (Wootton, 1959, 1962; O'Connor & Franks, 1960). Second, it was argued that it was not 'mother love' that mattered but rather a stimulating interaction between the child and other people (Casler, 1961, 1968) and the availability of readily discriminable effective contingencies in response to the child's behaviour so that adequate learning can take place (Gewirtz, 1968, 1969). Third, scepticism was expressed regarding the suggestion that the same mechanism was responsible for sequelae as varied as acute emotional distress, intellectual retardation, and antisocial behaviour (Rutter, 1972). Fourth, it was doubted that infancy constituted a critical period in the sense that experiences during that age period had effects that were not seen following comparable experiences at later ages (Clarke & Clarke, 1976). Finally, queries were raised with respect to the claim of permanent, irreversible effects stemming from experiences confined to the infancy period (Clarke & Clarke, 1976).

Testing of the environmental effect hypothesis

Animal studies provided the first critical test of the environmental effect hypothesis. Hinde and his colleagues undertook a series of well-planned investigations of the short- and long-term effects of separation experiences in rhesus monkeys under different conditions (Hinde & Spencer-Booth, 1971; Hinde & McGinnis, 1977). The results were clear-cut in showing that such experiences led to socio-emotional effects that could be quite long-lasting. Subsequent research by other workers has confirmed these findings (see e.g. Mineka & Suomi, 1978; Levine, 1982; Capitanio *et al.*, 1986). Both acute separation experiences and long-term patterns of rearing (as shown by cross-fostering experiments – Suomi, 1987) influence emotional reactivity in infant monkeys.

These findings provided convincing evidence of experimentally induced effects on emotional responsiveness but did not address the 'maternal deprivation' postulate that disrupted discontinuous parenting leads to seriously impaired social relationships ('affectionless psychopathy' in their extreme form). The studies by Harlow and his colleagues (Harlow & Harlow, 1969; Ruppenthal *et al.*, 1976) of rhesus monkeys reared in social isolation showed that this grossly abnormal pattern of rearing led to severe abnormalities in sexual and parenting behaviour in adult life. It was clear that a total lack of responsive parenting (the isolated monkeys had mechanical surrogate 'mothers') did indeed have a devastating effect in the development of social relationships. Of course, such isolation constitutes a grossly abnormal experience without any direct parallels with the patterns of rearing usually included under 'maternal deprivation'. Moreover, as Hinde has emphasised repeatedly, although animal studies are useful because they can demonstrate mechanisms or processes that may be applicable to humans, the extrapolation to other species must be tested directly, rather than assumed. Nevertheless, the animal research certainly made clear that stressful or otherwise adverse experiences *could* give rise to many of the effects hypothesised to follow 'maternal deprivation'.

It has proved more difficult to test the environmental effect hypothesis directly in humans in terms of the specific experiences provided by the parent and outcomes subsumed under the original 'maternal deprivation' concept. However, a substantial body of research has tested environmental effects on different aspects of development.

The findings are, perhaps, most clear cut with respect to cognitive development (Rutter, 1985a). Five main types of evidence provide the most critical test. First, the intellectual development of children from severely disadvantaged homes who are adopted into socially superior homes has been compared with that of their biological half-siblings. Schiff & Lewontin (1986) found that the IQ of the latter was a dozen points below that of the former – providing convincing evidence of a causal effect stemming from the difference in rearing conditions. The data from other studies (Scarr & Weinberg, 1976; Horn, 1983) point to the same conclusion. Second, the same basic design allows testing of environmental effects by means of parent–child correlations in the adoptive families. These tend to be appreciably lower than the comparable correlations in biological families (Rutter, 1985a), where the correlation reflects both genetic and environmental effects. Nevertheless, the presence of significant effects associated with the social class of adoptive parents (Duyme, 1988) points to a substantial environmental effect. Third, the comparison of siblings and half-siblings reared apart and together also allows a teasing apart of genetic and environmental effects (Teasdale & Owen, 1984). Again, a substantial environmental effect is evident, albeit greater for scholastic performance than on IQ. Fourth, the intellectual recovery of children following rescue from extremely adverse conditions of rearing indicates a major environmental influence (Skuse, 1984). Fifth, the beneficial effects of the experimental introduction of family and preschool interventions also attest to environmental effects on cognitive performance (Garber & Heber, 1982; Lazar & Darlington, 1982; Ramey, MacPhee & Yeates, 1982; Berrueta-Clemont *et al.*, 1984; Ramey & Campbell, 1984; Garber, 1988; Lee, Brooks-Gunn & Schnur, 1988). We may conclude that the deleterious effects of markedly adverse rearing conditions on cognitive performance have been confirmed and do indeed represent an environmental influence.

Similar research designs could be used to test the environmental hypothesis with respect to social deficits and behavioural disturbance but fewer rigorous investigations have clearly separated genetic and environmental effects. Nevertheless, some findings again point to a substantial environmental effect. Thus, adoption studies have shown that antisocial behaviour is more prevalent in individuals reared by lower social class adoptive parents than in those reared by middle-class adoptive parents (Cloninger *et al.*, 1982; van Dusen *et al.*, 1983; Cadoret, Troughton & O'Gorman, 1987). The finding provides strong evidence that the association between social class and antisocial behaviour is in substantial part environmentally mediated (the evidence that there is also an association with the social class of the biological parent indicates that there is an additional genetic effect: van Dusen *et al.*, 1983). Similarly, within genetic-risk groups (at risk because of birth to a criminal parent), adverse experiences as indexed by early institutional rearing, family discord, or disorder in the adoptive parents are associated with a raised rate of delinquency (Crowe, 1974; Cadoret & Cain, 1980; Mednick, Gabrielli & Hutchings, 1987). In all these studies, the environmental risk factor cannot have been genetically mediated because it did not apply to the biological family environment; however, the strength of the environmental mediation inference is dependent on both exclusion of selective placement effects and identification of the relevant genetic risk factor.

A somewhat comparable approach can be used within non-adoptive samples through 'control' for the genetic factors by taking a sample defined in terms of a genetic risk. Thus, in our own prospective studies of the children of mentally ill parents, we found that marital discord was associated with conduct disturbance in the children, even within a subgroup all of whom had a parent with a long-standing personality disorder (Rutter & Quinton, 1984). Similarly, we found that among institution-reared girls, disrupted parenting in infancy was associated with a worse outcome in adult life even after controlling for the presence of deviance (as indexed by criminality, mental illness or drug/alcohol abuse) in the biological parents (Quinton & Rutter, 1988).

In each of these studies the possibility that the supposed environmental variable represented some unmeasured genetic risk factor cannot be ruled out entirely. Thus, the disrupted parenting or marital discord could represent some genetic risk that is not adequately tapped by the presence of manifest disorder in the parent (although there is no evidence that this is likely to be the case). An alternative approach is to take environmental variables that could not themselves be genetically mediated. For example, Roy (1983) compared institution-reared and family-fostered children of similar biological background and found that hyperactivity was more frequent in the institutional group. Hodges & Tizard (1989a, b), in a prospective study extending from infancy to age 16 years of children all of whom spent their first few years in a residential nursery, compared those who were adopted late and those who were restored to their biological parents. The restored children had a substantially higher rate of antisocial behaviour at 16 years. Also, Reitsma-Street, Offord & Finch (1985) found that delinquent boys differed from their non-delinquent brothers in their experience of more negative child relationships.

None of these studies is decisive on its own but they all add up to a considerable weight of evidence in favour of substantial environmental effects, particularly when taken in conjunction with the animal findings. Of course, that does not mean that genetic effects are not also very important. Indeed, there is evidence that they are (Rutter *et al.*, 1990a). However, with respect to most of the disorders usually associated with 'maternal deprivation', the genetic evidence suggests that much of the variance is accounted for by environmental factors. On the other hand, a limited amount of evidence points to the possibility that susceptibility to environmental adversities may be greater in genetic-risk groups (Crowe, 1974; Cadoret & Cain, 1980; Cloninger *et al.*, 1982; Mednick *et al.*, 1987). Certainly, that possibility warrants further study (see Plomin, De Fries & Fulker, 1988).

A concern rather separate from the issue of genetic mediation is the possibility that the causal arrow runs in the opposite direction; namely, that behaviourally disordered children create abnormal environments for themselves (Scarr & McCartney, 1983). Since Bell (1968) first systematically raised the possibility that some supposed socialisation effects might represent child effects on parents, rather than the other way round, the evidence in favour of child effects has gradually accumulated (Bell & Harper, 1977; Lerner & Spanier, 1978; Brunk & Henggeler, 1984; Bell & Chapman, 1986).

Four main strategies may be employed to test whether the causal arrow runs from parent to child, rather than (or in addition to) the other way round. First, longitudinal studies may be used to determine whether parental deviance or family disturbance has consequent effects on children's behaviour when the children were not born or were behaviourally normal at the time the deviance/disturbance was first measured. Richman, Stevenson & Graham

(1982) showed that children, behaviourally normal at age 3 years, who experienced family adversity or marital discord at that age, were two to three times as likely to show emotional/behavioural disorder at age 8 than children who did not have these experiences. Predictive effects from before the children were born are evident in long-term follow-ups of children born after requests for abortion have been refused (David *et al.*, 1988) and of children born to adolescent mothers (Furstenberg, Brooks-Gunn & Morgan, 1987). For example, in the Prague study of children born to women twice denied abortion for the same pregnancy, the rate of adult criminality in the offspring was twice that in their pair-matched controls and the level of social maladaptation was significantly worse.

Second, longitudinal studies may be used to determine the effects on children's behaviour of a change in their experiences that could not have been a result of their own behaviour. This design provides a clear demonstration that the emotional distress seen in many young children admitted to hospital is indeed a result of the hospital admission and factors associated with it (see Rutter 1979, 1981a). The same applies to the effects of parental remarriage following divorce (Hetherington, 1988) and to the reduction in delinquency associated with a move away from inner London (West, 1982).

Third, intervention strategies focused on changing parental behaviour may be examined in terms of their effects on the children's behaviour. Thus, if it could be shown that reductions in family discord, following marital therapy, resulted in a diminution in antisocial behaviour in the children, this would provide good evidence of a parent-to-child effect. However, although there is evidence of child benefits associated with family-focused interventions (see Patterson, 1982; Rutter & Giller, 1983), and some evidence of associations between change in parental behaviour and child benefits (Patterson & Chamberlain, 1988), no studies provide a clean test of the type suggested. Moreover, once conduct disorders in children become well established, response to modest improvements in family functioning is limited (Patterson, 1982; Richman *et al.*, 1982), although benefits may follow major changes for the better (Rutter, 1971).

The fourth strategy is different in so far as it focuses on non-familial environments. Rutter *et al.* (1979) examined pupils' scholastic attainment, behaviour and attendance at the end of their period at secondary school; school effects were determined after controlling for the children's background and personal characteristics at the time they entered the school at the age of 11–12 years. It was found that the pupils' outcomes differed markedly according to the school they attended, that this still held after controlling for intake variables, and that the variation was systematically associated with the qualities of the schools as social organisations. Other studies of schools

(Rutter, 1983) and of different forms of institution (see Rutter *et al.*, 1979) have given rise to similar findings. A recent study by Mortimore *et al.* (1988) of primary schools in inner London, in which pupils' progress was followed from school entry to leaving, has added a variety of improvements in methodological rigour, with a similar demonstration of substantial school effects – especially on scholastic attainment but also on behaviour. School effects at secondary level have also been confirmed by Smith and Tomlinson (1989) in a systematic longitudinal study of pupils attending 25 geographically scattered schools.

Of course, school studies cannot provide a direct test of 'maternal deprivation' effects, not only because they do not concern the family but also because they deal with other aspects of childrens' experiences. Nevertheless, they are informative in demonstrating the results of experiential effects on childrens' cognitive performance and behaviour – effects that cannot be attributed to genetic influences or the impact of the childrens' characteristics. The evidence on the environmental mediation hypothesis has been discussed at some length because the criticism that the supposed effects of 'maternal deprivation' might all be a consequence of genetic influences loomed large in the more thoughtful academic critiques of Bowlby's views (see Wootton, 1959, 1962; O'Connor & Franks, 1960) and because at the time of my 1972 appraisal of the field it was noted that the evidence on this possibility was 'not very satisfactory' (Rutter, 1972, p. 119). The need critically to examine the possibility that the supposed ill-effects of 'maternal deprivation' are artefactual is also emphasised by the growing ascendancy of so-called biological psychiatry (Guze, 1989). This ascendancy is backed by real and important advances in knowledge but there has crept in on the tide a regrettable tendency to replace the old fault of 'brainlessness' in some branches of psychiatry by the new fault of 'mindlessness' (see Eisenberg, 1986 on this issue). In other words, in some quarters, the failure to take account of possible organic factors has been replaced by a failure to appreciate that people are thinking beings likely to be influenced by the processing of the experiences they undergo. Of course, the dichotomy is artificial. Hinde has long argued that a biological approach must encompass psychosocial influences (see e.g. Hinde, 1987). It is as necessary to recognise that *Homo sapiens* is a social animal (and liable to be influenced by social forces) as it is to accept that the brain is the organ of the mind (Rutter, 1986). While an enormous amount has still to be learned about the interplay between genetic and environmental influences (an interplay that extends well beyond statistical interaction effects – see Rutter, 1983; Rutter & Pickles, 1990), the evidence is now sufficient to conclude with confidence that the seriously adverse experiences encompassed within the concept of 'maternal deprivation' may indeed influence childrens' development.

The 'maternal love' hypothesis

The second major area of controversy concerned the notion that the critical element in 'maternal deprivation' experiences was the lack of 'mother love' – meaning a lack of a warm, intimate and continuous relationship with the mother or mother-substitute. The postulate was most important in its focus on affectional aspects of parent–child interactions (as distinct from, say, cognitive stimulation, or disciplinary elements) and, especially, in its claim that the enduring continuity of the parent–child relationship was crucial. To begin with, this was accompanied by a somewhat unfortunate preoccupation with the supposed risks associated with brief mother–child separations as such, even though Bowlby's own research soon led him to conclude that the dangers of separation had been overstated (Bowlby *et al.*, 1956). Hinde's experimental studies of separation experiences in rhesus monkeys did much to clarify the issues (Hinde, 1977; Hinde & McGinnis, 1977). The results showed that separations did lead to emotional disturbance in infant monkeys, but also that they did so largely because they were associated with tension and disruption of the mother–infant relationship.

Research with children led to similar conclusions (Rutter, 1981a). Thus, Rutter (1971) found that whereas obviously stressful separations (those associated with family discord or psychopathology) were associated with emotional/behavioural disturbance, this did not apply to less stressful ones (such as those associated with a prolonged holiday or convalescence from an illness). Moreover, several large-scale studies showed that the psychiatric risks associated with parental divorce were substantially greater than those that followed parental death. Attention shifted from physical separation as such to separation as a non-specific indicator of possible family discord and conflictful or disrupted relationships. More recently, the importance of this distinction has been shown with respect to the long-term risks for depression in adult life that may be associated with early parental loss (Harris, Brown & Bifulco, 1986; Breier *et al.*, 1988; Birtchnell, Evans & Kennard, 1988). It is clear that it is not the loss *per se* that creates the risk but rather the inadequate affectional parental care that it may bring about. Poor parental care and poor family relationships were associated with an increased risk for later psychiatric disorders irrespective of whether there was any loss; conversely, loss had *no* effect on psychiatric risk unless it was associated with poor care or relationships. The findings on the risk for adult mental disorder are in keeping with those that apply to psychiatric disturbances in childhood. Many studies have shown that serious family discord constitutes an important risk variable (Emery, 1982; Rutter, 1985b). Longitudinal studies have also been important in demonstrating that the rate of emotional/behavioural disturbance in children rises *before* parental divorce occurs

339

(Block, Block & Gjerde, 1986) and before children go into group foster care (St Clair & Osborne, 1987). Family break-up may aggravate the situation if it is associated with a worsening in relationships or in patterns of child care (Hetherington, 1988) but it seems that it is the chronic disturbance in intimate family relationships that creates the main risk and not the acute separation or loss as such (although the latter may add to the risk).

These findings have served to clarify some aspects of the issue but have left many questions unanswered. One key difficulty is that disturbed family relationships frequently form part of a more complex set of psychosocial difficulties with the consequent uncertainty as to which adversity is chiefly responsible for the psychiatric risk to the children (Rutter, 1979; Kolvin *et al.*, 1988). Family discord may constitute less of a risk factor when not associated with other adversities (Emery, 1982). Nevertheless, it does seem to constitute part of the set of risk mechanisms. Thus, Rutter & Quinton (1984) found that the psychiatric risks to the children of being reared by a mentally ill parent were mainly attributable to the associated family discord and disruption. Fendrich, Warner & Weissman (1990) have recently confirmed this finding with respect to the development of conduct disturbance in the offspring of depressed mothers (see also Rutter, 1990a).

One important distinction is between the risks associated with actively negative relationships and those resulting from a lack of positive ones. Bowlby's (1951) WHO monograph placed emphasis on the latter, drawing attention to the psychiatric problems shown by children placed in group foster homes or other institutions. Of course, children going into institutions have frequently experienced many other adversities and it is not easy to partial out their separate effects. Moreover, many of the early studies dealt with institutions of generally poor quality. We need to turn to more recent studies of institutions where the general quality of care is good but where the turnover of staff has meant a severe lack of continuity in caregiving. Barbara Tizard's follow-up of children who spent their first years in residential nurseries constitutes a good example of this kind, as the care provided was known to be good (Tizard, 1977), apart from an extremely high turnover of caregivers. The results are striking in showing that in both infancy and middle childhood the institutional children had difficulties in social relationships (Tizard & Tizard, 1971; Tizard & Rees, 1974; Tizard & Hodges, 1978). Similarly, Roy (1983) found that institution-reared children tended to differ from family-fostered children in showing a higher rate of inattention and poorly modulated social behaviour. Our own follow-up into adult life of institution-reared girls (Quinton & Rutter, 1988) also showed that the outcome for social functioning in adult life was particularly poor for the small group who were admitted to Group Homes in infancy and who remained there through adolescence. The finding is striking because their institutional rearing had largely 'protected' them from daily discord, albeit at the price of a lack of continuity in personalised parent–child relationships (i.e. a lack of relationships that are particular to each child and that involve the same parental figure over time). Other studies, too, have shown rather similar long-term risks associated with both parental abuse and neglect (see Rutter, 1989a).

In so far as research has been able to disentangle the risk factors involved in 'maternal deprivation', it seems that the postulate that a lack of continuity in loving committed parent–child relationships is central has received substantial support. The further specification that it has to be with the mother has, however, had to be qualified (Lamb, 1982; Campos *et al.*, 1983; Parke & Tinsley, 1987). Children's relationships with their mothers are often particularly close but most children have more than one loving relationship that provides security, and other family relationships must also be taken into account in considering the effects of 'maternal deprivation'. Moreover, it would be going much too far to claim that continuity in secure loving relationships constitutes the only important element. Many other facets of parental behaviour are also likely to have important effects on children's development (Maccoby & Martin, 1983).

'Love' is no longer the term that predominates in discussion of parent–child relationships. Hinde's monkey research drew attention to the importance of attachment characteristics and to the ways in which the balance of initiative in the mother–infant relationship altered as infants grew older (Hinde & Spencer-Booth, 1967). Most particularly, he emphasised the ways in which relationships grew out of interactions, how such relationships involved a variety of different components and facets, how each relationship was necessarily embedded in a broader context of other relationships and how one relationship may serve to influence other relationships (Hinde & Spencer-Booth, 1971; Hinde & Stevenson-Hinde, 1988). Attention has shifted from 'mother-love' as such to the growth of social relationships. However, within the latter topic, the concept of attachment has come to dominate both theory and empirical research (see Bowlby, 1969, 1973, 1980; Bretherton & Waters, 1985; Bretherton, 1987). The basic idea is that children have a natural propensity to maintain proximity with a mother figure, that this leads to an attachment relationship and that the quality of this relationship in terms of security/insecurity serves as the basis for later relationships (Ainsworth, 1967, 1982). Some of the unresolved issues involved in this concept are discussed further below but it is mentioned here because its relevance to discussion of the mechanisms involved in the effects of 'maternal deprivation'.

Heterogeneity of effects

Little space need be spent on the third area that gave rise to early controversy; namely, the supposition that there was a single syndrome of maternal deprivation with all aspects due to the same basic mechanism. Much evidence points to several rather different outcomes associated with different risk factors (Rutter, 1981a). Possibly, distinctions should be drawn between some half a dozen principal patterns or syndromes. First, acute distress reaction is shown by many young children admitted to hospitals or residential nurseries. It seems that this is largely a function of: (i) acute separation from all people to whom the child is attached; (ii) a lack of opportunity to form new attachments during the separation (because caregivers keep changing); and (iii) an unpleasantly strange and frightening environment. Separation experiences that lack these qualities are less likely to give rise to distress. Also, this type of reaction is particularly common in preschool children after the early infancy period.

Second, there are conduct disorders or antisocial problems. These differ from acute distress reactions in their lack of age-specificity, their association with chronic psychosocial adversities rather than acute separation experiences, and their tendency to persist over years rather than weeks or months. Much empirical evidence shows an association with family discord, disruption and disorganisation and points to the likely causal role of these disturbed family relationships (Emery, 1982; Rutter & Giller, 1983; Rutter, 1985b; Patterson & Bank, 1989). Family break-ups and parent–child separations as such do not seem to play a crucial role because longitudinal studies have shown that the children's behavioural disturbance frequently precedes the separation (Lambert, Essen & Head, 1977; Block *et al.*, 1986; St Clair & Osborne, 1987), and because family conflict is associated with conduct disturbance even in the absence of separation or family break-up (Rutter, 1971). However, considerable problems remain in sorting out just which aspects of family discord predispose to conduct disturbance. The difficulty arises because it is usual for family adversities to occur as part of clusters of multiple risk factors rather than in isolation (McCord, 1979; Farrington, 1986; Kolvin *et al.*, 1988). Thus, for example, Patterson emphasised poor parental discipline, supervision and monitoring as well as a coercive, emotionally negative style of family interaction (Patterson, 1982; Patterson & Dishion, 1988; Patterson & Bank, 1990); and Farrington (1986) added the effects of antisocial attitudes shown by criminal parents; whereas Greenberg & Speltz (1988) argued that insecure attachment deriving from insensitive, non-responsive caregiving is basic. The available evidence does not allow a clear differentiation between these possibilities, and it is likely that more than one type of family risk factor plays a part in the causal processes that are involved. Nevertheless, the evidence that the quality of parent–child relationships distinguishes delinquent and non-delinquent boys within the same family (Reitsma-Street *et al.*, 1985) suggests that poor family relationships constitute an important element in the causal mechanisms. This is also evident from the findings that a good relationship with one parent serves as a protective factor (Rutter, 1971; Kolvin *et al.*, 1988) and that disrupted parenting in infancy and an institutional upbringing that lacks continuity in caregiving predisposes to antisocial behaviour (Quinton & Rutter, 1988; Rutter *et al.*, 1990b). However, it should be noted that the findings on institution-reared children suggest that a *lack* of personalised caregiving, as well as the *presence* of discordant family relationships, is important.

Third, there is cognitive impairment as an outcome of deprivation experiences. Research findings are consistent in indicating that the key risk feature is a lack of active learning experiences, rather than discordant personal relationships (Rutter, 1985b). As Sroufe (1988) has underlined, neither theoretical expectations nor empirical findings suggest that early parent–child attachments make a major impact on cognitive development. Of course, cognitive performance is influenced by social context and effective learning is likely to be facilitated by a style of personal interactions and relationships that promotes self-confidence and an interest in learning (Rutter, 1985a). Moreover, the long-term benefits stemming from successful early childhood educational programmes may stem as much from the adaptive social processes set in motion as from the learning input as such (Woodhead, 1985, 1988). Nevertheless, the evidence suggests that the crucial factor promoting cognitive development concerns active learning experiences rather than harmonious personal relationships. Institution-reared children, raised in good quality Group Homes, who are particularly at risk for socio-behavioural problems, do not usually have intellectual impairment (Rutter, 1981a).

The fourth syndrome that has been associated with 'maternal deprivation' is what was once termed 'affectionless psychopathy' (Bowlby, 1946), meaning an inability to make lasting relationships, associated with recidivist delinquency and a lack of guilt. The concept has rather gone out of fashion but elements of it have been revived as a result of recent findings. The early research on this hypothesised syndrome was consistent in noting the particular frequency with which it was found in children who had been reared in residential nurseries with a very high turnover of caregivers or who had suffered from 'pillar to post' ever-changing caretaking arrangements outside of institutions (see Rutter, 1981a). Accordingly, interest has focused on the social development of institution-reared children. As already noted, Barbara Tizard's small, well-studied sample of children who spent most of their preschool years in a residential nursery provides the best data on the outcome of an institutional rearing, with clinging and diffuse attachments at 2 years, and attention-seeking, indiscriminately friendly behaviour at 4 years. Most of the residential nursery children who were then adopted at this relatively late age succeeded in forming deep relationships with their adoptive parents, but, even so, at 8 years of age they continued to show the same social and attentional problems at school as did those who had remained in the institution (Tizard & Hodges, 1978). Hodges & Tizard (1989 a, b) have now followed the children up to 16 years of age, with striking findings. In general, as would be expected from their currently good social circumstances, the adopted children were functioning much better than those who were restored to their biological parents (and hence usually to disorganised families facing many adversities). Nevertheless, both the adopted and restored children differed from their controls in being more adult-orientated in their relationships; more likely to have difficulties in peer relationships; less likely to have a special friend; less likely to turn to peers for emotional support when anxious; and less likely to be selective in choosing friends. Half the ex-institutional children showed at least four out of these five characteristics compared with only one (4%) of the comparison group. Adolescents with these characteristics were significantly more likely to show other psychological problems but the 'syndrome', in so far as it could be considered as such, was characterised more by an unusual pattern of peer relationships that seemed to lack depth and selectivity rather than by overt psychiatric disorder as usually recognised. Nevertheless, the pattern does seem to reflect the outcome of some aspect of the earlier institutional experiences, of which the lack of continuity in caregiving seems the most relevant. In view of this, it has been included in the latest WHO (1989) psychiatric classification, albeit with the explicit recognition that there is a need for much more evidence on its validity and that its inclusion is experimental (Rutter, 1989c).

A fifth pattern of behaviour that has come to be recognised is what has been termed a reactive attachment disorder (American Psychiatric Association, 1987; WHO, 1989). It represents an unusual pattern of insecure attachment, associated with serious maladaptive patterns of behaviour, seen in young children who have been subjected to physical abuse or severely deviant forms of parenting (Crittenden, 1985, 1988; Radke-Yarrow *et al.*, 1985; Main & George, 1985). Data on the diagnostic characteristics of this pattern are sparse and little is known on its validity. Nevertheless, the evidence suggests that the distinctive features are strongly contradictory or ambivalent attachment behaviour, together with unusual forms of emotional disturbance (such as aggressive responses to their own or others' distress) and sometimes by fearful hypervigilance that is relatively unresponsive to comforting.

The last pattern differs in that it refers, not to a disorder as such, but rather to an hypothesised vulnerability to disorder. From early on, Bowlby (1973, 1980, 1988) postulated causal connections between early insecurity in attachment relationships and the later development of phobias, depression, suicide, parenting problems and other psychiatric conditions. The general proposition is that the qualities of a person's early attachment relationships serve as the basis for 'internal working models' of the self and of relationships with others. When early parenting experiences have been stressful, it is supposed that the models that develop include features of insecurity, helplessness, ambivalence and conflict that create a psychiatric vulnerability, perhaps especially in conjunction with the occurrence of stressors and adversities encountered in later life. A lack of affectionate care in childhood is associated with an increased risk for affective disorders in adult life (Adam, 1982; Harris *et al.*, 1986; Breier *et al.*, 1988; Birtchnell *et al.*, 1988; Tennant, 1988), so that it may be accepted that 'maternal deprivation' may sometimes predispose to a long-term psychological susceptibility, although the same evidence suggests that the risk stems from chronically inadequate parental care rather than from parental loss *per se*. It is also not unreasonable to suppose that the continuities reside in some form of cognitive and affective set that is subsequently reinforced or modified by later experiences (Bretherton & Waters, 1985; Bretherton, 1987). However, little is known of the mechanisms involved and even less on how to recognise the vulnerability before disorder develops.

Although it is all too evident that much has to be learned on the heterogeneous sequelae of the experiences once subsumed under the general rubric of 'maternal deprivation', it is clear that several rather different psychological processes are involved. It is primarily for that reason that the term is now little used. It served its purpose in drawing attention to an important set of phenomena but it has become replaced by a more differentiated set of concepts.

Infancy as a sensitive period

Although early concepts of 'maternal deprivation' (Bowlby, 1951) included the notion that infancy constituted a sensitive period, with the ill-effects of adverse parental care relatively immutable, this view has been dropped by almost all leading theorists (see Bowlby, 1988; Sroufe, 1988). This is because of the very extensive evidence that major life experiences at all age periods make a substantial impact on psychological functioning and that the sequelae of infantile experiences are greatly dependent on what happens during the course of later development (Rutter, 1981a). Even young children subjected to the most severely depriving experiences usually show a remarkable degree of recovery when rescued from their appalling circumstances (Skuse, 1984). Findings such as these led to a severe downgrading of the importance of the infancy years for later development and to an increased emphasis on the role of current (rather than past) life experiences by some influential writers (Clarke & Clarke, 1976; Kagan, 1984a). Clearly, the empirical evidence required rejection of the view that experiences in infancy have an overriding importance in fixing personality development regardless of what follows. It should be added that the concepts of imprinting and of critical periods that led to these early 'maternal deprivation' views have become outdated and do not coincide with those now held by animal researchers (Bateson 1979; Hinde, 1987).

Nevertheless, the downgrading of infancy does not mean that infants are unaffected by their early family experiences. Visual cliff experiences show that 1-year-old infants are highly sensitive to their mothers' facial expressions (Sorce, Emde & Frank, 1982; Sorce *et al.*, 1985). Observational data from the studies of Radke-Yarrow and her colleagues have shown that 2-year-olds are very sensitive to both adult conflict and distress (Cummings, Zahn-Waxler & Radke-Yarrow, 1981, 1984; Radke-Harrow, Zahn-Waxler & Chapman, 1983; Zahn-Waxler *et al.*, 1984; Cummings, Lanott & Zahn-Waxler, 1985). Also, severe maternal depression was found to be associated with an unusual variety of resistant/avoidant attachment (Radke-Yarrow *et al.*, 1985). An apparently comparable type of attachment insecurity has been found in physically abused toddlers (Crittenden, 1985, 1988; Main & George, 1985). It is evident from these and other findings that infants are certainly reactive to social and emotional stimuli and that they may show psychological disturbance when exposed to family pathology.

Dispute has centred on the questions of whether or not such disturbance persists into later childhood or adult life and of whether experiences in infancy have effects that differ qualitatively from those seen in older age groups. Kagan (1984a, b) has argued persuasively that a person's cognitive processing of experiences plays a major role in determining their longer-term effects. In that connection, he has pointed to the likely importance of the growth of self-awareness and appreciation of adult standards (Kagan, 1981). The careful and systematic naturalistic studies of family interaction at home undertaken by Judy Dunn, working in Hinde's MRC Unit, have provided vivid evidence of how children's social understanding increases during the second and third year of life (Dunn, 1988). It is clear that from about 18 months onwards, children understand how to comfort or hurt other people, show increasing sensitivity to the goals and intentions of others, appreciate social rules, and are beginning to reflect on other's mental states. Of course, their concepts at that age are much less well developed and less differentiated than they will be when they are older; nevertheless, toddlers and young children exhibit a surprising degree of social understanding.

By the end of the second year infants are able to process their experiences in ways that are likely to influence later functioning. What remains unclear is whether there is comparable cognitive processing (albeit at a more immature level) by infants younger than 18–24 months. Bretherton (1987) has suggested that primitive 'internal working models' of relationships may be present from earlier ages; Stern (1985) has postulated comparable processes in the development of 'internal representations of interactions'. However, we lack data on whether these are operative before 18 months. It should be added, too, that it remains uncertain how important such cognitive processing is for the persistence of effects of adverse early experiences. It seems plausible that the effects may be different when children can think about their experiences and develop concepts about what is happening to them but that hypothesis has not yet been tested adequately. Nevertheless, the demonstrations, on the one hand, that infants *are* affected by their experiences and, on the other, that their capacity for social understanding and for appreciating social meaning grows during the preschool years, has led many psychoanalysts to alter their views on the role of experiences in development. Thus, Bowlby (1988) has urged the importance of paying attention to the effects of real-life experiences, rather than focusing on fantasies, and Stern (1985) has similarly argued that infants are affected by reality and that, contrary to the traditional psychoanalytic position, reality experiences precede fantasy distortions in development, the capacity for defensive mechanisms being a later-developing feature. Both theorists place an emphasis on the developmental importance of social relationships and, in so doing, reject psychoanalytic notions of the supposedly crucial role of psychosexual stages. It is striking that 'maternal deprivation' concepts arose primarily from psychoanalysis but that the empirical studies to which they gave rise led to a major shift in focus in what psychoanalysts think is important in early development.

The notion that experiences in early life have effects that are different in degree or kind from those that follow similar experiences at a later age has proved quite difficult to test for a host of methodological reasons concerned with the uncertainties of comparability between age periods and with the rarity of experiences at one age that are independent from those at other ages. Children's reactions to hospital admission constitute one of the few examples where it has been possible to test the hypothesis of age-related differences in susceptibility (because the event is acute and because it has no necessary connection with ongoing experiences). The findings show that distress reactions are less likely in the first 6 months of life and during the years of schooling than they are in the intermediate age period (Vernon *et al.*, 1965; Rutter, 1979). Single short admissions to hospital have no detectable effect on emotional or behavioural disturbance some years later but there are effects from *repeated* hospital admissions provided the first admission took place during the preschool years (Douglas, 1975; Quinton & Rutter, 1976). As already discussed, this increased susceptibility during the early years of life (but post early infancy) is likely to be a consequence of the combined importance of developing attachment relationships at that age and a limited ability to understand the meaning of separation experiences and to maintain relationships during an absence (Rutter, 1987a).

It is quite likely that there may be other age-related differences in children's responses to acute life events but the matter has been little investigated up to now. For example, the demonstrated age differences in the quality of children's peer relationships (Hartup, 1983) might well mean that adolescents will be more affected than toddlers by rebuffs from peers. Also, it might be thought that children's ability to suffer from the experiences of failure or disappointment might increase with age in parallel with an increasing capacity to experience feelings of helplessness and guilt. Whether or not either is in fact the case is not known but the possibility serves as a reminder that it is unhelpful to consider vulnerability to stress as some homogeneous quality that is likely to be greater at one age period than another; rather, it is probable that maturational changes will tend to increase susceptibility to some types of stress and decrease susceptibility to others.

Age differences in response to persistent life experiences are necessarily more difficult to study as they require the occurrence of chronic adversities at one age but their absence at other ages (or the use of methods of statistical analysis that partial out the effects of experiences at different ages). Some attempt has been made, however, to investigate the matter with respect to cognitive development. For example, Bradley, Caldwell & Rock (1988) used a partial correlation approach to their longitudinal study data to compare the relative effects of the home environment at age 6 months, 2 years and 10 years. On the whole, the effects on 10-year-old cognitive measures were greater for the current environment than for the past one and, within the past experiences, the effects from those at 2 years exceeded those at 6 months. However, as the authors point out, the data set was not ideal for the purpose and the findings were in any case complex. Nevertheless, both correlational data from longitudinal studies (Yeates *et al.*, 1983) and data from intervention studies (Ramey & Campbell, 1981, 1984; Ramey *et al.*, 1982) suggest that the home environment at age 2 years onwards has a greater effect on later cognitive levels than does the environment in early infancy. On the other hand, adoption studies show that the IQ scores of late-adopted children tend to be slightly lower than those of children adopted in infancy (Dennis, 1973); also, that the rise in cognitive level associated with early adoption is not seen with adoption after the age of $4\frac{1}{2}$ (Hodges & Tizard, 1989a). There are methodological problems in using the adoption data to examine age differences in susceptibility to family influences on cognitive development (see Rutter, 1985a) and no strong conclusions are unwarranted. Even so, the few available data are compatible with the suggestion that such influences may be relatively greater during the preschool years after early infancy than either earlier or later in childhood. The hypothesis warrants further study.

The data on age differences regarding influences on social development are even more rudimentary, but they raise interesting possibilities. First, in his study of children in institutional care, Wolkind (1974) found that the characteristics of indiscriminate friendliness and lack of social inhibition were especially evident in those admitted before the age of 2 years. The implication was that a lack of continuous personal parenting in early childhood may have social sequelae that are not seen following a similar lack at later ages. The same age difference was *not* found for other forms of psychological disturbance. Second, Hodges and Tizard (1989a, b) found that, whereas other aspects of behavioural functioning were more a function of children's current family circumstances than their pattern of experiences in infancy, children who spent their first few years in a residential nursery tended to show a similar pattern of non-confiding peer relationships regardless of their later experiences. Again, the data are too sparse for firm conclusions but the implication is that the opportunity to form secure continuous attachment relationships is particularly important in the first few years of life and that the effects of a lack of such opportunities tend to be relatively persistent even if their later family experiences are much improved. The developmental implications are provocative and the matter clearly should be investigated further.

We may conclude that, although the idea of infancy as a period that is generally characterised by a heightened susceptibility to psychosocial influences with effects that are critical for later development must be rejected, the notion that there are important age-related differences in susceptibility to environmental experiences is far from dead. It is unlikely that these will amount to any one age period being one of globally increased vulnerability and it is probable that different age periods will be important for different effects or different types of experiences. Nevertheless, there is a substantial remaining potential for the study of age-related variations in response to particular types of life experiences.

Michael Rutter

Persistence of effects of experiences in infancy

The fifth source of controversy regarding the initial claims on the effects of 'maternal deprivation' concerned the suggestion that the effects were relatively immutable and not reversible by later experiences. The early evidence was flawed by its failure to take account of environmental influences in later childhood and adolescence. Most children who suffer from early psychosocial adversities also experience later environments that are hazardous and the impression of persistence of effects resulting from experiences in infancy is misleading because the damaging experiences have themselves persisted. If the effects of experiences in infancy were to be separated from those in later childhood it seemed necessary to search out examples of early damaging experiences that were followed by later beneficial ones (see Rutter, 1981 a). There are not many well-documented studies of children who have been exposed to sharply contrasting environments at different ages as a consequence of a highly unusual discontinuity in upbringing but both late adoption and rescue from conditions of extreme deprivation provide opportunities to separate infancy from late childhood experiences. The findings showed that greatly improved circumstances were usually followed by a substantial degree of recovery, but there was also evidence of slight residual effects in some cases. A review of the evidence 8 years ago concluded that although '...the long term effects of early deprivation depend heavily on whether or not the deprivation continues, it would be premature to conclude that infantile experiences are of no importance in their own right' (Rutter, 1981 a, p. 197).

The question being tackled then was whether there were *direct* effects from infancy experiences that were independent from later ones. It now appears that that may not have been the most relevant question to pose. Although there had been suggestions that new phases of biological maturation or new experiences might wipe clean the slate of what had gone before (Kagan, 1981), the evidence did *not* prove that development was a largely discontinuous process (Hinde, 1982; Rutter, 1982; Hinde & Bateson, 1984). Certainly, it was clear that earlier views of strong and inevitable connectedness in the developmental process were mistaken (see Kagan, 1984a, b), but it was also evident that linkages could be detected across developmental transitions. Necessarily, development must involve a mixture of continuities 1 discontinuities (Hinde, 1988). What was becoming increasingly apparent, however, is that both the continuities and discontinuities arise because so many effects are *indirect*, rather than direct (Rutter, 1987a, 1989b). For example, intergenerational transmission of parenting breakdown seems to arise from a chain that extends from breakdown in parenting in one generation which predisposes to institutional rearing of the children; this is often followed by a return in adolescence to a discordant family environment when the young people leave the institution; the family stresses then predispose to a marriage to 'escape' what are felt to be intolerable circumstances; the hasty marriage all too often leads either to marital breakdown or to an unhappy, unsupportive marital relationship; the marital strains and lack of support make it more likely that there will be generalised social difficulties; these social difficulties in turn predispose to parenting breakdown and the cycle is complete (Quinton & Rutter, 1988). Numerous possible mediating factors may be involved in these chains of indirect linkages that underlie developmental continuities and discontinuities. These include: genetic mechanisms; effects on the biological substrate; shaping of the environment by a person's own behaviour or actions; the acquisition of cognitive and social skills; effects on self-esteem and self-efficacy; the establishment of habits, cognitive sets and copy styles; and links between experiences so that one bad (or good) experience makes another one more likely (Rutter, 1989b). Research attention has moved from the study of direct effects that are entirely separate from later experiences (an unusual situation in real life) to the investigation of chain effects over time in which the goal is to analyse each link in the chain, to determine how the links interconnect and to study how changes in life trajectory come about. In this way, life transitions have to be considered both as end products of past processes and as instigators of future ones.

These considerations have led to a growing interest in what have been termed 'turning points' in a person's development (Elder, Caspi & Burton, 1988; Rutter, 1989b,d; Maughan & Champion, 1990; Pickles & Rutter, 1990). By this is meant everyday events or happenings that bring about a potential for long-term psychological change. The potential comes about in two main ways (Pickles & Rutter, 1990). First, experiences open up or close down opportunities; going to university and dropping out of school constitute examples of this kind. Second, events may involve a radical lasting change in circumstances – as from key subtractions or additions to a person's nexus of intimate family relations (as with divorce or marriage); from alterations in life pattern (as by transition to parenthood or by being made redundant in mid-life); or from a major social change stemming from a geographical move (as with immigration or a move from the inner city to the countryside). Changed experiences of these kinds in adolescence or adult life are indeed followed by changes in psychological functioning. What is new, however, is the realisation in recent years that has stemmed from disparate longitudinal studies that these later experiences are not independent from what has gone before. To an important extent, whether or not a person *has* some beneficial or damaging experience in later life will have been influenced by their past behaviour or experiences. For example, we found that girls who experienced an institutional rearing were much more likely than other girls to make an unhappy marriage (Quinton & Rutter, 1988). The *effects* of an unhappy marriage on social functioning were statistically independent from past experiences but the *experience* of being in an unhappy marriage was not. The empirical findings suggest a dynamic model involving interlinked chain effects both before and after the turning point (Rutter, 1987a, b, 1989a, b). While the testing of such models involves a variety of statistical and conceptual problems that are only partially resolved (Pickles & Rutter, 1990) their testing clearly constitutes one of the key challenges for future research in this area.

Individual differences in outcome

It has been apparent from the very outset of 'maternal deprivation' research that children differ in their responses. At first, little attention was paid to individual differences but a review in 1972 concluded that their study should prove rewarding (Rutter, 1972). Since then, evidence on the topic has gradually accumulated (Rutter, 1981a, 1987b, 1989d). It cannot be claimed that this has led to a good understanding of the mechanisms underlying variations in children's reactions to what appear to be comparable experiences, but there are leads on some directions to follow.

Research into individual differences has mainly focused on temperamental characteristics, so that the literature on this topic is now very considerable (Kohnstamm, Bates & Rothbart, 1989). A number of studies have shown that certain temperamental patterns are associated with a substantially increased risk of psychological/psychiatric disturbance in childhood (Garrison & Earls, 1987). However, only a very few investigations have considered the role of temperament as a possible explanation for variations in children's reactions to any of the types of psychosocial adversity that might be included in concepts of 'maternal deprivation', and little is known of the mechanisms by which temperamental features may represent a psychological risk or protective factor (Rutter, 1989d). Traditionally, two main processes have been thought to be operative. First, it could be that certain temperamental qualities *directly* create an increased vulnerability to certain psychopathological disorders, as is thought to be the case with the trait of extreme behavioural inhibition and anxiety disorders (Kagan, Reznick & Snidman, 1987; Kagan *et al.*, 1988). Second, the temperamental qualities might operate indirectly, through rendering the individual more susceptible to psychosocial adversities (Maziade *et al.*, 1985; Maziade, 1989). Intuitively, the latter possibility appears likely to be operative. Thus, it is well demonstrated that individuals differ in their physiological reactivity to stress situations and it would seem reasonable to postulate a psychological equivalent. Unfortunately, there is a paucity of good evidence on the extent to which this is actually the case. Part of the difficulty has lain in the lack of theoretical clarity on which individual characteristics were supposed to interact with which risk environments to predispose to which disorders; part in the rather simplistic conceptualisation of person–environment interactions (Rutter, 1983; Bateson, 1987); and part in the limited availability of the appropriate statistical techniques to test for the hypothesised interactions (Kendler & Eaves, 1986). Even so, some evidence within the field of antisocial disorders suggests that those who are genetically at risk are also most likely to be affected by adverse patterns of rearing (Cadoret, 1982, 1985). Clearly, this is a possibility that needs to be investigated further.

Of course, the demonstration that some individuals have an increased susceptibility to psychosocial adversity does not explain how that susceptibility operates. One possibility is that it resides in an unusually marked immediate reaction of a kind that leads on to psychopathology – as, perhaps, with a fear response to a frightening situation or a depressive reaction to loss or a sense of insecurity or helplessness following poor parenting. Data linking variations in intensity of initial responses with later outcome are largely lacking, and are much needed. Nevertheless, this is not the only means by which an increased susceptibility can come about. For example, in our study of children being reared by mentally ill parents we found that those with adverse temperamental characteristics were particularly likely to be the target of parental criticism and hostility (Rutter, 1978a). Thus, it appears that children's personal qualities made them more or less likely to be *exposed* to negative features in the environment, through their effects on other people. It is necessary to recognise that, to an important extent, people act in ways that help shape their environment (Scarr & McCartney, 1983) and that for many aspects of psychosocial development, these personal non-shared elements of the environment have a greater influence than the overall family circumstances (Plomin & Daniels, 1987).

In that connection, it is relevant that the same temperamental features may be both risky and protective, according to the situation. As Hinde (1982) has emphasised, the notion that certain traits are adaptive in all circumstances is not in keeping with biological understanding. Thus, the so-called 'difficult' temperament is one that is associated with psychiatric risk. However, De Vries (1984) found that during famine conditions in Africa it was associated with survival – probably because infants with these characteristics demanded and received more attention and food. Similarly, Maziade *et al.* (1987) found that, in upper (but not lower) social status families, difficult temperament in infancy was associated with higher IQ at $4\frac{1}{2}$ years. The data are too sparse, and the findings too inconsistent across studies, for any conclusion on the importance or generality of interactions of this kind. Nevertheless, it does seem important to examine temperamental effects in relation to a range of possible mechanisms involving person–environment interactions, and not just in terms of direct vulnerability processes (Rutter, 1989d).

Similar considerations arise with respect to gender differences in children's response to psychosocial stress and adversity (Rutter, 1970, 1982; Zaslow & Hayes, 1986). Many studies have shown that boys tend to react more adversely to some types of psychosocial stress and adversity than do girls. The increased vulnerability of males does not apply to all situations, however. For example, it has not been found in relation to institutional rearing (Wolkind, 1974; Rutter, Quinton & Hill, 1990b) or head injury (Rutter, Chadwick & Shaffer, 1983). This suggests that although, to some extent, males may be generally psychologically more vulnerable than females, in parallel with their greater psychological vulnerability (Rutter, 1970; Eme, 1979; Earls, 1987), that is most unlikely to constitute the whole explanation. Several further mechanisms have been suggested (Zaslow & Hayes, 1986). Thus, the stress situation may have greater salience for boys. For example, when parents separate, the children usually remain with the mother so that whereas the boys lack a same-sexed parent, the girls do not. Alternatively, it may be that boys experience greater exposure to the stress. Thus, it seems that parents were more likely to quarrel in front of their sons than their daughters (Hetherington & Camara, 1984). However, it is unlikely that the greater male exposure applies to all stress circumstances. For example, Radke-Yarrow, Richters & Wilson (1988) reported that some depressed mothers tended to use their daughters as 'comfort objects', so engulfing them in their negative mood. Probably boys and girls tend to elicit somewhat different patterns of behaviour from their parents but in each case this may be either protective or the reverse, depending on the consequences.

The sex difference in susceptibility may reside as much in the sequences that follow exposure to stress/adversity as in the pattern of exposure itself. For example, when exposed to discord, boys are more likely than girls to respond with aggressive or oppositional behaviour (Cummings *et al.*, 1985); a difference in keeping with a general tendency for aggressive responses to be characteristic of males and distress responses of females (Maccoby & Jacklin, 1974; Eme, 1979; Earls, 1987). Probably, the latter are likely to elicit a more sympathetic reaction from parents. There is some evidence (reviewed by Zaslow & Hayes, 1986) that adults are more likely to perceive negative affects in babies as anger if the infant is male and distress if female (Condry & Condry, 1976; Haviland & Malatesta, 1981), and that parents are more likely to provide comfort and help to daughters than sons (Lambert, Yackley & Heir, 1971; Fagot, 1974, 1978).

These findings refer to immediate responses but longitudinal data indicate that the same applies to longer time sequences. For example, Buss (1981) found that high activity was associated with positive interactions between fathers and sons but negative interactions between fathers and daughters; Maccoby, Snow & Jacklin (1984) found that mothers tended to back away from difficult sons whereas the reverse applied with girls; and Hinde & Stevenson-Hinde (1987b; Stevenson-Hinde, Hinde & Simpson, 1986) found that shyness in boys was associated with largely negative interpersonal interactions whereas in girls the correlates were largely positive (Radke-Yarrow *et al.*, 1988 showed much the same). We may conclude that it is crucial to consider both gender and temperamental differences in interactional, as well as individual, terms (see also Stevenson-Hinde, Chapter 13). Individual differences in responsivity to 'maternal deprivation' may derive from the adaptive or maladaptive cycles of interpersonal interactions that are set up, as much as from biological variations in psychological vulnerability as such. Unquestionably, this consideration greatly complicates the investigation of individual differences but the need for such a complication derives from the empirical findings available so far.

One further aspect of individual differences that has come to prominence in recent years is the need to consider protective mechanisms (Rutter, 1987 b, 1989d). The issue first arose, perhaps, through a recognition that children's responses to one stress or adversity needed to be considered in the context of other positive and negative features of their environment (Rutter, 1978b). It was found that children were more likely to be resilient if the stress experience was an isolated one and/or if it was accompanied by environmental strengths (particularly the presence of one or more good close relationships) as well as by the hazards (Rutter, 1985c). This was followed by an appreciation that if protection was conceptualised in this way it amounted to little more than a measure of the degree of overall risk, with positive influences simply the counterpoint of negative ones. However, this did not seem to be the whole story in that there were circumstances in which the supposed protective factors operated only in the presence of risk variables (Rutter, 1987b, 1990b). For example, in our follow-up of girls reared in institutions we found a protective effect of positive school influences that was not found in the control group (Quinton & Rutter, 1988). Protection needs to be defined in terms of a modification of a person's response to a risk situation – an interactive process rather than a positive influence *per se*.

These considerations have led to a renewal of interest in the concept of 'steeling' effects from stress experiences (Rutter, 1981 b). The phenomenon is well established with respect to physical stressors (such as electric shock), where these may bring about lasting structural and functional changes in the neuroendocrine system that are protective against later stressors (Hennessy & Levine, 1979). Protection seems to derive from the adaptive changes that follow successful coping (Ursin, Baade & Levine, 1978). Similarly, in the field of immunology it is well known that resistance to infection comes from successful coping with the noxious infectious agent and not from avoidance of exposure or from positive health promotion as such. Indeed, the latter may sometimes involve unexpected risks; for example, secular trends suggest that improved household hygiene may have caused an increase in the risk of appendicitis (Barker *et al.*, 1988). We lack data on whether successful coping has a protective effect in relation to psychosocial stress and adversity but there is suggestive evidence that it may have – for example, Elder's (1974, 1979) finding that older children who took on additional family responsibilities during the Great Depression seemed to benefit thereby. It should be added that longitudinal studies bring out the further point that resilience may derive from what happens *after* the adverse experiences as well as from prior protective influences (Rutter, 1979, 1989d). Protection needs to be considered in terms of processes over time and not as something that resides in the chemistry of the moment of the stress experience.

One final consideration concerns the possibility that, in some circumstances, psychopathology or abnormal experiences may be protective. In medicine there are, of course, well-documented examples of this kind. The protection against malaria afforded by sickle cell disease is probably the best known but there are others (Rotter & Diamond, 1987). We do not know whether there are parallels in responses to 'maternal deprivation' but there may be. For example, Hinkle (1974) commented that adults who seemed most immune to stress had an almost 'sociopathic' flavour to their personality and somewhat similar observations have been made by others (Lieberman, 1975; Jenkins, 1979). Also, Farrington *et al.* (1988) have shown that social withdrawal may protect against delinquency.

It is apparent that research into individual differences has not so far provided firm answers to the question of why some children succumb to 'maternal deprivation' experiences whereas others do not. However, what it has shown is that it is seriously misleading to relegate individual differences to 'constitutional' factors of little interest because they are unalterable (Ainsworth, 1962). To the contrary, the investigation of individual differences leads straight to the heart of the interactive processes involved in the psychological damage deriving from 'maternal deprivation' experiences.

Attachment

Although the original focus of 'maternal deprivation' concepts was on the psychological damage brought about by disruptions in the early mother–child relationship, probably the greatest lasting impact stems from the theory of attachment to which the concepts gave rise (Bowlby, 1969/82, 1973, 1980) and from the extensive body of empirical research on attachment that followed (Campos *et al.*, 1983; Sroufe, 1983; Bretherton & Waters,

1985; Belsky & Nezworski, 1988). The essence of the theory lay in its giving primacy to the need to develop social relationships; in its differentiation of attachment from other qualities of relationships (so that, for example, anxiety intensifies attachment behaviour but inhibits play); in its emphasis on the importance of selectivity in attachments; in its suggestion that selective attachments provide emotional security; and in its postulate that these early attachment relationships provide the basis for later social relationships. The approach has been broadly supported by empirical evidence (Rajecki, Lamb & Obmascher, 1978; Rutter, 1981 a), although over the years there have been some modifications of the details as a result of research findings (such as a dropping of the parallel with the old notions of imprinting, a down-playing of sensitive period effects, abandonment of the notion of monotropy, and a recognition that social development is affected by later as well as earlier experiences: see Rutter 1981 a; Bowlby, 1988; Sroufe, 1988).

A major step forward in attachment research was the conceptualisation of different qualities of attachment in terms of security/insecurity and, especially, the provision of a means of measuring these qualities through the Strange Situation devised by Ainsworth (1967; Ainsworth *et al.*, 1978). Although the concept and its measurement have their limitations (Lamb *et al.*, 1984), the approach has generally paid off richly in its making sense of variations in relationship qualities and in its (moderate) power to predict later social functioning (Bretherton & Waters, 1985).

Nevertheless, for all the manifest strengths of attachment theory, many difficulties remain in the application of attachment concepts to developmental and clinical issues. One problem, as Hinde (1982) pointed out, has stemmed from using the same term (attachment) to refer to discrete patterns of behaviour (such as proximity-seeking), to a relationship, to a postulated inbuilt predisposition to develop specific attachments to individuals, and to the hypothesised internal controlling mechanisms for this predisposition. Although the need to differentiate between these features is now generally recognised (see Bowlby, 1988), the blurring in the past of the distinction between phenomena to be explained and the psychological processes hypothesised to account for the phenomena has meant that certain key questions remain largely unanswered.

For example, Hinde (1976, 1979; Hinde & Stevenson-Hinde, 1988) emphasised the need to determine how interactions are influenced by the qualities that each partner brings to the interactions and how interactions lead on to relationships. Because attachment research had its origins in 'maternal deprivation' concepts, the initial focus was on maternal influences and especially on sensitivity to the infants' signals as a source of security (Ainsworth *et al.*, 1978). At first, there was a reluctance to accept the possibility that infant temperament might affect attachment security because of the need to separate attachment as a *relationship* quality from dependency as an *individual* trait (Sroufe, Fox & Pancake, 1983). However, the available evidence now suggests that both maternal and infant characteristics contribute to attachment qualities and that, as Hinde (1980) argued, the dyadic relationship is also influenced by the broader social context (Belsky & Isabella, 1988). Probably, insecure attachments are more likely to develop when parents are depressed or exhibit personality difficulties, when the marital relationship is strained, when there are external stresses, and when there is a lack of social support. It seems likely that the infants' temperamental qualities are also influential (Thompson, Connell & Bridges, 1988) but the findings are inconclusive so far.

A further question concerns the process by which a relationship quality becomes transformed into an individual characteristic. That attachment security/insecurity is a relationship quality initially is shown by the repeated finding that the quality of the mother–infant relationship does not predict the quality of the father–infant relationship, or relationships with other caregivers (Bretherton & Waters, 1985). On the other hand, the finding that it does predict the character of later peer relationships indicates that some reflection of the attachment quality must be carried forward within the individual, unless the relationship continuity is merely a consequence of continuity in environmental influences. At least in the Hodges & Tizard (1989a, b) follow-up of residential nursery children, the continuity could not be an effect of this kind, because the links between relationships persisted in spite of a change in environment. However, the problem is not simply one of explaining how an insecure (or secure) attachment leads to some comparable quality in the individual that influences later relationships. The point is that children's relationships with key figures in their environment are likely to vary in their security qualities. The question then becomes one of how discrepant relationships become internalised. Does the most important relationship predominate, is there a balance between differing relationships, or does one secure relationship compensate for insecurities in others? Moreover, we need to ask how later relationship experiences alter the individual qualities, which clearly they do (Bretherton & Waters, 1985; Belsky & Nezworski, 1988; Hinde & Stevenson-Hinde, 1988). The prevailing view at the moment is that the mediation resides in some form of internalised representation, or working model, of relationships (Stern, 1985; Sroufe & Fleeson, 1986; Bretherton, 1987). At some level, this must be the case in that individuals will bring to their relationships both memories of past interactions and expectations of future ones. However, at least as presently conceptualised, the notion of internal working models is too all encompassing to have much testable explanatory power (Hinde, 1988). Moreover, at least in so far as the processes in infancy are concerned, the cognitive complexity involved in representing both sides of discrepant relationships seems beyond the cognitive capacity available at, say, one year of age (Dunn, 1988).

These issues constitute just one part of the broader question of how one relationship affects other relationships (Hinde & Stevenson-Hinde, 1988). That issue necessarily goes beyond the dyad. For example, it is necessary to explain why in some circumstances women in a discordant marital relationship show more involvement (albeit with less sensitivity) with their babies than do mothers in a harmonious relationship (Engfer, 1988); why marital relationships may alter after the birth of a first child (Belsky & Isabella, 1988); why dyadic interactions may be different when a third party is present (Clarke-Stewart, 1978; Corter, Abramovitch & Pepler, 1983); and why children who have a close relationship with their mothers tend to develop a hostile relationship with their next-born sibling (Dunn & Kendrick, 1982). While these compensatory and rivalry situations are in no way incompatible with attachment theory, it is not obvious that the theory provides an adequate explanation on its own. There is a need both to consider dyadic relationships in terms that go beyond attachment concepts (Hinde, 1976, 1979; Nash, 1988) and to consider social systems that extend beyond dyads.

Research into social relationships in childhood has primarily concentrated on parent–child relationships. However, it may be that more attention needs to be paid to peer relationships. It is striking, in the Hodges & Tizard (1989a, b) follow-up of late-adopted children reared initially in residential nurseries, that they *did* seem to develop attachments with their adoptive parents, but nevertheless their peer relationships still lacked intimacy and selectivity. It appeared that the main outcome of a lack of continuity in caregiving in infancy was to be found in friendship patterns rather than in later parent–child relationships. It is also evident that poor peer relationships in childhood predict later social malfunction and psychopathology (Parker & Asher, 1987). The findings raise questions on the connections and parallels between types of relationships (parent–child as experienced as a child, sibling–sibling, peer–peer, sexual love relationships, parent–child as experienced by the parent, etc.). What are the attachment components in each of these and how may security/insecurity qualities be conceptualised and measured in later childhood, adolescence and adult life? A useful start has been made (Main, Kaplan & Cassidy, 1985; Cassidy & Kobak, 1988; Main & Cassidy, 1988) but much more remains to be done.

One of the controversial claims associated with the initial 'maternal deprivation' concept was that caregiving outside the family was to be avoided and that group day care was especially likely to be damaging. Curiously, that issue is still not entirely resolved in spite of extensive empirical research. On the one hand, it is evident that most infants who experience good quality day care with continuity in caregiving showed no detectable ill-effects (Rutter, 1981 a; Zigler & Gordon, 1982). On the other hand, much day care lacks continuity and provides less personalised care than is desirable. In these circumstances, there are some risks, albeit not as great as originally stated. To a substantial extent such risks as there are derive from the poor quality of care rather than from the fact that it has been provided on a group basis (McCartney & Galanopoulos, 1988). However, it has been suggested that group day care may itself be difficult for babies under a year old when it is on a full-time basis while both parents are working (Belsky, 1988; Belsky & Rovine, 1988). The evidence is too fragmentary for firm conclusions. It is developmentally plausible that group day care might have different effects just when infants are developing their first selective attachments but it is not yet clear whether in fact this is so. Clearly, the risks were greatly overstated in the past but they cannot be entirely ruled out on the basis of present evidence. What is clear, regardless of that issue, is that the quality of day care and of the children's relationships with non-parental caregivers are important and may have implications for their later social functioning (Phillips, McCartney & Scarr, 1987; Oppenheim, Sagi & Lamb, 1988; Vandell, Henderson & Wilson, 1988).

Finally, it is necessary to consider disorders of attachment and the mechanisms involved in associations between attachment insecurity and psychopathology. These issues have been the focus of attention in infant psychiatry (Minde & Minde, 1986; Greenspan & Lieberman, 1988) but without an adequate resolution of how to classify relationship disturbances in early childhood (Sameroff & Emde, 1989). Indeed, as yet, we lack a good understanding of which disorders in childhood are, and which are not, related to insecure attachment (Bates & Bayles, 1988). Clearly, insecure attachment as measured by the Strange Situation cannot be regarded as synonymous with disorder, if only because of its high frequency in the normal population and its inconsistent association with psychopathology. The expansion of the Ainsworth A–B–C classification to include A/C and D categories that reflect avoidant/ambivalent and disorganised patterns has been helpful in picking out more obviously abnormal qualities (Main & George, 1985; Radke-Yarrow *et al.*, 1985; Crittenden, 1988). Nevertheless, it seems doubtful whether the Strange Situation procedure is sufficient on its own as a diagnostic tool; moreover, its validity is uncertain when used with infants with gross psychopathology or with older children. Thus, for example, in one study (Sigman & Ungerer, 1984) children with autism (the child psychiatric disorder with the most severe relationship deficit) did not stand out in terms of their responses as traditionally measured.

Also, in spite of important pointers (Belsky & Nezworski, 1988; Bowlby,

1988) it is not yet obvious how to make use of attachment concepts in therapeutic practice with older children or with adults. How, for example, may individuals who have experienced poor parenting be helped to overcome their early adversities? Main *et al.* (1985) have argued that it is important for healthy personality development to have access to memories of painful experiences in order to come to terms with them. The suggestion is certainly plausible but critical tests of the hypothesis have yet to be undertaken.

Undoubtedly attachment theory has been successful in casting crucial light on the importance of early parent–child relationships, in making helpful hypotheses on some of the processes involved in social development, and in drawing attention to the possible role of disordered relationships in psychopathology. However, its very success carries dangers. The boundaries of attachment theory need to be defined, indicating what it does *not* explain as well as what it does (Sroufe, 1988) and to place it in the context of the broader study of social relationships involving non-attachment, as well as attachment, features; and polyadic as well as dyadic qualities (Hinde, 1979; Hinde & Stevenson-Hinde, 1988).

Conclusions

Our understanding of child development, of parenting qualities, and of environmental influences on child psychopathology have advanced a long way since 'maternal deprivation' concepts were first put forward some 40 years ago. Many of the key features of those concepts have been confirmed through empirical research although they have had to be modified substantially. What has stood the test of time most of all has been the proposition that the qualities of parent–child relationships constitute a central aspect of parenting, that the development of social relationships occupies a crucial role in personality growth, and that abnormalities in relationships are important in many types of psychopathology. It is evident that, as knowledge has advanced, so the questions to be tackled have extended in range and complexity. Such is the way of science. As is also apparent from this review, many of those key questions have been most clearly formulated by Robert Hinde. Although he would not regard himself as a 'maternal deprivation' theorist, the fact that the field has developed so constructively over the years owes much to the clarity of his conceptualisations on developmental issues and on the study of social relationships.

References

Adam, K. S. (1982). Loss, suicide and attachment. In *The Place of Attachment in Human Behavior*, ed. C. M. Parkes and J. Stevenson-Hinde, pp. 269–94. London: Tavistock Publications.

Ainsworth, M. D. (1962). The effects of maternal deprivation: A review of findings and controversy in the context of research strategy. In *Deprivation of Maternal Care: A Reassessment of its Effects*. Public Health Papers No. 14. Geneva: World Health Organization.

Ainsworth, M. D. S. (1967). *Infancy in Uganda: Infant Care and the Growth of Love*. Baltimore, Maryland: Johns Hopkins Press.

Ainsworth, M. D. S. (1982). Attachment: retrospect and prospect. In *The Place of Attachment in Human Behavior*, ed. C. M. Parkes and J. Stevenson-Hinde, pp. 3–30. London: Tavistock Publications.

Ainsworth, M. D. S., Blehar, M. C., Waters, E. & Wall, S. (1978). *Patterns of Attachment: A Psychological Study of the Strange Situation*. Hillsdale, NJ: Erlbaum.

American Psychiatric Association (1987). *Diagnostic and Statistical Manual of Mental Disorders* (3rd edition, revised) – DSM-III-R. Washington, DC: American Psychiatric Association.

Baers, M. (1954). Women workers and home responsibilities. *International Labor Review*, **69**, 338–55.

Barker, D. J. P., Osmond, C., Golding, A. & Wadsworth, M. E. J. (1988). Acute appendicitis and bathrooms in three samples of British children. *British Medical Journal*, **296**, 956–8.

Bates, J. E. & Bayles, K. (1988). Attachment and the development of behavior problems. In *Clinical Implications of Attachment*, ed. J. Belsky and T. Nezworski, pp. 253–99. Hillsdale, NJ: Erlbaum.

Bateson, P. (1979). How do sensitive periods arise and what are they for? *Animal Behaviour*, **27**, 470–86.

Bateson, P. (1987). Biological approaches to the study of behavioural development. *International Journal of Behavioural Development*, **10**, 1–22.

Bell, R. Q. (1968). A reinterpretation of the direction of effects in studies of socialization. *Psychological Review*, **75**, 81–95.

Bell, R. Q. & Chapman, M. (1986). Child effects in studies using experimental or brief longitudinal approaches to socialization. *Developmental Psychology* **22**, 595–603.

Bell, R. Q. & Harper, L. V. (1977). *Child Effects on Adults*. Hillsdale, NJ: Erlbaum.

Belsky, J. (1988). Infant day care and socio-emotional development. The United States. *Journal of Child Psychology and Psychiatry*, **29**, 397–406.

Belsky, J. & Isabella, R. (1988). Maternal, infant, and social-contextual determinants of attachment security. In *Clinical Implications of Attachment*, ed. J. Belsky and T. Nezworski, pp. 41–94. Hillsdale, NJ: Erlbaum.

Belsky, J. & Nezworski, T. (ed.) (1988). *Clinical Implications of Attachment*. Hillsdale, NJ: Erlbaum.

Belsky, J. & Rovine, M. J. (1988). Nonmaternal care in the first year of life and the security of infant–parent attachment. *Child Development*, **59**, 157–67.

Berrueta-Clement, J. R., Schweinhart, L. J., Barnett, W. S., Epstein, A. S. & Weikart, D. P. (1984). *Changed Lives: the Effects of the Perry Preschool Program on Youths through age 19*. Ypsilanti, Michigan: High Scope Press.

Birtchnell, J., Evans, C. & Kennard, J. (1988). Life history factors associated with neurotic symptomatology in a rural community sample of 40–49-year-old women. *Journal of Affective Disorders*, **14**, 271–85.

Block, J. H., Block, J. & Gjerde, P. F. (1986). The personality of children prior to divorce: A prospective study. *Child Development*, **57**, 827–40.

Bowlby, J. (1946). *Forty-four Juvenile Thieves: Their Characters and Home Life.* London: Baillière, Tindall & Cox.

Bowlby, J. (1951). *Maternal Care and Mental Health.* WHO Monograph Series, No. 2. Geneva: World health Organization.

Bowlby, J. (1969). *Attachment and Loss, Vol. 1. Attachment* (2nd edition, 1982). New York: Basic Books.

Bowlby, J. (1973). *Attachment and Loss, Vol. 2. Separation, Anxiety and Anger.* London: Hogarth Press.

Bowlby, J. (1980). *Attachment and Loss, Vol. 3. Loss, Sadness and Depression.* London: Hogarth Press.

Bowlby, J. (1988). *A Secure Base: Clinical Implications of Attachment Theory.* London: Routledge & Kegan Paul.

Bowlby, J., Ainsworth, M., Boston, M. & Rosenbluth, D. (1956). The effects of mother–child separation: A follow up study. *British Journal of Medical Psychology*, **29**, 211.

Bowlby, J., Robertson, J. & Rosenbluth, D. (1952). A two-year-old goes to hospital. *Psychoanalytic Study of the Child*, **7**, 82–94.

Bradley, R. H., Caldwell, B. M. & Rock, S. L. (1988). Home environment and school performance: A ten-year follow-up and examination of three models of environmental action. *Child Development*, **59**, 852–67.

Breier, A., Kelsoe, J. R., Kirwin, P. D., Beller, S. A., Wolkowitz, O. M. & Pickar, D. (1988). Early parental loss and development of adult psychopathology. *Archives of General Psychiatry*, **45**, 987–93.

Bretherton, I. (1987). New perspective on attachment relations: Security, communication, and internal working models. In *Handbook of Infant Development*, 2nd edition, ed. J. D. Osofsky, pp. 1061–100. Chichester: John Wiley.

Bretherton, I. & Waters, E. (ed.) (1985). *Growing Points in Attachment Theory and Research. Monographs of the Society for Research in Child Development*, **50** (1–2, Serial No. 209).

Brunk, M. A. & Henggeler, S. W. (1984). Child influences on adult controls: An experimental investigation. *Developmental Psychology*, **20**, 1074–81.

Buss, D. M. (1981). Predicting parent–child interactions from children's activity level. *Developmental Psychology*, **17**, 59–65.

Cadoret, R. J. (1982). Genotype–environmental interaction in antisocial behavior. *Psychological Medicine*, **12**, 235–9.

Cadoret, R. J. (1985). Genes, environment and their interaction in the development of psychopathology. In *Genetic Aspects of Human Behavior*, ed. T. Sakai and T. Tsuboi, pp. 165–75. Tokyo: Igaku-Shoin.

Cadoret, R. J. & Cain, C. (1980). Sex differences in predictors of antisocial behavior in adoptees. *Archives of General Psychiatry*, **37**, 1171–5.

Cadoret, R. J., Troughton, E. & O'Gorman, T. W. (1987). Genetic and environmental factors in alcohol abuse and antisocial personality. *Journal of Studies on Alcohol*, **48**, 1–8.

Campos, J. J., Barrett, K., Lamb, M. E., Goldsmith, H. H. & Stenberg, C. (1983). Socioemotional development. In *Handbook of Child Psychology*, 4th edition, ed. P. H. Muse. *Vol. 2. Infancy and Developmental Psychobiology*, ed. M. M. Haith and J. J. Campos, pp. 783–915. New York: John Wiley.

Capitanio, J. P., Rasmussen, K. L. R., Snyder, D. S., Laudenslager, M. & Reite, M. (1986). Long-term follow-up of previously separated pigtail macaques: Group and individual differences in response to novel situations. *Journal of Child Psychology and Psychiatry*, **27**, 531–8.

Casler, L. (1961). Maternal deprivation: a critical review of the literature. *Monograph of Society of Research in Child Development*, **26**, 2.

Casler, L. (1968). Perceptual deprivation in institutional settings. In *Early Experience and Behaviour*, ed. G. Newton and S. Levine. Springfield, Ill: Chas C. Thomas.

Cassidy, J. & Kobak, R. R. (1988). Avoidance and its relation to other defensive processes. In *Clinical Implications of Attachment*, ed. J. Belsky and T. Nezworski, pp. 300–323. Hillsdale, NJ: Erlbaum.

Clarke, A. M. & Clarke, A. D. B. (ed.) (1976). *Early Experience: Myth and Evidence*. London: Open Books.

Clarke-Stewart, K. A. (1978). And Daddy makes three: The father's impact on mother and young child. *Child Development*, **49**, 466–78.

Cloninger, C. R., Sigvardsson, S., Bohman, M. & von Knorring, A. L. (1982). Predisposition to petty criminality in Swedish adoptees. II. Cross-fostering analysis of gene–environment interaction. *Archives of General Psychiatry*, **39**, 1242–7.

Condry, J. & Condry, S. (1976). Sex differences: A study of the eye of the beholder. *Child Development*, **47**, 812–19.

Corter, C., Abramovitch, R. & Pepler, D. (1983). The role of the mother in sibling interactions. *Child Development*, **54**, 1599–605.

Crittenden, P. M. (1985). Maltreated infants: Vulnerability and resilience. *Journal of Child Psychology and Psychiatry*, **26**, 85–96.

Crittenden, P. M. (1988). Relationships as risk. In *Clinical Implications of Attachment*, ed. J. Belsky and T. Nezworski, pp. 136–74. Hillsdale, NJ: Erlbaum.

Crowe, R. R. (1974). An adoption study of antisocial personality. *Archives of General Psychiatry*, **31**, 785–91.

Cummings, E. M., Lanott, R. J. & Zahn-Waxler, C. (1985). Influence of conflict between adults on the emotions and aggression of young children. *Developmental Psychology*, **21**, 495–507.

Cummings, E. M., Zahn-Waxler, C. & Radke-Yarrow, M. (1981). Young children's responses to expressions of anger and affection by others in the family. *Child Development*, **52**, 1274–82.

Cummings, E. M., Zahn-Waxler, C. & Radke-Yarrow, M. (1984). Developmental changes in children's reactions to anger in the home. *Journal of Child Psychology and Psychiatry*, **25**, 63–74.

David, H. P., Dytrych, Z., Matejcek, Z. & Schuller, V. S. (ed.) (1988). *Born Unwanted: Developmental Effects of Denied Abortion*. New York: Springer-Verlag.

Dennis, W. (1973). *Children of the Creche*. New York: Appleton-Century-Crofts.

De Vries, M. W. (1984). Temperament and infant mortality among the Masai of East Africa. *American Journal of Psychiatry*, **141**, 1189–94.

Douglas, J. W. B. (1975). Early hospital admissions and later disturbances of behaviour and learning. *Developmental Medicine and Child Neurology*, **17**, 456–80.

Dunn, J. (1988). *The Beginnings of Social Understanding*. Oxford: Blackwell.

Dunn, J. & Kendrick, C. (1982). *Siblings: Love, Envy and Understanding*. Cambridge, Mass.: Harvard University Press.

Duyme, M. (1988). School success and social class: An adoption study. *Developmental Psychology*, **24**, 203–9.

Earls, F. (1987). Sex differences in psychiatric disorders: origins and developmental influences. *Psychiatric Developments*, **5**, 1–23.

Eisenberg, L. (1986). Mindlessness and brainlessness in psychiatry. *British Journal of Psychiatry*, **148**, 497–508.

Elder, G. H. (1974). *Children of the Great Depression*. Chicago: University of Chicago Press.

Elder, G. H. (1979). Historical change in life patterns and personality. In *Life Span Development and Behavior, Vol. 2*, ed. P. B. Baltes and O. G. Brim. New York: Academic Press.

Elder, G. H., Caspi, A. & Burton, L. (1988). Adolescent transitions in developmental perspective: Sociological and historical insights on adolescence. In *Minnesota Symposia on Child Psychology*, ed. M. R. Gunner. Hillsdale, NJ: Erlbaum.

Eme, R. F. (1979). Sex differences in childhood psychopathology: A review. *Psychological Bulletin*, **86**, 574–95.

Emery, R. E. (1982). Interparental conflict and the children of discord and divorce. *Psychological Bulletin*, **92**, 310–30.

Engfer, A. (1988). The interrelatedness of marriage and the mother–child relationship. In *Relations Between Relationships*, ed. R. A. Hinde and J. Stevenson-Hinde. Oxford: Oxford University Press.

Ernst, C. (1988). Are early childhood experiences overrated? A reassessment of maternal deprivation. *European Archives of Psychiatry and Neurological Sciences*, **237**, 80–90.

Fagot, B. I. (1974). Sex differences in toddlers' behavior and parental reaction. *Developmental Psychology*, **10**, 554–8.

Fagot, B. I. (1978). The influence of sex of child on parental reactions to toddler children. *Child Development*, **49**, 495–65.

Farrington, D. P. (1986). Stepping stones to adult criminal careers. In *Development of Antisocial and Prosocial Behavior: Research, Theories and Issues*, ed. D. Olweus, J. Block and M. Radke-Yarrow, pp. 359–84. New York: Academic Press.

Farrington, D. P., Gallagher, B., Morley, L., St Ledger, R. & West, D. J. (1988). Are there any successful men from criminogenic backgrounds? *Psychiatry*, **51**, 116–30.

Fendrich, M., Warner, V. & Weissman, M. (1990). Family risk factors, parental depression and childhood psychopathology. *Developmental Psychology*, **26**, 40–50.

Furstenberg, F. J., Brooks-Gunn, J. & Morgan, S. (ed.) (1987). *Adolescent Mothers in Later Life*. Cambridge: Cambridge University Press.

Garber, H. (1988). *The Milwaukee Project: Preventing Mental Retardation in children at Risk*. Washington, DC: American Association on Mental Retardation.

Garber, H. & Heber, R. (1982). Modification of predicted cognitive development in high-risk children through early intervention. In *How and How Much Can Intelligence be Increased?*, ed. M. K. Detterman and R. J. Sternberg, pp. 121–37. Norwood, NJ: Ablex Publishing.

Garrison, W. & Earls, F. (1987). *Temperament and Child Psychopathology*. Newbury Park: Sage.

Gewirtz, J. L. (1968). The role of stimulation in models for child development. In *Early Child Care: The New Perspectives*, ed. L. L. Dittman. New York: Atherton Press.

Gewirtz, J. (1969). Mechanisms of social learning: some roles of stimulation and behaviour in early development. In *Handbook of Socialization Theory and Research*, ed. D. Gostin, pp. 57–212. New York: Rand McNally.

Gottfried, A. E. & Gottfried, A. W. (ed.) (1988). *Maternal Employment and Children's Development, Longitudinal Research*. New York: Plenum Press.

Greenberg, M. T. & Speltz, M. L. (1988). Attachment and the ontogeny of conduct problems. In *Clinical Implications of Attachment*, ed. J. Belsky and T. Neyworski, pp. 177–218. Hillsdale, NJ: Erlbaum.

Greenspan, S. I. & Lieberman, A. F. (1988). A clinical approach to attachment. In *Clinical Implications of Attachment*, ed. J. Belsky and T. Nezworski, pp. 387–424. Hillsdale, NJ: Erlbaum.

Guze, S. B. (1989). Biological psychiatry: Is there any other kind? *Psychological Medicine*, **19**, 315–23.

Harlow, H. F. & Harlow, M. K. (1969). Effects of various mother–infant relationships on rhesus monkey behaviours. In *Determinants of Infants Behaviour, Vol. 4*, ed. B. M. Foss. London: Methuen.

Harris, T., Brown, G. W. & Bifulco, A. (1986). Loss of parent in childhood and adult psychiatric disorder: The role of lack of adequate parental care. *Psychological Medicine*, **16**, 641–59.

Hartup, W. W. (1983). Peer relations. In *Handbook of Child Psychology, Vol. 3. Socialization, Personality and Social Development*, ed. E. Hetherington, Series ed. P. Mussen, pp. 103–96. New York: John Wiley.

Haviland, J. J. & Malatesta, C. Z. (1981). The development of sex differences in non-verbal signals: Fallacies, facts and fantasies. In *Gender and Non-verbal Behavior*, ed. C. Mayo and M. M. Henley, pp. 183–208. New York: Springer-Verlag.

Hennessy, J. & Levine, S. (1979). Stress, arousal and the pituitary–adrenal system: A psychoendocrine hypothesis. In *Progress in Psychobiology and Physiological Psychology*, ed. J. M. Sprague and A. N. Epstein, pp. 133–78. New York: Academic Press.

Hetherington, E. M. (1988). Parents, children and siblings: 6 years after divorce. In *Relationships Within Families: Mutual influences*, ed. R. A. Hinde and J. Stevenson-Hinde. Oxford: Clarendon Press.

Hetherington, E. M. & Camara, K. (1984). Families in transition. The processes of dissolution and reconstitution. In *Review of Child Development Research: The Family*, ed. R. D. Parke, R. N. Emde, H. P. McAdoo and G. P. Sackett. Chicago: University of Chicago Press.

Hinde, R. A. (1976). Interactions, relationships and social structure. *Man* **11**, 1–17.

Hinde, R. A. (1977). Mother–infant separation and the nature of inter-individual relationships: experiments with rhesus monkeys. *Proceedings of the Royal Society of London, B*, **196**, 29–50.

Hinde, R. A. (1979). *Towards Understanding Relationships*. London: Academic Press.

Hinde, R. A. (1980). Family influences. In *Scientific Foundations of Developmental Psychiatry*, ed. M. Rutter, pp. 47–66. London: Heinemann Medical.

Hinde, R. A. (1982). *Ethology*. Oxford: Oxford University Press.

Hinde, R. A. (1987). *Individuals, Relationship and Culture: Links Between Ethology and the Social Sciences*. Cambridge: Cambridge University Press.

Hinde, R. A. (1988). Continuities and discontinuities: conceptual issues and methodological considerations. In *Studies of Psychosocial Risk: The Power of Longitudinal Data*, ed. M. Rutter. Cambridge: Cambridge University Press.

Hinde, R. A. & Bateson, P. P. G. (1984). Discontinuities versus continuities in behavioural development and the neglect of process. *International Journal of Behavioural Development*, **7**, 129–43.

Hinde, R. A. & McGinnis, L. (1977). Some factors influencing the effect of temporary mother–infant separation: some experiments with rhesus monkeys. *Psychological Medicine*, **7**, 197–212.

Hinde, R. A. & Spencer-Booth, Y. (1967). The behaviour of socially living rhesus monkeys in their first 2½ years. *Animal Behaviour*, **15**, 169–96.

Hinde, R. A. & Spencer-Booth, Y. (1971). Effects of brief separation from mother on rhesus monkeys. *Science*, **173**, 111.

Hinde, R. A. & Stevenson-Hinde, J. (1987a). Interpersonal relationships and child development. *Developmental Review*, **7**, 1–21.

Hinde, R. A. & Stevenson-Hinde, J. (1987b). Implications of a relationships approach for the study of gender differences. *Infant Mental Health Journal*, **8**, 221–35.

Hinde, R. A. & Stevenson-Hinde, J. (ed.) (1988). *Relationships Within Families: Mutual Influences*. Oxford: Oxford University Press.

Hinkle, L. E. (1974). The effect of exposure to culture change, social change, and changes in interpersonal relationships on health. In *Stressful Life Events: Their Nature and Effects*, ed. B. S. Dohrenwend and B. P. Dohrenwend. New York: John Wiley.

Hodges, J. & Tizard, B. (1989a). IQ and behavioural adjustment of ex-institutional adolescents. *Journal of Child Psychology and Psychiatry*, **30**, 53–75.

Hodges, J. & Tizard, B. (1989b). Social and family relationships of ex-institutional adolescents. *Journal of Child Psychology and Psychiatry*, **30**, 77–97.

Horn, J. M. (1983). The Texas adoption project: adopted children and their intellectual resemblance to biological and adoptive parents. *Child Development*, **54**, 28–275.

Jenkins, C. D. (1979). Psychosocial modifiers of response to stress. *Journal of Human Stress*, **5**, 3–15.

Kagan, J. (1981). *The Second Year: The Emergence of Self-Awareness*. Cambridge, Mass.: Harvard University Press.

Kagan, J. (1984a). *The Nature of the Child*. New York: Basic Books.

Kagan, J. (1984b). Continuity and change in the opening years of life. In *Continuities and Discontinuities in Development*, ed. R. N. Emde and R. J. Harmon, pp. 15–39. New York: Plenum Press.

Kagan, J., Reznick, J. S. & Snidman, N. (1987). The physiology and psychology of behavioural inhibition in children. *Child Development*, **58**, 1459–73.

Kagan, J., Reznick, J. S., Snidman, N., Gibbons, J. & Johnson, M. O. (1988). Childhood derivatives of inhibition and lack of inhibition to the unfamiliar. *Child Development*, **59**, 1580–9.

Kendler, K. S. & Eaves, L. J. (1986). Models for the joint effect of genotype and environment on liability of psychiatric illness. *American Journal of Psychiatry*, **143**, 279–89.

Kohnstamm, G. A., Bates, J. E. & Rothbart, M. K. (ed.) (1989). *Temperament in Childhood*. Chichester: John Wiley.

Kolvin, I., Miller, F. J. W., Fleeting, M. & Kolvin, P. A. K. (1988). Risk/protective factors for offending with particular reference to deprivation. In *Studies of Psychosocial Risk: The Power of Longitudinal Data*, ed. M. Rutter, pp. 77–95. Cambridge: Cambridge University Press.

Lamb, M. E. (ed.) (1982). *Non-traditional Families: Parenting and Child Development*. Hillsdale, NJ: Erlbaum.

Lamb, M. E., Thompson, R. A., Gardner, W., Charnov, E. L. & Estes, D. (1984). Security of infantile attachment as assessed in the 'Strange Situation': Its study and biological interpretation. *Behavioral and Brain Sciences*, **7**, 127–47.

Quinton, D. & Rutter, M. (1976). Early hospital admissions and later disturbances of behaviour: an attempted replication of Douglas' findings. *Developmental Medicine and Child Neurology*, **18**, 447–59.

Quinton, D. & Rutter, M. (1988). *Parental Breakdown: The Making and Breaking of Intergenerational Links*. Aldershot: Avebury.

Radke-Yarrow, M., Cummings, E. M., Kuczynski, L. & Chapman, M. (1985). Patterns of attachment in two and three year old normal families and families with parental depression. *Child Development*, **56**, 884–93.

Radke-Yarrow, M., Richters, J. & Wilson, W. E. (1988). Child development in the network of relationships. In *Relationships Within Families: Mutual Influences*, ed. R. A. Hinde and J. Stevenson-Hinde, pp. 48–67. Oxford: Clarendon Press.

Radke-Yarrow, M., Zahn-Waxler, C. & Chapman, M. (1983). Children's prosocial dispositions and behavior. In *Handbook of Child Psychology, Vol. 4. Socialization, Personality, and Social Development*, ed. P. H. Mussen. New York: John Wiley.

Rajecki, D. W., Lamb, M. E. & Obmascher, P. (1978). Toward a general theory of infantile attachment: A comparative review of aspects of the social bond. *Brain and Behavioral Sciences*, **2**, 640–3.

Ramey, C. T. & Campbell, F. A. (1981). Educational intervention for children at risk for mild retardation: a longitudinal analysis. In *Frontiers of Knowledge in Mental Retardation, Vol. 1. Social, Educational and Behavioral Aspects*, ed. P. Mittler, pp. 47–57. Baltimore, Md.: University Park Press.

Ramey, C. T. & Campbell, F. A. (1984). Preventive education for high risk children: Cognitive consequences of the Carolina Abecedarian project. *American Journal of Mental Deficiency*, **88**, 515–24.

Ramey, C. T., MacPhee, D. & Yeates, K. (1982). Preventing developmental retardation: A general systems model. In *Facilitating Infant and Early Childhood Development*, ed. L. Bond and J. Joffe. Hanover, NH: University Press of New England.

Reitsma-Street, M., Offord, D. R. & Finch, T. (1985). Pairs of same-sexed siblings discordant for antisocial behaviour. *British Journal of Psychiatry*, **146**, 415–23.

Richman, N., Stevenson, J. & Graham, P. J. (1982). *Preschool to School: A Behavioural Study*. London: Academic Press.

Rotter, J. I. & Diamond, J. M. (1987). What maintains the frequencies of human genetic diseases? *Nature*, **329**, 289–90.

Roy, P. (1983). Is continuity enough?: Substitute care and socialization. Paper presented at the Spring Scientific Meeting, Child and Adolescent Psychiatry Specialist Section, Royal College of Psychiatrists, London, March.

Ruppenthal, G. C., Arling, G. L., Harlow, H. F., Sackett, G. P. & Suomi, S. J. (1976). A 10-year perspective of motherless-mother monkey behavior. *Journal of Abnormal Psychology*, **85**, 341–9.

Rutter, M. (1970). Sex differences in children's responses to family stress. In *The Child in His Family*, ed. E. J. Anthony and C. Koupe, pp. 165–96. Chichester: John Wiley.

Rutter, M. (1971). Parent–child separation: Psychological effects on the children. *Journal of Child Psychology and Psychiatry*, **12**, 233–60.

Rutter, M. (1972). *Maternal Deprivation Reassessed*. Harmondsworth, Middlesex: Penguin.

Rutter, M. (1978a). Family area and school influences on the genesis of conduct disorders. In *Aggression and Antisocial Behaviour in Childhood and Adolescence*,

Journal of Child Psychology and Psychiatry, Book Supplement 1, ed. L. A. Hersov and M. Berger with D. Shaffer. Oxford: Pergamon Press.

Rutter, M. (1978b). Protective factors in children's responses to stress and disadvantage. In *Primary Prevention of Psychopathology, Vol. 3. Social Competence in Children*, ed. M. W. Kent and J. E. Rolf, pp. 49–74. Hanover, NH: University Press of New England.

Rutter, M. (1979). Separation experiences: A new look at an old topic. *Journal of Pediatrics*, **95**, 147–54.

Rutter, M. (1981a). *Maternal Deprivation Reassessed*, 2nd edition. Harmondsworth, Middlesex; Penguin.

Rutter, M. (1981b). Stress, coping and development: Some issues and some questions. *Journal of Child Psychology and Psychiatry*, **22**, 323–56.

Rutter, M. (1982). Continuities and discontinuities in socio-emotional development: Empirical and conceptual perspectives. In *Continuities and Discontinuities in Development*, ed. R. Emde and R. Harmon. New York: Plenum Press.

Rutter, M. (1983). School effects on pupil progress: research findings and policy implications. *Child Development*, **54**, 1–29.

Rutter, M. (1985a). Family and school influences on cognitive development. *Journal of Child Psychology and Psychiatry*, **26**, 683–704.

Rutter, M. (1985b). Family and school influences on behavioural development. *Journal of Child Psychology and Psychiatry*, **26**, 349–68.

Rutter, M. (1985c). Resilience in the face of adversity: Protective factors and resistance to psychiatric disorder. *British Journal of Psychiatry*, **147**, 598–611.

Rutter, M. (1986). Child Psychiatry: Looking 30 Years Ahead. *Journal of Child Psychology and Psychiatry*, **27**, 803–40.

Rutter, M. (1987a). Continuities and discontinuities from infancy. In *Handbook of Infant Development*, ed. J. Osfosky, pp. 1256–96. New York: John Wiley.

Rutter, M. (1987b). Psychosocial resilience and protective mechanisms. *American Journal of Orthopsychiatry*, **57**, 316–31.

Rutter, M. (1989a). Pathways from childhood to adult life. *Journal of Child Psychology and Psychiatry*, **30**, 23–51.

Rutter, M. (1989b). Intergenerational continuities and discontinuities in serious parenting difficulties. In *Child Maltreatment*, ed. D. Cicchetti and V. Carlson. New York: Cambridge University Press.

Rutter, M. (1989c). Child psychiatric disorders in ICD-10. *Journal of Child Psychology and Psychiatry*, **30**, 499–513.

Rutter, M. (1989d). Temperament: Conceptual issues and clinical inplications. In *Temperament in Childhood*, ed. G. A. Kohnstamm, J. E. Bates and M. K. Rothbort, pp. 463–79. Chichester: John Wiley.

Rutter, M. (1990a). Commentary: Some focus and process considerations regarding effects of parental depression on children. *Developmental Psychology*, **26**, 60–7.

Rutter, M. (1990b). Psychosocial resilience and protective mechanisms. In *Risk and Protective Factors in the Development of Psychopathology*, ed. J. E. Rolf, A. S. Masten, D. Cicchetti, K. Nuechterlein and S. Weintraub. New York: Cambridge University Press.

Rutter, M., Chadwick, O. & Shaffer, D. (1983). The behavioural and cognitive sequelae of head injury. In *Developmental Neuropsychiatry*, ed. M. Rutter, pp. 83–111. New York: Guilford Press.

Rutter, M. & Giller, H. (1983). *Juvenile Delinquency: Trends and Perspectives*. Harmondsworth, Middlesex: Penguin.

Rutter, M., MacDonald, H., Le Couteur, A., Harrington, R., Bolton, P. & Bailey, A. (1990a). Genetic factors in child psychiatric disorders: II. Empirical findings. *Journal of Child Psychology and Psychiatry*, **31**, 39–83.

Rutter, M., Maughan, B., Mortimore, P. & Ouston, J. with Smith, A. (1979). *Fifteen Thousand Hours: Secondary Schools and Their Effects on Children*. London: Open Books and Cambridge, Mass.: Harvard University Press.

Rutter, M. & Pickles, A. (1990). Person–environmental interactions: Concepts, mechanisms and implications for data analysis. In *Conceptualization and Measurement of Organism–Environment Interaction*, ed. T. D. Wachs and R. Plomin. Washington, DC: American Psychological Association.

Rutter, M. & Quinton, D. (1984). Parental psychiatric disorder: Effects on children. *Psychological Medicine*, **14**, 853–80.

Rutter, M., Quinton, D. & Hill, J. (1990b). Adult outcome of institution-reared children: Males and females compared. In *Straight and Devious Pathways from Childhood to Adulthood*, ed. L. Robins and M. Rutter. New York: Cambridge University Press.

St Clair, L. & Osborne, A. F. (1987). The ability and behavior of children who have been 'in-care' or separated from their parents. *Early Child Development Care*, *28*, No. 3 Special Issue.

Sameroff, A. J. & Emde, R. N. (ed.) (1989) *Relationship Disturbances in Early Childhood: A Developmental Approach*. New York: Basic Books.

Scarr, S. & McCartney, K. (1983). How people make their own environments: A theory of genotype → environment effects. *Child Development*, **54**, 424–35.

Scarr, S. & Weinberg, R. A. (1976). IQ test performance of black children adopted by white families. *American Psychologist*, **31**, 726–39.

Schiff, M. & Lewontin, R. (1986). *Education and Class: The Irrelevance of IQ Genetic Studies*. Oxford: Clarendon Press.

Sigman, M. & Ungerer, J. (1984). Attachment behaviors in autistic children. *Journal of Autism and Development Disorders*, **14**, 231–44.

Skuse, D. (1984). Extreme deprivation in early childhood – II. Theoretical issues and a comparative review. *Journal of Child Psychology and Psychiatry*, **25**, 543–72.

Smith, D. J. & Tomlinson, S. (1989). *The School Effect: A Study of Multi-Racial Comprehensives*. London: Policy Studies Institute.

Sorce, J. F., Emde, R. N., Campos, J. & Klinnert, M. D. (1985). Maternal emotional signaling: Its effects on the visual cliff behavior of 1-year-olds. *Developmental Psychology*, **21**, 195–200.

Sorce, J. F., Emde, R. N. & Frank, M. (1982). Maternal referencing in normal and Down's syndrome infants: A longitudinal analysis. In *The Development of Attachment and Affiliative Systems*, ed. R. N. Emde and R. J. Harmon, pp. 281–92. New York: Plenum Press.

Sroufe, L. A. (1983). Infant–caregiver attachment and patterns of adaptation in the preschool: The roots of competence and maladaptation. In *Minnesota Symposia in Child Psychology*, *Vol. 16*, ed. M. Perlmutter, pp. 41–83. Hillsdale, NJ: Erlbaum.

Sroufe, L. A. (1988). The role of infant–caregiver attachments in development. In *Clinical Implications of Attachment*, ed. J. Belsky and T. Nezworski, pp. 18–38. Hillsdale, NJ: Erlbaum.

Sroufe, L. A. & Fleeson, J. (1986). Attachment and the construction of relationships. In *Relationships and Development*, ed. W. Hartup and Z. Rubin, pp. 51–71. Hillsdale, NJ: Erlbaum.

Sroufe, L. A., Fox, N. & Pancake, V. (1983). Attachment and dependency in developmental perspective. *Child Development*, **55**, 17–29.

Stern, D. N. (1985). *The Interpersonal World of the Infant: A View from Psychoanalysis and Developmental Psychology*. New York: Basic Books.

Stevenson-Hinde, J., Hinde, R. A. & Simpson, A. E. (1986). Behavior at home and friendly or hostile behavior in preschool. In *Development of Antisocial and Prosocial Behavior: Research, Theories and Issues*, ed. D. Olweus, J. Block and M. Radke-Yarrow. New York: Academic Press.

Suomi, S. J. (1987). Genetic and maternal contributions to individual differences in rhesus monkey biobehavioral development. In *Perinatal Development: A Psychobiological Perspective*, ed. N. A. Krasnegor, E. M. Blass, M. A. Hofer and W. P. Smotherman, pp. 397–419. New York: Academic Press.

Teasdale, T. W. & Owen, D. R. (1984). Heredity and familial environment in intelligence and educational level – a sibling study. *Nature*, **309**, 620–2.

Tennant, C. (1988). Parental loss in childhood. *Archives of General Psychiatry*, **45**, 1045–50.

Terr, L. C. (series editor) (1989). Resolved: Day care is the best care for children under age 5 of working Americans. *Journal American Academy Child and Adolescent Psychiatry*, **28**, 130–5.

Thompson, R. A., Connell, J. P. & Bridges, L. J. (1988). Temperament, emotion and social interactive behavior in the Strange Situation: A component process analysis of attachment system functioning. *Child Development*, **59**, 1102–10.

Tizard, B. (1977). Varieties of residential nursery experience. In *Varieties of Residential Experience*, ed. J. Tizard, I. Sinclair and R. V. G. Clark, pp. 102–21. London: Routledge & Kegan Paul.

Tizard, B. & Hodges, J. (1978). The effect of early institutional rearing on the development of eight-year-old children. *Journal of Child Psychology and Psychiatry*, **19**, 99–118.

Tizard, B. & Rees, J. (1974). A comparison of the effects of adoption, restoration to the natural mother and continued institutionalization on the cognitive development of four-year-old children. *Child Development*, **45**, 92–9.

Tizard, J. & Tizard, B. (1971). The social development of 2 year old children in residential nurseries. In *The Origins of Human Social Relations*, ed. H. E. Schaffer. London: Academic Press.

Ursin, H., Baade, E. & Levine, S. (1979). *Psychobiology of Stress: A Study of Coping Men*. New York: Academic Press.

Vandell, D. L., Henderson, V. K. & Wilson, K. S. (1988). A longitudinal study of children with day-care experiences of varying quality. *Child Development*, **59**, 1286–92.

van Dusen, K. T., Mednick, S. A., Gabrielli, W. F. & Hutchings, B. (1983). Social class and crime in an adoption cohort. *Journal of Criminal Law and Criminology*, **74**, 249–69.

Vernon, D. T. A., Foley, J. M., Sipowicz, R. R. & Schulman, J. L. (1965). *The Psychological Responses of Children to Hospitalization and Illness*. Springfield, Ill: Chas. C. Thomas.

West, D. J. (1982). *Delinquency: Its Roots, Careers and Prospects*. London: Heinemann.

Wolkind, S. (1974). The components of 'affectionless psychopathy' in institutionalized children. *Journal of Child Psychology and Psychiatry*, **15**, 215–20.

373

Woodhead, M. (1985). Pre-school education has long term effects: But can they be generalized? *Oxford Review of Education*, **11**, 133–55.

Woodhead, M. (1988). When psychology informs public policy: The case of early childhood intervention. *American Psychologist*, **43**, 443–54.

Wootton, B. (1959). *Social Science and Social Pathology*. London: Allen & Unwin.

Wootton, B. (1962). A social scientist's approach to maternal deprivation. In *Deprivation of Maternal Care: A Reassessment of its Effects*. Geneva: World Health Organization.

World Health Organization Expert Committee on Mental Health (1951). *Report on the Second Session 1951*. Geneva: WHO.

World Health Organization (1989). *ICD-10 1988 Draft of Chapter V: Categories F00–F99, Mental, Behavioral and Developmental Disorders. Clinical Descriptions and Diagnostic Guidelines*. Geneva: WHO.

Yeates, K. Q., MacPhee, D., Campbell, F. A. & Ramey, C. T. (1983). Maternal IQ and home environment as determinants of early childhood intellectual competence: a developmental analysis. *Developmental Psychology*, **19**, 731–9.

Zahn-Waxler, C., Cummings, E. M., McKnew, D. H. & Radke-Yarrow, M. (1984). Altruism, aggression and social interactions in young children with a manic-depressive parent. *Child Development*, **55**, 112–22.

Zaslow, M. J. & Hayes, C. D. (1986). Sex differences in children's response to psychosocial stress: Toward a cross-context analysis. In *Advances in Developmental Psychology, Vol. 4*, ed. M. E. Lamb, A. L. Brown and B. Rogoff, pp. 285–337. Hillsdale, NJ: Erlbaum.

Zigler, E. F. & Gordon, E. W. (ed.) (1982). *Day Care: Scientific and Social Policy Issues*. Boston, Mass.: Auburn House.

—15—

Relationships and behaviour: the significance of Robert Hinde's work for developmental psychology

Judy Dunn

Developmental psychology – perhaps even more than other social sciences – has grown through its links with a wide range of other sciences. If we think of the individuals who have asked the most provocative and generative questions in developmental psychology, or who have changed the framework of enquiry in an illuminating way, that list must include individuals whose backgrounds arc in biology, in psychoanalytic theory, in philosophy, in child psychiatry, in epidemiology, in behaviour genetics, and in ethology. Robert Hinde has, in my view, a special place on that list, and in this chapter I want to take just one issue that he has studied, to substantiate that claim. The issue is our understanding of the nature and developmental significance of children's relationships – a topic with a central place in the grand theories of human development, yet one on which clear critical thought and rigorous systematic enquiry are still urgently needed.

Hinde's work has, I believe, transformed our appreciation of that central idea: that children's relationships have a role of crucial significance in their development. To spell out how and why, let me begin by borrowing from a famous Hinde slide, a figure that appears in his books (e.g. Hinde, 1982), and that has been shown to many audiences, initially baffling some, finally illuminating many. The figure sets out an ambitious scheme, representing the relations between individuals, interactions, relationships and social structure. These 'levels' of analysis are represented in tiers, with the top level representing social structure, the middle, relationships, and at the lower levels interactions and finally individuals. Figure 1 shows a version.

We can use his scheme, I suggest, to highlight the different ways in which he himself has clarified the study of relationships and development, by beginning at the most abstract level with his discussions of the differences between disciplines in the social sciences, and then moving 'down' to respect of social psychologists, such as Henri Tajfel, whose work he discussed. I was lucky enough to be at Madingley when the book was being completed and was published, and it was, educationally, a marvellous experience. It brought centrally to my attention, as it did to many other child psychologists, the importance of appreciating and recognising the perspective of sociologists, anthropologists and social psychologists. It has taken developmental psychologists a long time to build that appreciation into their research endeavours, but for many developmental questions it is a very important widening of perspective – a point to which I shall return.

Theoretical models and research questions

Hinde's ideas on the distinctive usefulness of the approaches of different disciplines to the study of relationships have been brought together in integrative models of considerable power. That famous figure on the relations between interactions, relationships and social structure is part of the story, but consider too the implications of the simpler version in Hinde, 1982 (Figure 32). He has, as a distinguished colleague of ours put it, 'raised the consciousness' of developmental psychologists about the importance of other social sciences in the study of relationships, and his theoretical writing is very widely cited indeed (see, for instance, the recently published *Handbook of Personal Relationships* edited by Duck, 1988).

Perhaps most important for developmental psychologists has been the way that he has set out in an orderly manner the distinctions between interactions and relationships, the dimensions of interactions that characterise the latter, and the nature of the connections between the properties of individuals and those of the relationships in which they are involved. The chapter entitled 'What do we mean by a relationship' and the discussion of the content, diversity, and patterning of interactions in the 1979 book provide a framework for those working on children and their peers, on parents and children, on friendship between adults, indeed on relationships at any stage of the life span. He takes, in his argument and in the description and classification he sets out, an essential first step towards an analysis of the processes by which relationships affect development.

A second feature of his work, at this level of theoretical models, that stands out is the power of his critical judgement. For me, a particularly important recent illustration of this (sometimes devastating) pin-pointing of careless or illogical thought, this refusal to let vagueness win the day, occurred during the conference on 'Relations among relationships' organised by Robert and Joan Stevenson-Hinde in 1987 (see Hinde & Stevenson-Hinde, 1988). The issue was this. In puzzling over the mechanisms by which children's experiences with their mothers during the first year of life could possibly influence their own adult relationships years later, the idea of 'internal working models' has been developed, first from Bowlby's seminal work (Bowlby, 1969, 1973), and later through much innovative theoretical writing (e.g. Bretherton, 1985). At first sight this is an enticing idea, conveniently inclusive in its explanatory sweep, linking recent research on the development of social understanding with the attachment paradigm. But it is a construct that is fraught with problems, and Hinde would not let anyone off the hook by feeling comfortable that they had 'explained' the underlying processes with this metaphor (Hinde, 1989).

Specific studies of interaction and relationships

It is at the next level 'down' – the level of particular studies – that the significance of Hinde's work for developmental psychologists is perhaps easiest to illustrate. A particularly striking example comes from his studies of mother–infant rhesus monkeys. This research has had a profound influence on a whole domain of theoretical enquiry: it set out a number of principles with elegance and precision, and these principles have guided much of the work of developmental psychologists on mothers and their very young children. Two examples must suffice as illustrations.

First, his analysis of the dynamics of mother–infant interaction in the monkeys first brought centrally to attention the *reciprocal* nature of influence between mother and infant, and showed how investigators could tease apart the relative responsibility of mother and infant in the changing relationship between them. 'Who determines what?' was the question as he raised it in *Towards Understanding Relationships*, and he showed us how to answer it. The research was with baby rhesus monkeys and their mothers, yet the principles were very much those that we applied, following his research, to a subsequent study of the changing patterns of relationships between firstborn children and their mothers following the birth of a second child (Dunn & Kendrick, 1982). We were able to show both *general* patterns, and *individual differences* in the patterns of changing relationships that were of developmental and clinical importance. For instance, one general change in the interaction between mother and firstborn child that was revealed was this: a dramatic decrease in maternal attention and responsiveness following the sibling birth (important in contributing to the disturbed behaviour shown by the majority of the children following their siblings' birth), and an increase in the children's own demands and role in initiating interaction. The analysis of individual differences showed that in families in which the firstborn children responded to the sibling birth by withdrawing, the level of interaction and disturbances in their behaviour, but the form of disturbance, its extent, and its prognostic significance differ widely between families. When we began our research, no systematic prospective studies had been done that could clarify why some children were more vulnerable than others, or what might help children to cope with what was a major change in their lives.

What our research showed was that, just as in the Hinde and Spencer-Booth monkey studies, the quality of the mother–firstborn relationship before the 'event,' and the disturbance in the mother–child relationship following the 'event' were of major importance (along with other factors) in accounting for these differences in children's outcome (Dunn & Kendrick, 1982). And a review of the impact of other 'normative' but potentially stressful events in children's lives, such as starting and changing schools, moving house, periods away from the parents, as well as that of the stresses of divorce and parental separation that are increasingly common, further reinforced the view that the quality of children's relationships with parents and siblings plays a major role in the nature of their reaction to those events (Dunn, 1988 b). We come, again and again, to the clinical implications of the monkey mother–infant studies and Hinde's consideration of the relationship between mother and infant. For instance, in these experiments, every independent variable that affected infant rhesus depression also affected mother–infant interaction (Hinde & McGinnis, 1977). And now, in work on depression in children, on suicide attempts in childhood, and on the effects of divorce and bereavement we find, yet again, that it is long-term changes in family interaction patterns that are implicated in the links between initial events and child outcome (Hetherington, Cox & Cox, 1976; Rutter, 1981; Dunn, 1986; Hetherington, 1987).

That relationships are now recognised as important in individual development seems obvious when we are considering children's social and emotional development. Hartup (1986) set out particularly clearly and succinctly the ways in which relationships are important in the emotional and social development of individuals – a chapter, incidentally, that he wrote while on sabbatical at Madingley and which he considers to reflect, clearly, the extensive conversations which he had with Robert over that period (W. Hartup, personal communication). He points out that relationships are, first, the contexts in which most of socialisation takes place, in which communication skills develop, and which the development of the self-system and the regulation of the emotions have their origins. Second, relationships provide the bases from which children are able to function as independent individuals – whether these are attachment relationships to parents, or friendships with peers. Third, he argues, relationships in childhood are the models on which later relationships are based – a central issue, as we have noted, in attachment theory.

It is now, however, increasingly widely appreciated that the significance of social relationships and the social context in individual development is much broader than this emphasis on socialisation and attachment would suggest. Not only social and emotional development, but cognitive and linguistic development – the development of children's minds and their grasp of language – take place *because* children grow up as members of a social world, and *through* their interactions and relationships with others in that social world (see, for example, Vygotsky, 1962; Donaldson, 1978; Trevarthen, 1978; Bruner, 1983). In my own work on the development of social understanding in children, the point is, I think, particularly clear, and I will comment briefly next on this research because it illustrates both how valuable a 'naturalistic' approach to studying children's development can be, how important it is for us to have a framework for studying relationships if we are to make progress in studying individual development, *and* how important Hinde's influence and perspective has been in focusing attention on that point.

Relationships and the development of social understanding in early childhood

The work to be considered has focused on the beginnings of children's understanding of the feelings, needs and interests of others who share their social world, and of the social rules and roles of that social world. At first sight, these might seem to be a set of issues rather far from those that Robert Hinde has pursued in his own empirical research and writing (with the exception of an edited volume: Hinde, Perret-Clermont & Stevenson-Hinde, 1987). Yet the findings, and the new theoretical perspective developed in this research, are quite directly products of the ethological approach, and of a consideration of the connections between relationships and the wider social world; the links with Hinde's work are, in this sense, clear and direct.

In the study of young siblings and their mothers that Carol Kendrick and I carried out from Madingley we had focused upon the developing relationship between young siblings, and its connection with other family relationships. The study, which involved long observations in the children's homes, developed in an unexpected direction. Watching the jokes, fights and games between the siblings, and their reactions to the other members of their families, I became fascinated with the glimpses of understanding that much of the children's behaviour appeared to reflect. These very young children appeared to have a considerable practical grasp of how to annoy, tease, comfort, and provoke the other family members, and of how to disrupt, compete with or join the interactions between others. The observations suggested powers of understanding in these children well beyond those that

383

from Hinde's powers of rigorous clarification, and his enthusiasm and excitement over developmental issues. I am extraordinarily lucky to have been his student and his colleague.

References

Belsky, J. (1988). The 'effects' of infant daycare reconsidered. *Early Childhood Research Quarterly*, **3**, 235–72.

Bowlby, J. (1969). *Attachment and Loss, Vol. 1. Attachment*. London: Hogarth Press.

Bowlby, J. (1973). *Attachment and Loss, Vol. 2. Separation*. London: Hogarth Press.

Bretherton, I. (1985). Attachment theory: Retrospect and prospect. In *Growing Points of Attachment Theory and Research. Monographs of the Society for Research in Child Development*, *50*, ed. I. Bretherton and E. Waters, pp. 1–2.

Bruner, J. (1983). *Child's Talk*. New York: Norton.

Clarke-Stewart, S. K. (1989). Infant day care: Maligned or malignant? *American Psychologist*, **44**, 266–74.

Donaldson, M. (1978). *Children's Minds*. London: Fontana.

Duck, S. (1988). *Handbook of Personal Relationships*. New York: John Wiley.

Dunn, J. (1977). Patterns of early interaction: continuities and consequences. In *Studies in Mother–Infant Interaction*, ed. H. R. Schaffer. London: Academic Press.

Dunn, J. (1986). Stress, development and family interaction. In *Depression in Young People: Developmental and Clinical Perspectives*, ed. M. Rutter, C. E. Izard and P. B. Read. New York: Guilford Press.

Dunn, J. (1988a). *The Beginnings of Social Understanding*. Oxford: Basil Blackwell/ Cambridge, Mass.: Harvard University Press.

Dunn, J. (1988b). Normative life events as risk factors in childhood. In *Studies of Psychosocial Risk*, ed. M. Rutter. Cambridge: Cambridge University Press.

Dunn, J. & Kendrick, C. (1982). *Siblings: Love, Envy and Understanding*. Cambridge, Mass.: Harvard University Press.

Dunn, J. & Munn, P. (1987). Development of justification in disputes with mother and sibling. *Developmental Psychology*, **23**, 791–8.

Hartup, W. W. (1986). On relationships and development. In *Relationships and Development*, ed. W. W. Hartup and Z. Rubin. Hillsdale, NJ: Erlbaum.

Hetherington, E. M. (1987). Parents, children and siblings: Six years after divorce. In *Relationships Within Families*, ed. R. A. Hinde and J. Stevenson-Hinde. Oxford: Oxford University Press.

Hetherington, E. M., Cox, E. M. & Cox, R. (1976). Divorced fathers. *Family Coordinator*, **25**, 417–28.

Hinde, R. A. (1979). *Towards Understanding Relationships*. London: Academic Press.

Hinde, R. A. (1982). *Ethology*. Oxford: Oxford University Press.

Hinde, R. A. (1987). *Individuals, Relationships and Culture: Links Between Ethology and the Social Sciences*. Cambridge: Cambridge University Press.

Hinde, R. A. (1989). Continuities and discontinuities: conceptual issues and methodological considerations. In *Studies of Psychosocial Risk: The Power of Longitudinal Data*, ed. M. Rutter. Cambridge: Cambridge University Press.

Hinde, R. A. & McGinnis, L. (1977). Some factors influencing the effects of temporary mother–infant separation – some experiments with rhesus monkeys. *Psychological Medicine*, **7**, 197–212.

Hinde, R. A., Perret-Clermont, A. & Stevenson-Hinde, J. (ed.) (1987). *Social Relationships and Social Cognition*. Cambridge: Cambridge University Press.

Hinde, R. A. & Spencer-Booth, Y. (1970). Individual differences in the responses of rhesus monkeys to a period of separation from their mothers. *Journal of Child Psychology and Psychiatry*, **11**, 159–76.

Hinde, R. A. & Stevenson-Hinde, J. (1988). *Relationships within Families: Mutual Influences*. Oxford: Clarendon Press.

Howes, C., Rodning, C., Galluzo, D. C. & Myers, L. (1988). Attachment and child care. Relationships with mother and caregiver. *Early Childhood Research Quarterly*, **3**, 403–16.

Rutter, M. (1972). *Maternal Deprivation Reassessed*. Harmondsworth: Penguin Books.

Rutter, M. (1981). Stress, coping and development: Some issues and some questions. *Journal of Child Psychology and Psychiatry*, **22**, 323–56.

Trevarthen, C. (1978). Descriptive analyses of infant communicative behaviour. In *Studies in Mother–Infant Interaction*, ed. H. R. Schaffer. London: Academic Press.

von Cranach, M., Foppa, K., Lepenies, W. & Ploog, D. (ed.) (1979). *Human Ethology: Claims and Limits of a New Discipline*. Cambridge: Cambridge University Press.

Vygotsky, L. S. (1962). *Thought and Language*. New York: John Wiley.

—16—

The individual and the environment in human behavioural development

Marian Radke-Yarrow

'Boy, age six, head large at birth. Thought to have had brain fever. Three siblings died before his birth. Mother does not agree with relatives and neighbors that child is probably abnormal. Child sent to school . . . diagnosed as mentally ill by teacher. Mother is angry . . . withdraws child from school, says she will teach him herself.'

'Boy, senior year secondary school, has obtained certificate from physician stating that nervous breakdown makes it necessary for him to leave school for six months. Boy not a good all-around student, has no friends . . . teachers find him a problem . . . Spoke late . . . Father ashamed of son's lack of athletic ability . . . Poor adjustment to school. Boy has odd mannerisms, makes up own religion, chants hymns to himself . . . Parents regard him as "different".'

'Girl, age sixteen, orphaned, willed to custody of grandmother by mother, who was separated from alcoholic husband . . . Mother rejected the homely child, who has been proven to lie and to steal sweets. Swallowed penny to attract attention at five . . . Four young uncles and aunts in household cannot be managed by the grandmother . . . Grandmother resolves to be more strict with granddaughter since she fears she has failed with own children. Dresses granddaughter oddly. Refused to let her have playmates, put her in braces to keep back straight . . .[1]

Goertzel and Goertzel, 1962, pp. xii–xiii.

Individual behavioural development continues to present intriguing and perplexing questions to the various scientific disciplines involved in its study. The course of development is not easily projected and not always readily explained. Nor is the unpredicted outcome of development limited to the

---

[1] The first child is Thomas Edison, the second is Albert Einstein, and the third is Eleanor Roosevelt.

lone 'outlier'. In the early study by Spitz & Wolf (1946), of institutionalised infants who had been deprived of mothering, only some developed severe life-threatening depression. Later in the studies by Sigman & Parmelee (1979), many infants with neurological problems, for whom the future appeared to hold considerable risk, did not fulfil predictions of psychological problems in childhood. Problems in adolescence are not invariably preceded by troubled developmental histories.

Another side to the state of our knowledge is very encouraging. Many predictions hold up well on average (e.g. Robins, 1966; Ledingham & Schwartzman, 1984), explanations of aetiologies are not fanciful (e.g. Block, Block & Keyes, 1988), and our interventions to head off developmental disasters or potentiate capabilities have shown successes (Kellam *et al.*, 1975). Nevertheless, differences and unpredictabilities in developmental paths present considerable amounts of variance to be explained and many challenges to theory and research.

Because human development is of interest to many different disciplines from cultural anthropology to genetics, it is not surprising that theorists and investigators differ considerably in where they place their emphasis, how they frame their questions and obtain their evidence, and how they interpret their findings. A common core of shared perspectives is only at a high level of abstraction: it is generally agreed that behaviour and development are multiply determined, that simple, single relations between an antecedent condition and an outcome are unlikely, and that multideterminism is an important reason for our difficulties in understanding human development.

Kagan (1984, p. xi) finds our limited knowledge of development 'embarrassing': '. . . we have a less satisfying explanation of human psychological development than of the life cycle of the fruit fly.' Whether the present state of understanding is regarded as embarrassing, discouraging, or challenging, advancement in knowledge requires a perspective that deals effectively with the inherent complexity of the processes involved. Such a point of view does prevail among theorists in developmental psychology and psychiatry. Thus, models have been elaborated in which behaviour and development are viewed as functions of continuing interaction and mutual influences between child and environment (e.g. Sameroff & Chandler, 1975; Sameroff & Fiese, 1982; Magnusson, 1985). A view of behaviour and development as qualitative reorganisations among and within behaviour systems has been summarised by Cicchetti & Schneider-Rosen (1986) (building on Werner, 1957, and many others). Wachs (1983) focuses on the dynamic nature of the environment in its role in individual development, with different aspects of environment having different effects on different patterns of behaviour at different periods. In their conceptualisation of interrelated relationships, Hinde & Stevenson-Hinde (1987) have described the multiple levels and complicated lines of influence on the individual. Rutter (1983) has called attention to genetic expression in relation to environment at different times in development, an issue that has not figured prominently in developmental research.

These conceptualisations reflect the thinking of developmentalists in recent years. Very similar positions were eloquently pleaded decades earlier. Lewin (1931) half a century ago stressed the interdependence between person and environment. The person was viewed as a part of his own environment. The behaviour of the person, he said, could only be understood in context, in relation to its embeddedness in multiple and overlapping situations. Barker (1968) and Bronfenbrenner (1979) continued the argument for ecological validity in behavioural assessment. Sears (1951) urged an approach to the child in terms of dyadic relationships, and, following this lead, Bell (1968) wrote his influential paper on 'child effects', in which he argued the bi-directional influences of child and caregiver on each other. In summary, these formulations represent the developmental process as one in which the young organism is changing, and is part of, and is encountering, a multifaceted and constantly changing environment. The child brings its unique endowments to the environment, makes a difference in the environment, and is modified by it. All in all, a formidable formulation of processes.

Models and methods

Why this parade of positions and conceptualisations? It is because they constitute a strong consensus, a critical theoretical mass, that creates a tension in research on development. These are accepted perspectives and conceptualisations, yet their implications are rarely realised in research designs, assessment procedures, and interpretations of findings.

Behavioural research on children, for the most part, is not geared to investigating transactions, encompassing a multiplicity of influences, measuring environment in non-static and developmental terms, addressing developmental questions developmentally, or accounting for individual differences in development. Cairns (1986) has made this point in a critical review of research methods:

Nondevelopmental concepts and the statistical procedures associated with them have been permitted to become dominant for the field, even though they may blur the diversity and individuality of behavioural development. Some procedures may actually retard psychological understanding – partly because of the distance created between the concepts of investigators and the phenomena they wish to explain

(Cairns, 1986, p. 99).

Appelbaum & McCall (1983) see a similar crisis of methods:

the most macroscopic framework, environment is dealt with in ways that have been assumed to require virtually no measurement – none at a direct level. It is inferred from a macrostructural characteristic, such as social class, single-parented families, birth order, or institution- versus home-reared. These broad contexts are assumed to organise a set of stable and predictable conditions and experiences that impinge similarly on all children within them; hence, they need not be measured. From this perspective, environment is dealt with as a static characteristic of experience, and variance is drastically compressed. While this approach is informative about average group differences, issues of process cannot be clarified. There is no way of knowing which conditions or subsets of variables within the classifying concepts are responsible for any behavioural differences that are found, leaving the door open to speculative interpretation.

Environment is also studied experimentally. A situation is devised or utilised that is assumed to represent some larger complex of experience. In many laboratory experiments, environment has been defined in terms of a single dimension of adult behaviour (such as contingent responding, affection, or control techniques), in a specific setting or task (e.g. mother is observed playing with her 2-year-old, or behaving according to an experimental plan by varying her facial expression, or enforcing a prohibition). Labelled as analogue studies of child rearing, the findings of these 'environments' have been interpreted as generalisable to family rearing processes. Although they deal with processes of influence, such miniaturised and sanitised environments have come under criticism as lacking ecological validity and being conceptually simplistic. These procedures differentiate among parents, but relatively little is known about the predictive value of the observed differences. Rarely in these designs has a developmental perspective been adopted.

Environment has been measured in a third way: in order to sample parental behaviour more broadly and to take rearing history into account, investigators, for a long time, have chosen to measure environment indirectly, through mothers' reports. These reports tend to provide trait-like characteristics of parents, without reference to interactive patterns of behaviour and specific contexts.

In contrast to the preceding methods are a number of endeavours in which the complex and dynamic characteristics of environment are recognised and incorporated in research questions. Family systems research (e.g. Reiss, 1981; Minuchin, 1988) and research on relationships (e.g. Hinde 1979, Hinde & Stevenson-Hinde, 1987) represent such approaches. They begin to take into account the embeddedness of behaviour and its multiple determinants.

And finally, methods of dealing with environment or context include its being ignored or regarded as of little or no relevance to understanding the behaviour being investigated. For example, many comparisons of boys' and girls' behavioural dispositions have been 'environment-free' (e.g. studies of moral reasoning, language development, emotional expression). Likewise, maternal psychiatric illness and children's problem behaviours have been linked, with little attention to the interactional contexts of these associations. At a more microscopic level, many investigations of associations between maternal caregiving qualities (e.g. sensitivity to child's needs, protectiveness, physical affection) and child characteristics have been conspicuously inattentive to the possible influences of the research contexts or environmental circumstances in which measurements are made.

Methods explored

We may now ask, regarding these methods, how well they meet objectives of measuring environment as a dynamic variable, and how well they permit us to assess different facets of the environment in relation to different patterns of child behaviour at different developmental stages. It is apparent that there are shortcomings. Measurement of environment may be brought somewhat closer to these objectives by considering the interdependent issues of how environment is conceptualised and how it is sampled.

Theoretically justified sampling. Let us begin with several facets of sampling. We are accustomed to thinking about the sampling of subjects; less accustomed to thinking about the sampling of environment.

A primary issue in sampling involves the necessary choices that investigators must make of contexts (situation, time, activity) in which to evaluate patterns of behaviour. Let us assume that the patterns of interest regarding maternal environment are mothers' 'sensitivities' to children's needs, or protectiveness or affection. The point at issue is: what assumptions underlie the selection of the particular samples of environmental conditions in which mother and child are observed? The field of infant research provides examples of sound sampling choices based on theoretical considerations. Thus, mothers are observed feeding the infant, soothing and quieting the tired child, and playing with the infant. Such combinations of settings and functions sample core maternal functions and experiences in caring for the infant. Another sampling success from infancy research is represented in the paradigm of the Strange Situation (Ainsworth *et al.*, 1978). Here the measurement of separations and reunions is an astute choice, based on theory, for indexing a basic mother–child relationship at this stage of development.

But in contrast to these examples, in much research, especially with children who are past infancy, the situation of measurement is not so likely of skills, knowledge, and understanding of self and social world, and providing affective meaning to interactions and relationships. These multi-dimensions need then to be observed simultaneously in relation to each other.

We have experimented with an approach that incorporates multi-dimensions. It is presented here as an example. It is an observational study (Radke-Yarrow, 1989) in which families are seen in the diversity of situations comprising the core rearing demands and experiences listed above. Semi-naturalistic and informal experimental methods are used, having families come to a home-like apartment for repeated half-day visits. Time is scripted to create a reasonably natural sequence of experiences designed to simulate at-home experiences. The apartment becomes familiar and comfortable to the families and they make use of it (e.g. its stocked refrigerator, TV, toys, couch) as if it were their own.

It is soon apparent in observing families in these activities that the specific maternal dimensions that we are accustomed to describing in isolation (e.g. affection, control, etc.) are not neatly separated from one another, nor do their effects appear to be uniform regardless of the matrix of rearing dimensions in which they occur. In the apartment, as in everyday life, parents' emotions and control techniques and information-giving, etc., 'happen' together and interdependently – in the routines of living, in dealing with unexpected events, and in stresses and pleasures.

Many examples in the data obtained from this study illustrate the dynamic nature of environment–child interaction. (i) The effects of a proximal environmental variable depend on its larger context. Thus, the correlation between positive mother–child relationship and children's compliance differs depending on the smooth or chaotic functioning of the family as a whole. Only in stable family contexts is there a significant positive correlation. (ii) Associations between negative qualities in maternal behaviour and problem behaviour in the child depend on the presence of combinations of maternal behaviour. For example, maternal qualities, such as frequent anger, deprecatory comments to child, poor control methods, when considered singly, are not strongly predictive of problematic child behaviour. However, when these qualities appear in combination, mothers with these characteristics are significantly over-represented among the most problematic children. (iii) Influences in the rearing environment are connected. Mother's behaviour not only influences the child directly; it has indirect consequences through its effects on other relationships within the family. As one example: the mothers' crescendo of insensitivity and irritability with her children mobilises an alliance between the siblings. They collaborate in devious actions against the mother. (iv) Maternal behaviour has different effects depending on the child's characteristics. Mothers' expressed negative emotions are not related to negative expression in boys, but are significantly associated with negative emotions in girls. (v) Child qualities, again gender, have different effects on the environment. Anger in little girls is less tolerated by mothers than is anger in little boys. (vi) Maternal qualities and child qualities influence each other. Mothers who are themselves emotionally needy tend to seek out the more needy of their children, drawing these children into anxious, depressed affect, with considerable stability in the developmental course of this process.

To sum up the explorations of measurement, environment needs to be made a first-class variable in developmental research, not inferred, not casually sampled, not given puny assessment. Sampling of environment needs to be theory-based. Multi-dimensional measures of rearing environments are needed to furnish data that more nearly meet the criteria of our conceptual models.

II. What is the course of development?

It is said that '... the longitudinal method is the life blood of developmental science. It is the only way researchers can study change within organisms over age' (Appelbaum & McCall, 1983, p. 441). It is also the only way researchers can examine developing and changing interdependencies between the individual and the environment. Longitudinal approaches make it possible to investigate how family environment and child affect each other differently at different ages, and affect each other cumulatively. How else, except with longitudinal data can one observe the evolution of a shy 2-year-old into a confident, sociable, and happy 11-year-old, in relation to the contexts or environments in which this child is developing?

Unfortunately longitudinal data form only a small portion of the information of developmental psychology. As an important method and a 'missing' method, longitudinal study becomes a candidate for exploration. There are the classic longitudinal studies in which psychological development is followed over childhood or the better part of a lifetime. Such are the studies of gifted children (Terman, 1925; Terman & Oden, 1947, 1959; Oden, 1968; Sears, 1979), the Berkeley studies of normal children (Macfarlane, Allen & Honzik, 1954), Olweus' study of aggression (1980), and others. More longitudinal investigations are short term, focused on particular developmental periods of theoretical significance (e.g. 0–3 years, 1–6 years, adolescence).

But longitudinal studies do not fully meet expectations. Generally the emphasis has been on the continuity of characteristics of the individual – rarely in relation to underlying processes. This orientation may be adequate for characteristics that are 'organism' characteristics, such as height, but not for behavioural or 'relationship' variables (see Stevenson-Hinde, 1988). Longitudinal studies of human development fall short, too, by being follow-up studies, with intervals of 6 months, 1 year, 5 years, and the like between measurements. Such studies provide a series of cross-sectional snapshots. To some extent, then, the necessary descriptive data of development as well as information regarding process fall between the checkpoints. Because of the potential wealth of information in the unmeasured intervals, there is reason to explore alternative longitudinal approaches.

Alternative approaches

The child whose bedroom is crowded with nature's wonders – tadpoles becoming frogs, caterpillars becoming cocoons becoming butterflies, shut-eyed kittens becoming alert frisky ones – is making the kinds of observations that provide truly longitudinal description. Are such observations possible or impractical in research on child development? Time, cost, and intrusiveness are considerable deterrents, but not ultimate barriers. While not seen as run-of-the-mill procedure, approaches involving close tracking of behaviour and environment at strategic points of inquiry can be uniquely informative. (We have stressed overt behaviour and environment. Underlying neurophysiological changes would also be primary drivers in the developmental course.)

Close tracking is valuable and well suited to the study of emerging functions and adaptations and rapidly changing organisations of behaviour. Indeed, there have been such studies in human development. A century ago, Preyer (1888–9, cited by Cairns, 1983) observed infants three times a day over a period of months to capture the emergence of the self (using the now familiar mirror technique). A contemporary example, also of infant behaviour, is Thoman's (1975) longitudinal study of sleep–waking patterns. Infants were observed for 7 hours once each week. Parents' infant diaries, too, qualify as continuous longitudinal accounts of development.

The young child's developing gender identity, the child's developing methods of coping with chronically stressful family relationships, the evolution of a mother–child relationship, the formation of a specific attitude or value orientation could profitably be the subject of longitudinal study. This approach might also be revealing when applied to a period like middle childhood which, from present methods, appears quiet and latent but which may not be so.

Close tracking of development would be very useful for understanding 'surprises' or discontinuities in development, which are not infrequent in follow-up studies. An instance of this sort is in our study of children of depressed parents (Radke-Yarrow, 1989). On multiple assessments, a number of 3-year-olds of manic depressive mothers appeared as cheerful, confident, uninhibited, and engaging children. When they returned for study at 5 years of age, they were withdrawn, anxious, and distressed. Was their bright confidence at 3 years a 'premature' maturity fostered by a chronically stressful experience? Were disturbed patterns of maternal behaviour not having an impact until 5 years? Were genetic factors being manifested at 5 years that were not expressed at 3? With assessments at the two separated points in time, investigators have little more to rely on than their own competing explanations. Given such puzzling and theoretically important findings, an intensive longitudinal study of a number of 'sparkling' 3-year-old offspring of affectively ill mothers would be a valuable next phase in research.

The more nearly continuous tracking of individual behaviour and environment can be implemented in many ways. In traditional longitudinal studies, the trust and relationship that develop between families and investigators make it possible to pursue intensive data collection, even with 'difficult' families. The many circumstances in which continuous contact with child and family are 'natural' can also be utilised for longitudinal studies. Such are the contacts of a paediatrician and family. Tracking need not always be in the form of direct observations by the investigator. Systematic interviewing and incident-reporting by an informant are workable techniques of monitoring.

Parents, too, are natural longitudinal observers. They can be trained and can become the extension of the investigator, thereby making accessible certain areas of child behaviour and environment and certain rare critical behavioural events that are otherwise not available to researchers. Parents were used in this way to study young children's emerging sensitivities to the feelings and emotions of other persons (Radke-Yarrow & Zahn-Waxler, 1984). Mothers were trained to observe and record (on audiotape, and according to a standard reporting schedule) their children's reactions to emotional incidents that occurred in everyday experiences and their responses to their children's reactions. Mothers' observing began when their children were 10, 15, or 20 months of age, and their monitoring continued for nine months. Their records provided a fine-grained account of developmentally changing reactions. For example, infants' concerned and furrowed expressions in response to someone's emotional distress were followed (developmentally) by tentative approaches to the 'victims'. Early reactions of confusion in locating the distress – in the other person or in self – slowly gave way developmentally to unambiguous approaches and attempts to comfort the other person. Individual differences in children's thresholds and tolerances for affective distress were also detectable along the developmental course. To check the validity and reliability of these procedures, periodic observations were made in the home by a staff member, and by subsequent testing in laboratory designs (Zahn-Waxler & Radke-Yarrow, 1982). Findings were strongly supportive of the trained mothers' observations.

In the sum, when relatively wide-spaced intervals of measurement limit understanding of development, strategic application of intensive longitudinal monitoring may yield exceptional additions to our knowledge.

III. Mutually interacting influences

The traditional and persistent formulation of research questions in terms of the effects of maternal variables on the child's outcome is joined and perhaps overtaken by another formulation in which the mutual influences of environment and child on each other are emphasised. This view is increasingly pressed, sometimes to the exaggeration of making the child the primary creator of his environment (Scarr & McCartney, 1983).

Almost no one has trouble with the concept of mutual influences. Such influences are commonly referred to in daily discourse. The teacher who carefully separates certain children from each other understands mutual influences: 'When those three boys are together, they go wild – and then the whole class is stirred up.' Folk wisdom regarding husband and wife becoming much like each other echoes the same process. The family therapist has no difficulty in finding examples of mutual effects. Relationship is a concept of mutual influences.

Almost everyone has difficulty with the measurement of mutual influences. The concept is not readily translated into research operations. Only approximations to such measurement exist. Differences in parental behaviour have been demonstrated in relation to differences in child characteristics such as gender (e.g. Condry & Condry, 1976), intelligence level (e.g. Scarr & McCartney, 1983), and temperament and personality (e.g. Rutter, 1987). Influences of relationships on other relationships have also been demonstrated (e.g. Hinde & Stevenson-Hinde, 1988). However, it seems fair to say that most often what we have in these findings are end products that speak eloquently of processes that have taken place. Generally missing are studies in which, for both parent and child, the influencing and the being influenced are observed as an ongoing course of influences over time. This process warrants study.

Methods explored

To measure the ongoing dialogue of influences (mother and child on each other) requires sequentially integrated sets of data (where 'sequence' is not necessarily, and is most often not, interpreted as the immediately following patterns of behaviour). Two approaches that undertake this task are noted.

Clinical studies.   One approach grows mainly out of clinical work and conditions of risk and pathology. Here the interplay of deviances is scrutinised. One example from this source is Patterson's (1982) well-known research on families with 'out-of-control' children. Through intensive and prolonged home observation, the negative pattern of interaction between mother and child is exposed as an upwardly spiralling course of aggression. Buying into each other's aggression, each participant becomes an altered stimulus to the other, and each moves into a changed state of readiness for subsequent encounters. The mutual effects are tracked. Processes like those in Patterson's aggressive families are captured, too, in family systems analyses and in data from family therapy (Reiss, 1981; Minuchin, 1988).

These observations of acutely stressed families might be thought of as speeded-up records of processes that are assumed to be present in slower motion in children's socialisation histories. Such progression in mutual influences over time is precisely the issue that is of fundamental concern in socialisation and development. The successful approaches in the clinical studies furnish valuable models to be extended to this longer time frame of development. The clinical approaches have been successful in analysing systems that have broken down. These approaches should be equally applicable and are equally important in following child–environmental transactions in the broader range of socialisation issues, including healthy and competent development. Such a transfer of clinical expertise into longitudinal studies of socialisation would produce the kinds of data needed for assessing transactional processes in the framework of development.

Multi-child families.   Reflection on the history of developmental research brings us to the consideration of a second avenue for gaining understanding of mutual influences. If, in research tradition, the question of socialisation had been 'how do parents influence their children?' instead of 'how does the parent influence the child?', we might have had evidence on intrafamilial similarities and differences in socialisation, and we might, long ago, have been alerted to mutual influences in children's development. As it is, we must now do a rerun by investigating the experiences of each child in the family, a procedure long advocated by behaviour geneticists (Plomin & Daniels, 1987) to help to clarify genetic and environmental contributions to child behaviour.

Study of multi-child families is a natural experiment in which to observe mutual influences at work, assuming that children in the same family have different endowments (e.g. temperament, physiology, intelligence, gender) that enter into interaction with the environment. We should expect to see child and mother having effects on each other's behaviour as they build a history together. The histories with different children should show different

generate hypotheses, modify conclusions and give direction to further research. The divisions between group and individual methods perhaps need not be as distinct and far apart as they have been.

V. The repertoire of questions and variables

In a way, the unknowns about behaviour have increased, and the hope of understanding development seems remote as research has shed more and more light on the complexities of behaviour. The research process itself has changed. Increasingly, developmentalists find themselves in territories that are beyond the problems and approaches that have traditionally defined their separate disciplines. They discover that the theories, concepts, tools, and fashions of other disciplines have new levels of relevance for their own research. For such mergings in science to be reciprocally enhancing, more than hit-and-miss borrowing of variables or techniques across disciplines is needed; expertise in the several disciplines is required. Since this is a large demand, met only occasionally by a single investigator, collaborations in research become essential. Collaborative research is likely to break ground with new research problems and to bring altered perspectives to many old questions.

Concluding comments

This essay began with discontent about the developmental disciplines moving on two courses: one proceeding toward conceptual clarification of behavioural and developmental processes, the other generating empirical data that poorly represent the phenomena purportedly measured. The purpose has been to prospect for methods that have capabilities of richer yields.

Environment (or context) was seen as a generally neglected or inappropriately assessed variable in developmental research. The case was made for conceptualising and measuring environment with the same scientific care that is given any other variable. It was observed that research methods only infrequently live up to the defining objective of the discipline, i.e. with truly developmental considerations. The strategic use of intensive longitudinal methods was explored. Mutual influences, attractive in conception and in tune with experience, prove to be difficult to measure directly. Possible approaches were noted for observing the developing mutual influences between parent and child. Yet another focus of change concerned the individual case. Perhaps developmental psychology and psychiatry cannot deal with individual prediction or even with the backward explanation of an Eleanor Roosevelt or a Thomas Edison. But neither can research continue to offer group differences and correlations as representative of all individuals and as ultimate explanations of processes. An important niche that prospective case studies can occupy is as sources of data for theoretical propositions about developmental processes, which then can be pursued in richer combination with group methods.

The history of research makes it evident that our understanding of human development is subject to change. 'Truths' are modified by new information; the reconstruction of information is much in the hands of the methods by which data are generated and analysed.

As guidelines for advancing knowledge of behavioural organisation and development, I have accepted the conceptualisations in which complexity and interdependencies of influences are stressed. I have argued for changes in research methods that would result in more harmony between theory and method. The changes advocated would require increased investment in investigative processes: they would alter the nature of the data obtained, and the time and effort needed to acquire the data. They would extend analyses and interpretations to include not only the 'universals' but also the processes involved in non-conforming findings. Such change is essential if the promise in the sophisticated conceptualisations of behavioural and developmental processes is to be attained.

References

Ainsworth, M. D. S., Blehar, M. C., Waters, E. & Wall, S. (1978). *Patterns of Attachment: A Psychological Study of the Strange Situation.* Hillsdale, NJ: Erlbaum.

Appelbaum, M. I. & McCall, R. B. (1983). Design and analysis in developmental psychology. In *Handbook of Child Psychology*, 4th edition, ed. P. H. Mussen. *Vol. 1. History, Theory, and Methods*, ed. W. Kessen. New York: John Wiley.

Barker, R. G. (1968). *Ecological Psychology: Concepts and Methods for Studying the Environment of Human Behavior.* Stanford, Calif.: Stanford University Press.

Bell, R. Q. (1968). A reinterpretation of the direction of effects in studies of socialization. *Psychological Review*, **75**, 81–95.

Block, J., Block, J. H. & Keyes, S. (1988). Longitudinally foretelling drug usage in adolescence: early childhood personality and environmental precursors. *Child Development*, **59**, 336–55.

Breznitz, Z. & Sherman, T. (1987). Speech patterning of natural discourse of well and depressed mothers and their young children. *Child Development*, **58**, 395–400.

Bronfenbrenner, U. (1979). *The Ecology of Human Development: Experiments by Nature and Design.* Cambridge, Mass.: Harvard University Press.

Brown, R. & Bellugi, U. (1964). Three processes in the child's acquisition of syntax. In *New Directions in the Study of Language*, ed. E. H. Lenneberg. Cambridge, Mass.: MIT Press.

Cairns, R. B. (1983). The emergence of developmental psychology. In *Handbook of Child Psychology*, 4th edition, ed. P. H. Mussen. *Vol. 1 History, Theory, and Methods*, ed. W. Kessen. New York: John Wiley.

Cairns, R. B. (1986). Phenomena lost: issues in the study of development. In *The Individual Subject and Scientific Psychology*, ed. J. Valsiner. New York: Plenum Press.

Cicchetti, D. & Schneider-Rosen, K. (1986). An organizational approach to childhood depression. In *Depression in Young People: Developmental and Clinical Perspectives*, ed. M. Rutter, C. E. Izard and P. B. Read. New York: Guilford Press.

Condry, J. & Condry, S. (1976). Sex differences: a study of the eye of the beholder. *Child Development*, **47**, 812–19.

Goertzel, V. & Goertzel, M. G. (1962). *Cradles of Eminence*. Boston, Mass.: Little, Brown and Co.

Hinde, R. A. (1979). *Towards Understanding Relationships*. London: Academic Press.

Hinde, R. A. & Stevenson-Hinde, J. (1987). Interpersonal relationships and child development. *Developmental Review*, **7**, 1–21.

Hinde, R. A. & Stevenson-Hinde, J. (1988). *Relationships Within Families: Mutual Influences*. Oxford: Clarendon Press.

Kagan, J. (1984). *The Nature of the Child*. New York: Basic Books.

Kazdin, A. E. (1981). Drawing valid inferences from case studies. *Journal of Consulting and Clinical Psychology*, **49**, 183–92.

Kellam, S. G., Branch, J. D. Agrawal, K. C. & Ensminger, M. E. (1975). *Mental Health and Going to School: The Woodlawn Program of Assessment: Early Intervention, and Evaluation*. Chicago: University of Chicago Press.

Ledingham, J. E. & Schwartzman, A. E. (1984). A 3-year follow-up of aggressive and withdrawn behavior in childhood: preliminary findings. *Journal of Abnormal Child Psychology*, **12**, 157–68.

Lewin, K. (1931). Environmental forces in child behavior and development. In *A Handbook of Child Psychology*, 2nd edition, ed. C. Murchison. Worcester, Mass.: Clark University Press.

Macfarlane, J. W., Allen, L. & Honzik, M. P. (1954). *A Developmental Study of the Behavior Problems of Normal Children between Twenty-one Months and Fourteen Years*. Berkeley: University of California Press.

Magnusson, D. (1985). Implications of an interactional paradigm for research on human development. *International Journal of Behavioral Development*, **8**, 115–37.

McClintock, C., Brannon, D. & Maynard-Moody, S. (1979). Applying the logic of sample surveys to qualitative case studies: the case cluster method. *Administrative Science Quarterly*, **24**, 612–62.

McGraw, M. (1935). *Growth: a Study of Johnny and Jimmy*. New York: Appleton Century.

Minuchin, P. (1988). Relationships within the family: a systems perspective on development. In *Relationships Within Families: Mutual Influences*, ed. R. A. Hinde and J. Stevenson-Hinde. Oxford: Clarendon Press.

Oden. M. H. (1968). The fulfillment of promise: 40-year follow-up of the Terman gifted group. *Genetic Psychology Monographs*, **77**, 3–93.

Olweus, D. (1980). Familial and temperamental determinants of aggressive behavior in adolescent boys: a causal analysis. *Developmental Psychology*, **16**, 644–60.

Patterson, G. R. (1982). Negative reinforcement and escalation. In *A Social Learning Approach to Family Intervention*, ed. G. R. Patterson and J. B. Reid. Eugene, Oregon: Castalia.

Piaget, J. (1930). *The Child's Conception of Physical Causality*. London: Kegan Paul.

Plomin, R. & Daniels, D. (1987). Why are children in the same family so different from one another? *Behavioral and Brain Science*, **10**, 1–60.

Preyer, W. (1888–9). *The Mind of the Child*. New York: Appleton.

Radke-Yarrow, M. (1989). Family environments of depressed and well parents and their children: issues of research methods. In *Family Social Interactions: Content and Methodological Issues in the Study of Aggression and Depression*, ed. G. R. Patterson and E. Blechman. NJ: Hillsdale, Erlbaum.

Radke-Yarrow, M. & Zahn-Waxler, C. (1984). Roots, motives, and patterns in children's prosocial behavior. In *Development and Maintenance of Prosocial Behavior*, ed. E. Staub, D. Bar-Tal, J. Karylowski and J. Reykowski. New York: Plenum Press.

Radke-Yarrow, M. & Sherman, T. (1990). Hard growing: children who survive. In *Risk and Protective Factors in the Development of Psychopathology*, ed. J. Rolf, A. Masten, D. Cicchetti, K. Neuchterlein, and S. Weintraub. Cambridge: Cambridge University Press.

Reiss, D. (1981). *The Family's Construction of Reality*. Cambridge, Mass.: Harvard University Press.

Robins, L. N. (1966). *Deviant Children Grown Up: A Sociological and Psychiatric Study of Sociopathic Personality*. Baltimore, Md.: Williams and Wilkins.

Rushton, P., Brainard, C. & Pressley, M. (1983). Behavioural development and construct validity: the principle of aggregation. *Psychological Bulletin*, **84**, 18–38.

Rutter, M. (1983). Stress, coping, and development: some issues and some questions. In *Stress, Coping, and Development in Children*, ed. N. Garmezy and M. Rutter. New York: McGraw-Hill.

Rutter, M. (1987). Temperament, personality and personality disorder. *British Journal of Psychiatry*, **150**, 443–58.

Sameroff, A. & Chandler, M. (1975). Reproductive risk and the continuum of care-taking causality. In *Review of Child Development Research, Vol. 4*, ed. F. D. Horowitz, M. Hetherington, S. Scarr-Salapatek and G. Siegel. Chicago: University of Chicago Press.

Sameroff, A. J. & Fiese, B. H. (1982). Transactional regulation and early intervention. In *Early Intervention: A Handbook of Theory, Practice, and Analysis*, ed. S. J. Meisels and J. P. Shonkoff. New York: Cambridge University Press.

Scarr, S. & McCartney, K. (1983). How people make their own environments: a theory of genotype → environmental effects. *Child Development*, **54**, 424–35.

Sears, R. R. (1951). A theoretical framework for personality and social behavior. *American Psychologist*, **6**, 476–83.

Sears, P. S. (1979). The Terman genetic studies of genius, 1922–1972. In *National Society for the Study of Education. The Gifted and the Talented: their Education and Development. Seventy-eight Yearbook*. Chicago: University of Chicago Press.

Sigman, M. & Parmelee, A. H., Jr (1979). Longitudinal evaluation of the pre-term infant. In *Infants Born at Risk*, ed. T. M. Field, A. M. Sostek, S. Goldberg and H. H. Shuman. New York: Spectrum Publications.

Spitz, R. & Wolf, K. (1946). Anaclitic depression. *Psychoanalytic Study of the Child*, *Vol. 2*, pp. 313–342.

Stevenson-Hinde, J. (1988). Individuals in relationships. In *Relationships Within Families: Mutual Influences*, ed. R. A. Hinde and J. Stevenson-Hinde. Oxford: Clarendon Press.

Stevenson-Hinde, J., Hinde, R. A. & Simpson, A. E. (1986). Behavior at home and friendly or hostile behavior in preschool. In *Development of Antisocial and Prosocial Behavior*, ed. D. Olweus, J. Block and M. Radke-Yarrow. New York: Academic Press.

Terman, L. M., assisted by B. T. Baldwin, E. Bronson, J. C. DeVoss, F. Fuller, F. L. Goodenough, T. L. Kelly, M. Lima, H. Marshall, A. H. Moore, A. S. Rauben-heimer, G. M. Ruch, R. L. Willoughby, J. B. Wyman, and D. H. Yates (1925).

Mental and physical traits of a thousand gifted children. *Genetic Studies of Genius, Vol. 1.* Stanford, Calif.: Stanford University Press.

Terman, L. M. & Oden, M. H. (1947). The gifted child grows up. *Genetic Studies of Genius, Vol. 4.* Stanford, Calif.: Stanford University Press.

Terman, L. M. & Oden, M. H. (1959). The gifted group at mid-life. *Genetic Studies of Genius, Vol. 5.* Stanford, Calif.: Stanford University Press.

Thoman, E. (1975). Sleep and wake behaviors in neonates: consistencies and consequences. *Merrill-Palmer Quarterley*, **21**, 295–314.

Valsiner, J. (1986). *The Individual Subject and Scientific Psychology.* New York: Plenum Press.

Wachs, T. D. (1983). The use and abuse of environment in behavior–genetic research. *Child Development*, **54**, 396–407.

Werner, H. (1957). The *Concept of Development: an Issue in the Study of Human Behavior*, ed. D. Harris. Minneapolis: University of Minnesota Press.

Zahn-Waxler, C. & Radke-Yarrow, M. (1982). The development of altruism in young children: a methodological analysis. In *The Development of Prosocial Behavior*, ed. N. Eisenberg-Berg. New York: Academic Press.

Commentary

—4—

The early ethologists had a certain prejudice against Psychology – a prejudice that, in so far as it was directed at the narrower forms of laboratory learning theory and at unscientific subjectivism, was perhaps not altogether unjustified. There were equal misgivings in the other direction – in so far as they were stimulated by some aspects of early ethological theory and by ethological popularisers, again perhaps not altogether unjustified. But we can all be glad that such internecine strife has largely disappeared, and the behavioural sciences are, at least in some areas, becoming more problem-oriented. I acquired an introduction to eclecticism from early contacts with Bill Verplanck, who also introduced me to the classic volume of Estes *et al.* (1954) on *Modern Learning Theory*. But my major lesson on this issue came from John Bowlby. As a psychoanalyst – a species not renowned for its eclecticism – it is the more remarkable that he should have gathered together a small but diverse group to focus on the mother–child relationship. The group included representatives of two varieties of psychoanalysis, two varieties of learning theorist, a Piagetian, an anti-psychiatrist, psychiatric social workers, myself as an ethologist, and so on, with nothing theoretically in common but all interested in the same problem – parent–child relationships. It was a tremendously important learning experience for me. And it was John Bowlby who helped me to set up the monkey colony at Madingley in order to study the effects of maternal deprivation experimentally – for me a stepping stone to developmental psychology.

It is proper that all six contributions to the section on developmental psychology should bring up conceptual or theoretical issues, derived from animal studies, that have been helpful in the study of humans. Bowlby's attachment theory, based on an improbable liaison between psychoanalysis, empirical data on forty-four thieves, ethology and, later, systems theory, is

411

the example *par excellence* of the fertility of an eclectic approach. Bowlby's chapter specifies the role that Harlow's (e.g. Harlow & Zimmerman, 1959) work on 'contact comfort' and the use of monkeys to assess the effects of separation played in his theorising. The subsequent development of attachment theory will provide a rich field for historians of science. For about two decades those using an attachment theory approach became the opposite to eclectic, and isolated themselves from outside influences as 'attachment theorists'. This was, perhaps, made necessary by the antagonism that they evoked from entrenched positions, and perhaps by the delicacy of their sensitive methodology. Now that attachment theory is emerging from that stage, its full potential, and the limitations of its applicability, are being realised. There seems little doubt that attachment theory has at least as much to say about behaviour in close relationships as any other theory, although it seems to me important at this stage that its progress should not be slowed by over-ambitious claims or irrefutable concepts.

Stevenson-Hinde's chapter will certainly play a part in the development of attachment theory, for it will help to lay to rest the sterile controversy, touched on also by Bowlby, that was developing between 'temperament' and 'attachment' theorists. She draws a parallel here with the sterile nature/ nurture controversy that caused ethologists and psychologists to bloody each others' pates over several decades. Stevenson-Hinde's chapter also links with other work on animals: she uses observational measures of fear that would gladden the heart of a classical ethologist.

Michael Rutter also writes about attachment theory. I confess that I would love to emulate Michael Rutter's encyclopaedic breadth – but many of us believe that he has a special corner of his cortex preadapted to store references with instant recall. Only the other day, needing access to the literature on two topics, I wrote to ask his advice and received by return two detailed reviews in press, both of course by Michael Rutter. I first got to know him through discussions over his earlier critique of attachment theory, and I have learned much from him over the years in many areas of developmental psychology and psychopathology. It is appropriate that he should here discuss an up-dated view of attachment theory, which can only profit from this hard-headed outside view. In the course of his chapter he discusses the relevance of animal work, and in particular mentions how the ethological concept of imprinting, not unimportant for early attachment theorising, is now being largely discarded. Here again is material for the historian of science – the imprinting concept originally seemed straight-forward, and was important in the early days of attachment theory (see Bowlby, Chapter 12), but ethologists too are now having to think hard about its nature (e.g. Bateson, 1966; Horn, 1985).

Associated with the imprinting concept was that of a 'critical period', and here there has been a sad lack of cross-fertilisation, for the debate has gone on independently in several different contexts. Many ethologists eschewed the critical period concept nearly thirty years ago (e.g. Hinde, 1962; Bateson, 1964; Bateson & Hinde, 1987) and came to recognise that the problem of age changes in sensitivity to experience is part of the problem of development itself. However, in the fields of child development and psychiatry the discussion has continued. Let us hope that Rutter has closed this issue with his conclusion that, while there are age-related changes in sensitivity to experience, the idea that infancy involves heightened susceptibility *critical* for later development must be rejected.

I am delighted that Marian Radke-Yarrow should be amongst the contributors to this book. I am a great admirer of her work – both for its methodology and for its conceptual sophistication. Here she discusses a host of conceptual, theoretical and practical problems and sets the scene for a new era in developmental research. Among the issues she raises is another in which communication between disciplines (and, as she points out, over the years within disciplines) has not been all that it should – namely, the conceptualisation of what goes on in development. She concludes that 'the young organism is changing, and is part of, and is encountering, a multifaceted and constantly changing environment. The child brings its unique endowments to the environment, makes a difference in the environment, and is modified by it.' Almost exactly the same words could be used to describe the manner in which a changing environment induces hormonal changes in a female canary, as a result of which her behaviour changes in a manner which changes that environment by building a nest, and stimuli from that changed environment cause further changes in her behaviour and endocrine state.

In mentioning this, I am not putting in a naïve claim that developmental psychologists would have made more rapid progress if they kept up with ethology. In any case, exactly the opposite could be said with equal justice. It is in the nature of science that similar ideas crop up in different places at the same time. And some issues, like the need to distinguish concepts that refer to observed behaviour, relationships, predispositions, and underlying mechanisms, crop up in every discipline. Though Rutter refers to such matters in the context of attachment theory, the same trails had to be followed in instinct theory, drive theory, reinforcement theory, and so on (e.g. Estes *et al.*, 1954; Miller, 1959). And as Fentress (Chapter 4) emphasises, we must also remember not only to distinguish the concepts, but to recognise their interrelations. But I am here again emphasising the fertility of bringing different perspectives together in problem-oriented research, as each of the contributors to this section has done.

It is interesting to note that one theme comes up in nearly every section and

413

in the majority of the chapters in this book – the importance of studying individual differences. This is emphasised here especially by Radke-Yarrow. It is in part because developmental psychologists have been content with comparing group means or with correlations that the contribution of developmental to clinical psychology has been less than it might have been. And, as Radke-Yarrow stresses, case studies can be an important step towards generalisations of wider applicability. Rutter makes a similar point. Although in tracing their origin to temperamental factors he takes a different view of temperament from that expressed by Stevenson-Hinde (Chapter 13), he emphasises that 'the investigation of individual differences leads straight to the heart of the interactive processes ...'. In our current work on the relations between preschoolers' behaviour at home and school, my colleagues and I are trying to make progress by first searching for general trends, and then carefully examining the exceptions to see what is odd about them. For instance, following Baumrind's (1971) lead, we find that two dimensions of mother–child interaction (maternal warmth and maternal control) are in combination moderately good predictors of aggressive behaviour in preschool. When children are plotted on these two dimensions, the more aggressive and less aggressive children tend to be in particular areas of the plot. But there are exceptions. One can then compare the few high aggressive children in the low aggressive area with the low aggressive children (and vice versa) and find out what is odd about the former. In principle, the process can be iterated. This procedure verges on a judicious fishing net strategy, and depends in part on replication for its success: how well it will work out remains to be seen. Anyway, it may prove to be another contribution to Marian Radke-Yarrow's important discussion of this theme.

Judy Dunn, who transferred from zoology to developmental psychology years before I did, and whose help in establishing studies of children at Madingley was crucial, takes up a conceptual issue that arose (at any rate for me) from work on animals in discussing levels of complexity. As we have seen, Thelma Rowell (Chapter 10) has evaluated an earlier version of this approach as applied to non-human species, and I am glad to see that Judy Dunn has found it useful in studies of children. It is my view that much of the research that she describes as having been helped by this approach would have happened anyway, but her chapter gives me an opportunity to say how much I admire her use of objective methods to get at such apparently intangible issues as interpersonal perception in children.

In her chapter, Judy Dunn takes up an issue raised also by Marian Radke-Yarrow – the question of understanding mutual influences. 'Are the processes of mutual influence inferred or measured?' she asks. Judy Dunn reports that her own work with children has been helped by phrasing the questions very precisely. This has certainly been the case with studies of monkeys and other species. With rhesus monkeys it is clear that the questions 'Who is primarily responsible for mother–infant proximity *over a short time span*?, 'Are *differences* between mothers or *differences* between infants primarily responsible for *differences* in mother–infant proximity?', and 'Is it *changes* in mothers or *changes* in infants that are primarily responsible for *changes* in mother–infant proximity?' are different questions and give different answers.

A final point concerns what I see as a central question, perhaps the central question in developmental research – how, to use Rutter's words, does a relationship quality become transformed into an individual characteristic? What does it mean to say that a relationship becomes internalised? Stevenson-Hinde addresses this at the conceptual level, considering the relation between individual characteristics and relationships as a continuous cycle operating throughout development. Radke-Yarrow meets it by treating parents' patterns of interaction with the child as its environment – a conceptualisation that has led her to focus on relationships in an elegant way, but in the long run in less sophisticated hands could lead to undervaluing of the dialectic relations between individual and relationship, the issue emphasised by Dunn. Bowlby used the metaphor of the internal working model of self, mother and others, and other workers have referred to internal working models of relationships (e.g. Bretherton, 1985). As a metaphor, this is extremely powerful, in fact too powerful, because it will explain almost anything (Hinde, 1989; Rutter, Chapter 14). If it is to be useful in the long run, and it may well be, much more detailed work will be necessary, and Bretherton (1985) is showing the way.

References

Bateson, P. (1964). Effects of similarity between rearing and testing conditions of chicks following avoidance responses. *Journal of Comparative and Physiological Psychology*, **57**, 100–3.

Bateson, P. (1966). The characteristics and context of imprinting. *Biological Reviews*, **41**, 177–220.

Bateson, P. & Hinde, R. A. (1987). Developmental changes in sensitivity to experience. In *Sensitive Periods in Development*, ed. M. H. Bornstein. Hillsdale, NJ: Erlbaum.

Baumrind, D. (1971). Current problems of parental authority. *Developmental Psychology Monographs*, **4** (1, Pt. 2).

Bretherton, I. (1985). New perspectives on attachment relations: security, communication, and internal working models. In *Handbook of Infant Development*, ed. J. Osofsky. New York: John Wiley.

Estes, W. K., Koch, S., McCorquodale, K., Meehl, P. E., Mueller, C. G., Schoenfeld, U. N. & Verplanck, W. (1954). *Modern Learning Theory*. New York: Appleton-Century-Crofts.

Harlow, H. F. & Zimmermann, R. R. (1959). Affectional responses in the infant monkey. *Science*, **130**, 421–32.

Hinde, R. A. (1962). Sensitive periods and the development of behaviour. *Little Club Clinic in Developmental Medicine*, 7. London: National Spastics Society.

Hinde, R. A. (1989). Reconciling the family systems and the relationship approaches to child development. In *Family Systems and Life-span Development*, ed. K. Kreppner and R. M. Lerner, pp. 149–64. Hillsdale, NJ: Erlbaum.

Horn, G. (1985). *Memory, Imprinting and the Brain*. Oxford: Clarendon Press.

Miller, N. E. (1959). Liberalization of S–R concepts. In *Psychology, a Study of a Science. Study 1, Vols 1 and 2*, ed. S. Koch. New York: McGraw Hill.

R.A.H.

VI
Aggression and war

—17—

An evolutionary perspective on human aggression

David A. Hamburg

Contributions of Hinde's ethology to understanding of human aggressiveness

Throughout his career, Robert Hinde has fostered the development of ethology as a discipline, and its fruitful interplay with related disciplines. As part of this enterprise, he has fostered research on animal behaviour in an evolutionary perspective. He has always been careful to avoid overreaching in evolutionary matters, being extremely sensitive to the limitations of evidence inherent in research dealing with events that occurred millions of years ago. In comparing the behaviour of non-human primates and human behaviour, he has been notable for his judicious assessments.

For the better part of a decade, his students and mine cooperated in conducting research on non-human primates in natural habitats and to some extent also in laboratory settings. These former students are continuing to make contributions and are becoming leaders in the field. One important focus of their work has been aggressive behaviour. To some extent, this reflects Hinde's influence and my own. He has long been concerned with understanding aggression and avoiding egregious or even dangerous misinterpretations of research on animal behaviour for contemporary aggression. Through deeply held humane values, he has been concerned about problems of prejudice and violence. He has effectively stimulated curiosity about the development of human behaviour and encouraged careful application of such knowledge to contemporary problems, including the avoidance of dangerous aggression.

In 1970 I had the privilege of helping to organise a UNESCO conference on human aggressiveness, one of the first to bring together the contributions of biologically oriented and socially oriented scholars of human behaviour to understand this critical problem. It was a complex, difficult and sensitive enterprise at the time. Robert Hinde's contributions there as elsewhere were exemplary (Hinde, 1971). He sought clarity of definition, and made distinctions of practical importance for research and social action. These distinctions were typically derived from careful observation of animal behaviour. Under the broad rubric of aggression as used in popular language, he distinguished those features which could legitimately be considered aggression in a scientific sense and those which should be handled by other concepts. He called attention to the drastic changes in human social environments characterising modern life compared with those of much earlier times and, indeed of different species. He pointed out the undesirable features of peace arrived at through rigid hierarchical control.

He highlighted the need in contemporary circumstances to diminish aggressive behaviour and sought ways in which insight might be obtained from the study of animal aggression to illuminate promising paths towards the control of aggression in contemporary circumstances. He clarified eliciting or precipitating factors in aggression as well as those of internal state that are predisposing factors. He also addressed augmenting factors such as frustration, pain and fear. In so doing, he related experimental observations to those in the natural habitat. He pointed out the severe limitations of the concept of 'instinct' in this context. He emphasised the complexity of aggression – e.g. the outcomes of aggressive encounters in relation to the subsequent likelihood of aggression. Above all, he called attention to the development of aggressive behaviour through the life span and the many influences that have a bearing upon this development: parental care; siblings and peers; cumulative effects of frustrating conditions; modelling by authority figures; previous experience in aggressive situations. He concluded with a fundamental orientation.

Understanding of these factors can lead to suggestions as to how aggression can be reduced – reduction in crowding, reduction in frustration, in improved conditions of rearing, and so on. If aggression is reduced, other constructive types of activity become possible. (Hinde, 1971)

Around the time of the UNESCO conference, there was a flurry of ethologically oriented popular books on aggression. These books had a welcome evolutionary orientation and included some valuable observations. But they also had serious disadvantages and were incisively criticised by Robert Hinde. They scarcely utilised studies of our closest living biological relatives – the non-human primates – or did so in ways that did not draw upon the most adequate studies. They were largely lacking in serious attention to developmental considerations. Their reflections on human behaviour were impressionistic, anecdotal, and inferential. There was little reliance on systematic research on humans, even where it was available in relative abundance.

The contributions of ethology to the study of human behaviour have been important – and Robert Hinde's part in this has been outstanding (Hinde, 1974, 1982, 1983a, b). One contribution of ethology has been to focus on natural habitats – as similar as possible to the habitat in which the organism evolved. Another contribution of ethology has been to study the relation of behaviour to ecological variability. It has been demonstrated that the same species does not behave in just the same way in different parts of its habitat; and the same animals do not behave in the same way in different seasons of the year. A third contribution of ethology has been its emphasis on the evolutionary view of behaviour, particularly on behaviour as adaptation. An orientation to adaptive tasks and strategies is helpful in studying human behaviour. By viewing the human species as a biological organism, ethology has established connections between biological and social sciences (Hinde, 1987).

Ethologists have been ingenious in conducting field experiments in the natural habitat; and also in designing laboratory experiments that are meaningful in relation to the natural habitat. They have been careful and systematic in their observational methods. Finally, there are advantages for students of human behaviour in animal studies *per se*. There are almost insurmountable ethical, financial, and technical difficulties about investigating in humans, for example, whether early mother/infant separation may permanently alter brain and endocrine function. In these circumstances, a constructive approach is to study non-human animals, including some that are closely biologically related to the human species; the results of such studies can tell us where to look in people (Hamburg, 1974). If we are interested in human problems, we must ultimately answer these questions in human subjects. Our justification for doing so is much stronger if we have first learned where to look by studying closely related species.

My own inquiries over several decades have been parallel to and influenced by ethology – especially the work of Robert Hinde. Like him, I have been deeply concerned with contemporary aggression and conflict resolution. I have sought insights from ethological perspectives. In this paper, I wish to summarise the main lines of this inquiry in which I have learned so much from collaborators in several biological and behavioural science disciplines as well as my own home base in medicine (Hamburg & McCown, 1979; Hamburg & Trudeau, 1981).

Before doing so, I want to say a word about the supreme dilemma of our time – how to manage international affairs without using weapons of virtually unimaginable destructive power. This terrible problem has been of great concern to Robert Hinde. In addition to considering how ethological research might be helpful in understanding aggression, he has worked in various ways with his characteristic thoughtful dedication to reduce the risk of nuclear war.

Contemporary human violence: the ultimate challenge

The central fact of the nuclear era is the destructive power of the weaponry, taken together with the inevitable and ubiquitous manifestations of human frailty. There are useful rules of thumb for the destructive power: one bomb, one city; one Trident-type submarine, one country. Never before in the long history of the human species, with all its extraordinary manifestations of destructiveness, has anything like this capability existed. In the past, no matter how ferocious, we could not destroy humanity, civilisation, the species itself even if we wanted to. Now we can.

Throughout human history, there are countless examples of destruction wrought by human error and in recent centuries by the interplay of human error with machine error. In the nuclear arena, the most vivid cases of recent years have fortunately not been in nuclear weapons but in nuclear energy: Chernobyl and Three Mile Island. Frightening though these episodes were, they are essentially child's play in relation to the explosion of nuclear weapons (Hamburg & George, 1984).

Thus, the beginning of wisdom in the nuclear era is to grasp the enormous, unprecedented, profound and pervasive consequences of nuclear war; and the likelihood that sooner or later human error, misjudgment, miscalculation, the interplay of personal and mechanical foibles – all this will eventually occur in the arena of nuclear weapons. These two sets of facts taken together go a long way toward explaining the deep unease in world populations about the adequacy of nuclear deterrence to keep the peace for the long term.

In this deadly context, the leaders of the superpowers take on a novel conjunction of attributes. They are the most powerful leaders in history. They are also potentially the most dangerous leaders in history. In the past few years, they have taken large steps forward, not least by making explicit the fundamental concept that nuclear war can never be won and must never be fought.

What can be done? We can reduce the number of weapons greatly and especially their capacity for a first strike. We can find ways to decrease the chance of accidental or inadvertent nuclear war; we can find additional safeguards against unauthorised launch and against serious miscalculation. We can also improve the political relations between the superpowers, partly through cooperative efforts in key fields bearing on the health and safety of humanity.

One useful way to advance all of these purposes is to combine the talents and experiences from diverse, pertinent sources in sustained efforts over the long term. Such efforts can benefit from the knowledge and judgment of people from many different fields, from the scientific and scholarly community as well as the policy community and other sectors, from people of different nations and different political orientations. The danger is so great in the long term, the puzzle so large and complex, that many different pieces are needed.

That is the spirit of this chapter. The scientific community has contributed a good deal to coping with the nuclear danger – and can contribute much more (Hamburg, 1986a). I believe that we have only begun to do what we are capable of doing in this crucial field. Among the many lines of inquiry that can be stimulating and lead to future insights regarding human aggressiveness and conflict resolution, research undertaken in an evolutionary and historical framework can be helpful. Ethology, in the wide-ranging spirit of Robert Hinde, can link with other lines of inquiry to achieve a deeper understanding of human behaviour that bears upon the ultimate problems of war and peace. The path is very difficult, the obstacles formidable, the haze covering ancient events virtually impenetrable. Yet we must try; because this ancient human organism has lately transformed its habitat and put itself in grave danger.

The study of non-human primates

In this chapter, I can explore only a very limited sample of recent research on human origins, and delineate a few of its implications for our current predicament. The ancient past is inaccessible to direct study. But by careful observation of monkeys and apes we can begin to understand the non-human primate heritage with which our ancestors took a route toward full humanity. In addition, interesting questions are raised by recent research on the way of life of the few remaining hunter-gatherers, who still follow basic subsistence patterns typical of almost all human experience. Several publications make available a great deal of documentation on these matters (Lee & DeVore, 1968, 1976; Hamburg & McCown, 1979; Konner, 1982; Price & Brown, 1985; Goodall, 1986; Smuts *et al.*, 1986).

Human ancestors have been separate from the apes for about five million years. For nearly all of that period, there were probably fewer than a million people on earth, all of whom subsisted by hunting and gathering in small, nomadic groups (Washburn & Harding, 1978). Agriculture and large, settled populations have existed for only about ten thousand of those five million years, and our technical world has been present for only a century or two – a moment on the time-scale of human evolution. The way we live today is, in important respects, a novelty for our species (Lenski & Lenski, 1987).

Such problems as excessive population growth, drastic impacts of urbanisation and industrialisation, serious environmental damage, resource depletion, and the profound risks of weapons technology have emerged since the industrial revolution – and especially in the twentieth century. In a very brief portion of evolutionary time, the human species has transformed its physical, biological, and social environments. Many of the changes are within the memory of living adults. Yet natural selection built the human organism over millions of years in ways that suited earlier environments. It is an open question and a matter of concern how well we are suited to the environment we have created so suddenly. To some extent, we are an old species in a new habitat.

Research on the evolution of behaviour, especially aggressive behaviour, is difficult for many reasons. The clues to the past are scanty and elusive (Binford, 1983). If reliable information is scarce, authority tends to substitute for evidence. Plausible conjectures are readily incorporated into political ideologies. A polemical tradition on this topic tends to impede rational problem-solving. Despite such difficulties, knowledge has been deepened in recent years, especially by the converging contributions of diverse disciplines (Hamburg & Trudeau, 1981; Archer, 1988; Groebel & Hinde, 1989).

What can we learn about the world of our ancestors? From what baselines of behaviour and environment have the recent changes taken off? To address such questions, it is useful to have firm evidence as to which living species are most closely related to our own. Methods of immunology and molecular biology have been added to traditional methods of comparing species and genera, such as comparative anatomy (Bendall, 1983; Ninio, 1983). These methods converge on finding that humans and African apes are closely related, sharing a common ancestor long after the separation of apes and monkeys (Simons, 1989). The newer behavioural work also supports the close relation of African apes and our own species (Washburn & McGown, 1978).

But do we know enough about non-human primate societies to give us any reasonable basis for constructing models of our prehuman ancestors? A direct comparison of two decades of experience provides encouragement. At the beginning of the 1960s, Sherwood Washburn and I made a proposal intended to strengthen a valuable institution and an emerging field of inquiry. The institution was the Center for Advanced Study in the Behavioral Sciences; the field was primate behaviour. Since its creation in 1954, the Center had invited only individual scholars, each completely free to pursue individual interests. The time seemed ripe to invite a cluster of scholars, especially young ones, with a set of shared interests. The possibility of creating a mutual aid ethic among a set of young scholars in the interest of strengthening a new, fascinating, and difficult field of scientific work was attractive.

One of the direct outputs of this 'primate project' was the book *Primate Behavior* (DeVore, 1965). It provided information, stimulation and guidance to students and scientists over the better part of two decades. As the twenty year mark approached, it occurred to me that it might well be useful to have a sort of 'primate behaviour revisited' project. Barbara Smuts, a young leader in the field, took up the role played two decades earlier by Irven DeVore. A set of excellent scholars was assembled. The most visible result of this cooperative enterprise is a recent volume presenting a comprehensive overview of research on primate societies (Smuts *et al.*, 1986). It contains a significant contribution by Hinde on the relevance of non-human primates for the understanding of human behaviour (Hinde, 1986).

Comparing the two volumes, one has to be struck by the progress that has been made. An upsurge of careful, systematic research has occurred during these two decades, much of it ingenious and creative. The leading scholars and field workers have related their work explicitly to the advancing body of knowledge in biological and behavioural sciences, especially in relation to evolution (Wrangham, 1986a). The new findings generally confirm and extend those of earlier workers.

At the time of our first primate project, reliable information on group composition, ranging, feeding, and social organisation was available for fewer than a dozen species; now it is more than a hundred. This in turn has made possible systematic interspecific comparisons and these have generated testable hypotheses. The growth of knowledge is reflected in the upsurge of field studies of much longer duration than those of the 1960s. These complex and difficult studies, sustained over many years at one field site, have documented the profound importance of long-term social relationships (Wrangham, 1983).

One of the fascinating features of the recent research is the light it casts on the richness and diversity of primate social behaviour: between individuals; in groups of many configurations; and in enduring patterns of organisation. Not only does the primate group typically include animals of different age, sex, kinship, and dominance status, but there are shifting sub-groups, temporary alliances, and long-term associations that cut across traditional demographic categories. All this provides opportunities for a wide range of ways in which social behaviour can contribute to strategies of survival and reproduction (Marler, 1976; Harcourt, 1979; Hinde, 1979; Tutin, McGrew & Baldwin, 1983; Ghiglieri, 1984; Wrangham, 1986b).

Of great interest is the documentation of long-term relationships among primates, in many different forms. A few pioneering long-term studies of individually recognised monkeys and apes have made clear that the mother–offspring bond generally continues through the juvenile period and in some species it persists through adulthood; this is particularly likely in the case of female offspring, since in most species females remain in their natal groups whereas males leave to join another group around adolescence. Moreover, close and enduring attachments may be observed among a variety of adult primates (Smuts, 1985).

Chimpanzees: closest biological relatives of the human species

One of the most fruitful of the long-term field stations was the Gombe Research Centre in Tanzania, established in 1960 by Jane Goodall, who shortly after became a graduate student working under Robert Hinde's guidance. During the 1960s and 1970s, it was my privilege to join in a variety of cooperative efforts with Goodall and Hinde to develop research at this site; and to stimulate scholars in the study of non-human primate behaviour and ecology, including its relevance for human evolution. It is important to be clear about the fact that chimpanzees are not early humans, nor are they the direct precursors of *Homo sapiens*. We and they are descended from a common ancestor, with the separation having occurred about five million years ago, or perhaps somewhat longer. Despite this evolutionary distance between chimpanzees and ourselves, they are the closest of all living creatures to our own species. So, chimpanzees are the best model of our ancestors among the non-human primates, whatever their limitations (Goodall & Hamburg, 1975).

A characteristic feature of our approach was to study chimpanzee social behaviour from multiple disciplinary perspectives in a natural habitat; and also in a semi-natural laboratory of behavioural biology utilising half-acre outdoor enclosures. Though such research can yield simple models of pre-human primate societies, it is no substitute for direct study of human societies, ancient and contemporary. When studying contemporary societies, it is useful to take into account what is known of the biological nature of human organisms, and the evolutionary history of human societies (Lenski & Lenski, 1987). Such knowledge enters into but cannot substitute for direct, systematic, quantitative study of contemporary societies.

The early phase of observations at Gombe in the 1960s was useful in several ways: in the habituation of the animals to human observers; description of behavioural components; building a history of individual relationships, especially in regard to kinship; stimulating interest in and demonstrating the feasibility of research on great apes.

When this phase was completed, a gradual change in research methods was introduced: (i) the construction of an interdisciplinary research group to bring fresh perspectives to bear on chimpanzee behaviour; (ii) a shift from general description to problems with a relatively sharp focus; (iii) extensive following of individuals 'beyond the provisioning area where food was provided to the far recesses of the forest, eventually covering the entire range of the study population; (iv) recording data in a systematic way in specified categories of behaviour and, as far as possible under the circumstances, taking a quantitative approach to the data; (v) systematically sampling each age/sex class; (vi) observing interactions between different communities and subcommunities. Utilisation of these new methods in the period 1970–5 extended earlier findings, modified some, and led to specific reformulations.

What can chimpanzees tell us about possible precursors of human aggressiveness and conflict resolution? Despite the inherent limitations of such evidence bearing upon ancient prehumans, there is much new information compared with two decades ago (Washburn & Hamburg, 1965, 1968; Smuts, 1986; Walters & Seyfarth, 1986). It is worth summarising here.

Chimpanzees live in societies that are very complex by non-human primate standards, possibly similar to the societies of *Australopithecus* but much smaller and simpler than twentieth-century human societies. There are 15–80 animals in a community, spread over about 15–20 square miles of forest, walking and climbing several miles per day in the food quest, subsisting mainly by gathering plants but also hunting small mammals whenever the opportunity arises. They interact with each other in predictable ways, apparently following implicit rules. Observers at Gombe following closely the long sequences of behaviour believe that such rules are learned during the years of growth and development. They cover conditions under which threat, attack, submissive, and reassurance patterns occur and the signals useful in their termination (van Lawick-Goodall, 1968, 1971; Goodall, 1986).

Patterns of threat, attack, and submission shared by a variety of other primates are similar to some of the aggressive patterns observed in our own species. These similarities are particularly striking in the case of chimpanzees who raise their arms in threat, hit, punch, and pound with the arms and kick with the legs in attack, brandish and throw objects to intimidate opponents, scream when frightened, crouch and whimper to express submission, and reach out to touch, pat, or embrace in order to reassure an uneasy subordinate (Goodall & Hamburg, 1975).

There are also some similarities between the contexts in which threat and attack behaviour occurs in non-human primates and humans (Hamburg, 1971 a). Monkeys and apes are particularly likely to engage in such behaviour in the following situations:

1. When competing for scarce and/or valuable resources that promote survival and reproductive success – e.g. food; and for males, access to fertile females.

2. In competition for high status within the group; severe aggression is particularly likely during periods of unstable dominance relationships.

3. When protecting close friends or relatives, and particularly infants, from threat or attack by other group members.
4. In response to threat or attack by higher-ranking animals; in this case redirection of aggression toward subordinates is common.
5. Toward strangers trying to enter the group and toward members of other groups, particularly when the groups are in competition for access to mates, territory, or high-quality, clumped foods.
6. Following the recent occurrence of other attacks.
7. In defending against potential predators.
8. In association with a presumably painful injury.
9. In some species, lower-ranking individuals may be attacked when they refuse to cooperate with the goals of higher-ranking animals, e.g. female chimpanzees who resist a male's attempts to mate.

Thus, the contexts in which aggression occurs most frequently are those in which an aggressive response seems likely to promote an individual's survival and reproductive success by (i) increasing access to resources; (ii) protecting relatives; (iii) defending relatives or 'friends' with whom the aggressor has affiliative bonds that promote cooperative efforts to achieve mutually beneficial goals. Similarly, submissive patterns of behaviour that often serve to inhibit attack can be viewed as adaptive responses by subordinates who would lose more through aggressive competition than they could gain.

Unlike most primates, the members of a chimpanzee group or community do not forage together as a single group, but instead wander about the community home range, alone or in small, flexible sub-groups or parties. These ranging patterns are probably an adaptation to the dispersed clumps of ripe fruit that form the main component of chimpanzee diet (Wrangham, 1986 a). Although all community members are rarely together at once, they are familiar to one another, linked by ties of kinship and friendship. When individuals meet in the forest after several days apart they often greet excitedly (Bauer, 1979).

In the early years of research on chimpanzees in natural habitats, the observations were almost entirely within-community behaviour. Valuable observations on aggressive behaviour were made (van Lawick-Goodall, 1968; Wrangham, 1974). Now there is substantial evidence on between-community interactions. These observations provide one of the most striking examples of the changes that have occurred in understanding chimpanzee social behaviour as a result of more systematic and long-term studies (Bygott, 1979; Nishida, 1979). They involve conjunction of findings from different sites.

It turns out that chimpanzee males are organised into distinct communities that occupy ranges. They defend these ranges against males from other communities. When males from different communities come into contact, violent fights may occur and individuals are sometimes severely injured. Females and infants are not immune to violent aggression by males from other communities (Bygott, 1972; Goodall *et al.*, 1979).

Moreover, several studies establish the systematic patrolling of community boundaries by groups of males who behave in distinctive and especially antagonistic ways in such encounters (Bygott, 1979). Males from a given community attempt to defend the community range when they hear or encounter males from other communities. They actively seek out such encounters during regular forays. Although females, usually in sexually receptive condition, sometimes accompany males on such journeys, they rarely take an active part in actual intercommunity encounters. While most aggressive encounters between communities involve males, females from other communities are also sometimes severely attacked, and in several cases infants have been killed during such attacks.

Males of one community (who are closely related since they remain in their natal group) regularly gather together to engage in such patrols. Moving silently and stealthily, in contrast to their normal noisy habits, these males move toward one edge of their range, frequently stopping to climb trees and peer into the distance, evidently looking and listening for signs of strange chimpanzees. If the males locate other chimpanzees, and if the party of strangers is outnumbered, the patrolling males move forward with extreme caution until they are just a few yards from the chimpanzees of the other community. At this point, they charge, hair fully erect and vocalising loudly in a cohesive display of aggressive intent. If the others do not manage to escape, they may be brutally attacked. The attackers pin an opponent to the ground, jump on him, pull out hair, hit, pound, kick and bite him, and twist his limbs with their strong arms.

On a number of occasions, males from one community at the Gombe Stream Reserve (the Northern Group) fatally wounded males from an adjacent community (the Southern Group) who were caught alone. Over a period of several years, the Northern group killed all the adult males of the Southern group, and then took over the latter's home range. The Northern males also killed an old female from the Southern community (she was probably past reproductive age), and on other occasions they attacked lone mothers from other groups, killing and eating the females' infants and seriously wounding the mothers (Bygott, 1979).

Goodall notes that the only fierce aggression between adult males at Gombe was between these two groups that had separated after once being part of the same community. They were thus not total strangers, though they were established in different, neighbouring communities. Beyond these male–male attacks by the Northern group on the Southern group, severe aggression in her experience has mainly been by males on females in another community (J. Goodall, personal communication).

Border patrols and intense aggression by males from different communities have been observed at both Gombe and another research site in the Mahali Mountains, suggesting that such violence may be characteristic of at least the East African populations of chimpanzees (Nishida, 1979; Nishida *et al.*, 1985).

What is the function of such intercommunity aggression? Some investigators have suggested that, by defending community range boundaries, a group of males achieves access to a greater number of females and other resources (Bygott, 1979; Wrangham, 1986b). The main difference between male territorial systems in other mammals and in chimpanzees is that the larger chimpanzee territory is established and defended by groups of males cooperating with one another, whereas in other species single males defend areas from all other males. This is consistent with other evidence from research on higher primates suggesting that the evolution of cooperative behaviour is related to the evolution of aggressive behaviour in primates (Nishida & Hiraiwa-Hasegawa, 1986).

Several distinctive features of chimpanzee violence deserve emphasis. First, in contrast to males in many other non-human primate species, male chimpanzees have rarely been observed to injure seriously other males from the *same* group. Elaborate charging displays and other forms of bluff are common, but within groups these rarely erupt into serious violence. Second, chimpanzee males systematically seek out vulnerable members of *other* groups; these attacks have been carefully observed and do not appear to be responses of alarm to accidental meetings. Third, females rarely participate actively in boundary patrols and attacks. Fourth, the intergroup attacks appear to be oriented toward seriously injuring or killing the opponents, in contrast to intergroup aggression in a variety of non-human primates in which the tendency is to intimidate or drive away opponents. Fifth, the most severe aggression – aggression that produces serious injuries in the victims – occurs when several individuals who share close bonds cooperate in attacking others. Sixth, male chimpanzees appear to benefit from successful attacks on other groups, since their home range may expand, increasing access to food, and to potential mates (Nishida *et al.*, 1985).

The systematic, organised, brutal, and male-dominated attacks of chimpanzees are the closest phenomenon to human warfare observed in any non-human primate – though a very long way from contemporary war. Chimpanzees are our closest living relatives, but there is no way of knowing whether the similarities between chimpanzee and human intergroup violence are a result of common ancestry, or instead merely represent superficially similar behaviour patterns that evolved independently. However, when the chimpanzee evidence is considered along with information on responses to strangers in a variety of non-human primate species, it appears likely that the human tendency to react with fear and hostility to relative strangers – as well as the related tendency to make in-group/out-group distinctions – has roots in the prehuman past.

Most human aggression no longer directly serves the reproductive interests of the aggressor. Yet throughout most of our evolutionary past, aggression probably contributed to the survival and reproductive success of appropriately aggressive individuals, just as it does under natural circumstances among non-human primates today. This is not meant to imply that aggressive behaviour is either desirable or inevitable – far from it (Bateson, 1989). The point is that human capacities for aggressive behaviour, and our tendencies to respond aggressively in particular situations, are partly the result of natural selection operating during our species' evolutionary past. The legacies of this past need to be taken into account in understanding how our species functions in the vastly different circumstances of today. Emotional response tendencies that may have been highly adaptive under ancient circumstances may become maladaptive when environmental conditions change drastically as they have in the most recent phase of human evolution.

Group membership and attachments between individuals

Monkeys and apes usually live in groups based upon strong and enduring bonds between individuals. These relationships may include various combinations of age and sex: not only between mothers and infants, but also between adults either of the same sex or of opposite sexes; between juveniles; and between adults (males or females) and young.

In a few remote areas in different parts of the world live people who subsist primarily, or totally, by hunting and gathering. These remnant populations are the only living representatives of a way of life that characterised all human populations until the invention of agriculture about ten thousand years ago. Hunter-gatherers are fully modern humans genetically, so they are different from our ancestors in important respects. However, they are the best models we have for reconstructing the way of life of the human hunting and gathering past. What problems do modern hunter-gatherers have to solve in order to survive and reproduce? How does their behaviour, including their social relationships, address these problems? Recent research has clarified these matters to some extent (Lee & DeVore, 1976; Konner, 1982). These societies show much variability as they adapt to widely differing ecological circumstances (Price & Brown, 1985). Yet they manifest certain core similarities in behaviour.

Hunter-gatherers usually live in small bands of about 20–50 members. Each member is typically well-known to every other member. Band size and composition is usually flexible, altering in response to social factors such as the desire to spend time with friends or relatives in another band; and also varying importantly with ecological circumstances.

Relationships within and between bands are based on reciprocity. Individuals are expected to share food with other band members, and large kills are shared between bands. Since membership in a band and access to food others have gathered or hunted is essential to an individual's survival, disapproval backed by the power to refuse to share in the future or by the threat of rejection from the band are powerful sanctions enforcing an ethic of group membership and mutual aid.

There are some striking similarities between higher non-human primates and hunter-gatherers in the mother–infant relationship (Nicolson, 1986). In both non-human primate societies and those of hunter-gatherers, the mother carries the infant from birth, and the two remain in physical contact much of the time until, or even after, the infant can move about on its own. The young infant suckles frequently and on demand, day and night. Weaning is accompanied by infant distress. The mother remains near the infant throughout the long period of gradually increasing independence, and the child is free to return to her for reassurance and protection when alarmed or in pain (Pusey, 1983). Bonds between mother and young persist long after the offspring has achieved the capacity to survive on its own.

Parallels also exist between non-human primates and living hunter-gatherers in the wider network of social relationships. The infant is introduced to the social universe through frequent interactions between other group members and the mother–infant pair. Infancy is followed by a relatively long period preceding sexual maturation during which the juvenile spends a large part of its time playing vigorously with peers and they become friends. During maturation, the child is surrounded and supported by close kin. Kinship bonds typically last a lifetime, although in many non-human primates this applies only to females. Relations among close kin are supplemented by the development of lasting relationships between less closely related individuals. In both higher primates and hunter-gatherers, most of an individual's social interactions are restricted to the small number of familiar individuals belonging to the same group, many of whom are familiar throughout the life span.

These observations suggest that patterns of attachment behaviour must have emerged over the course of millions of years of primate evolution because infants who formed close attachments to their mothers, and whose mothers reciprocated, were more likely to survive to pass on their genes to future generations than were infants who did not (Bowlby, 1969). It is reasonable to assume that attached infants were less likely to be caught by predators, less likely to get lost, to suffer from severe exposure, and to be injured by other members of their own species. The child's distress and attempts to re-establish contact upon separation are similar in principle to the infant's crying when hungry as well as shivering and crawling toward heat when cold. Indeed, patterns of attachment behaviour provide a fundamental underpinning for the adaptive properties of the human group – and, as we shall see, an important contributing factor in human aggressiveness.

The attachment between individuals so characteristic of non-human primates reaches a much more complex form in human societies (Parkes & Stevenson-Hinde, 1982). Although cooperation is important for non-human primates, it is rudimentary compared with that found in all human societies (Bateson, 1988). Adaptive features of human groups include: sharing of subsistence technology; organised joint efforts to find, harvest, or hunt food; cooperative building of shelters; caring for ill or aged group members; complex division of labour; pooling of resources; and trade. Thus, the human species builds upon and goes far beyond non-human primate ancestors in linking survival and reproduction of the individual to a sense of belonging in a group and behaving cooperatively within the group.

Small-scale, traditional societies manifest great variability in ways of life, diverse customs and social institutions – yet these societies share certain essential features (Goldschmidt, 1959). Traditional societies instil in their young certain guidelines for behaviour. These guidelines tend to be ones that were useful in the past of a particular society in meeting adaptive tasks under circumstances that, until very recently, probably did not change much for long periods of time. Such guidelines involve ways of conducting human relationships, ways of relating to environmental conditions, ways of coping with problems, ways of taking advantage of opportunities bearing directly on survival and reproduction. Such guidelines are typically learned early in life, shaped by powerful rewards and punishments, and invested with strong emotions supported by shared and highly valued social norms. This early learning tends to induce lifelong commitments to traditional ways of life. Thus, a sense of personal worth is predicated on one's sense of belonging to a valued group; a sense of belonging depends on the ability to undertake the traditional tasks of that society with skill and to engage in social interactions in ways that are mutually supportive. These experiences occur within the context of a small, face-to-face group that provides the security of familiarity, support in times of stress, and enduring attachments throughout the life span. Perhaps it is not surprising, then, that human devotion to the group can so readily take on a fierce character.

433

David A. Hamburg

Relationship between attachment and aggression

I shall argue that human capacities for attachment are linked fundamentally to our capacities for violence. Much of human aggression is in the service of attachment. We risk our lives and kill our enemies in the commitment to those we care about. In the name of love, duty and brotherhood, we carry out the threats and attacks that now constitute the ultimate peril to our species.

Knowledge of the human evolutionary background can help to understand this link between attachment and aggression. In non-human primates and humans alike, the first contexts in which distress, frustration, fear, and anger are experienced are those in which the bond to a primary caregiver is threatened. These emotional responses are adaptive for a primate infant whose relationship with the caregiver is jeopardised. Fear serves to promote the infant's attempts to re-establish contact with the caregiver, and anger heightens the infant's ability to overcome obstacles to achieving this goal. Similar emotions are also experienced later in life whenever intimate bonds are threatened.

In monkeys and apes, attachments to other group members are often developed and protected through aggression. One of the most frequent contexts of aggressive behaviour is protection of close relatives and friends. The prime example is mother's protection of her offspring, even against dangerous, high-ranking males. Usually, female macaques react with submission and deference to higher-ranking animals. But in defence of close kin, a female will threaten or even attack a more dominant animal; this, in fact, is the only context in which she will routinely do so. A female monkey who does not protect her offspring and other close relatives risks losing her genetic representation in future generations. For a male baboon, the development of close bonds with unrelated females is an important determinant of his reproductive activity. In order to maintain these bonds, he must be willing to protect his female friends and their offspring from attacks by other males (Smuts, 1985). Since developing and maintaining a network of close relationships is generally crucial to an individual's survival and reproductive success, it is likely that such aggressive responses would have been favoured by natural selection.

In addition to the strong bonds that develop between particular individuals, non-human primates are attached to the social group itself. With few exceptions, opportunities to make contact with other members of the species and to become part of a social group are pursued with great determination. In the wild, monkeys and apes accidentally separated from their groups often become agitated, vocalising loudly and repeatedly. They appear to be searching persistently for their lost companions. Many indications of excitement and pleasure have been observed in varied species of monkeys and apes upon reunion after brief separations. These pleasurable emotions are the positive counterpart to the negative emotions of anger, fear, and grief experiences when contact is disrupted. Such evidence is strong in studies of chimpanzees.

Thus, research on non-human primates and hunter-gatherer human societies foreshadows research on modern human societies that demonstrates the power of distinctions between in-groups and out-groups. Before summarising such evidence, it is important to sketch the immense transformation of the most recent era in human evolution.

The most recent phase of human evolution: a world in process of drastic transformation

Our ancient ancestors lived in small groups in which they learned the rules of adaptation for survival and reproduction. They used simple tools to cope with the problems of living. For the most part, they were vulnerable to the vicissitudes of nature – food, water, weather, predators, infections, other humans. Their world began to change with the onset of agriculture. An acceleration of momentous changes occurred with the industrial revolution two centuries ago, and then with its pervasive implementation in the twentieth century. Science and technology have played – and continue to play – a profound role in this transformation.

So, in a moment of evolutionary time, the human species has drastically changed the world of its ancestors. We have rapidly changed our technology, our diet, our activity patterns, the substances of daily use and exposure, patterns of reproductive activity, tension relief, and human relationships. These changes are laden with new benefits and new risks, and the long-term consequences are poorly understood. Natural selection over millions of years shaped our ancestors in ways that suited earlier environments. How well are we now suited to the world our species has so quickly made?

The historical record clearly shows that once humans developed agriculture, settled in larger numbers, accumulated goods, and came to rely on exclusive areas for growing food and grazing animals, intergroup hostility became common (Lenski & Lenski, 1987). Patterns of intragroup violence and intergroup warfare in pre-industrial people have been described in detail (McNeill, 1982). Two points deserve emphasis here. Whatever the evolutionary background and its biological legacy, the historical record makes it clear that aggressive behaviour between individuals and between groups has been a prominent feature of human experience for a very long time. Such behaviour has been easily learned, practised in play, encouraged by custom, and rewarded by most human societies for at least several thousand years.

Second, it appears that everywhere in the world aggression towards other people is facilitated by a pervasive human tendency toward harsh dichotomising between positively valued 'we' and negatively valued 'they'. Even among the !Kung San, a relatively peaceful hunter-gatherer group that has been well studied, members of one's own group are referred to by terms that translate as 'human', and members of other groups by terms that connote strangeness and lack of fully human qualities. This tendency is very widespread in human societies, whatever their form of organisation (Levine & Campbell, 1972). Dehumanisation of the adversary plays an important role in justifying violent behaviour that might be considered 'inhuman' were it directed towards members of one's own group.

When we view our current conflict predicament in the very long-range perspective of history and human evolution, we see a radical discontinuity in technology (Brodie & Brodie, 1973). Within the most recent moment of evolutionary time, there has occurred a vast change in destructive power available to the human species: nuclear war above all, but other modes as well. This change has occurred very rapidly indeed and is still accelerating. For example, recent calculations indicate that one of the new Trident submarines will carry explosive capacity several times greater than all the explosions of the Second World War combined.

We necessarily rely on existing capabilities to cope with this vastly expanded destructive power. These capabilities are fundamentally the human organism and human institutions that have evolved slowly over a long period of time. If the human organism and its institutions carry over some characteristics or tendencies from the past, what are the risks? Are they serious? What would we have to change from patterns of the past in order to avoid unprecedented disaster – or even species extinction?

This point of view can affect our way of thinking about many problems. The human organism and its societies have been shaped by our long evolutionary and historical past. Humans present now, after this long evolution, have incorporated biobehavioural patterns that have worked in survival and reproduction in the past. These patterns are transmitted both by genes and by culture. Among these are linked patterns of attachment and aggression. For millennia, it has evidently been important to belong to a group, to believe in a group, to be loyal to a group, and to be ready to defend one's group. In the process, it has been common to dehumanise members of other groups. All this is so because the human and prehuman group has been an essential feature of adaptation among the higher primates. Aggression has been used in implementing adaptive requirements.

It is possible to identify some prominent patterns of human behaviour and organisation over millennia (McNeill, 1971). A convergence of evidence from a variety of evolutionary and historical disciplines makes it possible to identify some of the factors influencing human conflict that are relevant to our current predicament. They are important components of the human legacy that, however transmitted, we must cope with in the transformed circumstances of contemporary life.

1. Fear of strangers – and aggression towards strangers, especially if no escape is available. A particular conjunction of circumstances provides a powerful instigator to aggression: crowding of strangers in the presence of valued resources (Hamburg, 1971 b).
2. Dominance and scapegoating; redirection of aggression to vulnerable individuals or groups.
3. Attachment and cooperation of males within a group, and a tendency to severe aggression between groups. Among the non-human primates, these patterns are almost unique to the chimpanzee and gorilla, the species that are biologically most closely related to the human (Fossey, 1983). (Some other species show similar patterns – e.g. howler monkeys and lions.)
4. In-group/out-group distinctions associated with fear and hostility.
5. Semi-closed, small, face-to-face groups in which the individual spends most or all of the life span.
6. Direct observation of norms and rules, including regulation of aggression; such observation is readily available to the developing youngster.
7. Drastic changes in environmental conditions mostly occur slowly – on a time-scale of centuries or millennia. Now major changes in the human environment are being produced by human activity at a rate that has little precedent in the record of life's evolution.
8. Power relations in historical times. Recent historical scholarship has been illuminating with respect to recurrent themes and emerging trends that bear on human violence in the historical record (Barraclough, 1967; McNeill, 1971, 1982; Bigelow, 1972; Garraty & Gay, 1972; Brodie & Brodie, 1973; Howard, 1976; Thomas, 1980; Robbins, 1985; Brown, 1987; Craig & George, 1990). These include the following:
   (a) The ubiquity of war throughout human history.
   (b) Recurrent powerful instigators to war, such as prejudice-ethnocentrism and areas in which population growth puts groups into intense competitive pressure for survival-relevant resources.
   (c) Interactive cycles: threat of loss in war leads to an increase in the number of weapons, and innovation in the nature of weapons, in the belief that such a move can have definitive significance with respect to potential enemies; but usually this turns out not to be the case and then there are further moves interactively involving

437

two or more nations; so there is a fallacy-of-the-last-move frequently observed in these interactive cycles.

(d) The growing role of science and technology in war over several centuries and accelerating markedly in the twentieth century.

(e) The emergence of what amounts to a military–industrial complex long before such a term existed.

(f) Serious errors of judgment by leaders – not only in the fog of war but in planning war, in the decision to begin, in implementation, in settlement, and in follow-up after a war.

(g) Complacency, avoidance, and denial with respect to the life-threatening issues of war; leadership decision making has often manifested a tendency to avoid unpleasant facts, to deny the significance of such facts when they cannot be avoided, and to remain complacent in the face of grave dangers.

(h) Attachments, group loyalty, and warfare; these are intimately linked throughout history. We risk our lives and inflict great damage in the service of devotion to a valued group, most recently the nation state.

(i) A tendency to use most of the destructive power available sooner or later; technology that permits a wider scale of violence may lie dormant for a time, but within decades of advent it is usually employed to the maximum extent possible.

(j) Limitations of international restraint; international institutions are characteristically weak and readily overtaken by events, especially in technology as applied to ambition and hostility among nations.

9. Acceleration of major change in very recent times. The metric for major technological changes and their powerful social impact has shifted in the course of evolution from millennia to centuries to decades and now even in some cases to single years.

10. This time-scale is relevant to contemporary circumstances; 45 years without a nuclear war is a moment in evolutionary time. It is not an impressive criterion if species survival is the issue. Not only is the technology of destructive power accelerating rapidly in this century, but other exacerbating factors are evident as well. For example, massive social dislocations affect the probability of fear, hostility and war – e.g. huge and uprooting migrations, the crowding of strangers, fear of the unknown and unpredictable, threat and loss of previous supports, and contagion of violence through mass media. The institutional restraints on aggression are weak. Institutional adaptation is altogether slow and difficult compared with technological change. Thus, the general problem of contemporary

438

circumstances is how to achieve judicious and humane use of technological capability – above all with respect to weapons.

11. A rapid shift from the small primary group of human evolution to the mass society of contemporary times.

12. Emergence, for the first time, of a species-wide intimate interdependence on a world-wide basis. Now there is no escape from interdependence, however attractive a nostalgic view of past small communities may be. Today, the old biology and customs are set in a new technological and social context. It is as if we were ancient humans in the twenty-first century.

13. In the past, a great deal of individual, institutional and even national learning has been stimulated by scrutiny of serious mistakes. Now, in the instance of nuclear war, for the first time ever we cannot afford one serious mistake. The opportunity to learn from disaster and near-disaster is much diminished in comparison with the past. Indeed, for the first time ever, we probably have the capacity to make the human species extinct.

Development of aggressive behaviour in the individual life span

The fact that aggression occurs in similar contexts and takes similar forms across a wide variety of primates by no means implies rigid genetic determination of aggressive behaviour. In fact, a great deal of evidence suggests that many aspects of aggression are learned – in non-human primates as well as in humans. There are several contexts in which learning of aggression and submission seems particularly likely. The earliest context is the mother–infant relationship. Weaning conflict contains many components of later aggressive/submissive interactions.

Aggression also appears to occur in the context of frustrated desires (Fossey, 1979). In infancy, temper tantrums develop in response to loss of maternal proximity, and later as an apparent consequence of a failure in mastering a given situation. Such perceived deprivation may involve failure to obtain premium food or reassurance from a higher-ranking animal. The behaviour of these tantrums is similar in chimpanzees and humans; the contexts of occurrence are similar also (Hamburg & Goodall, 1974).

Play is another context that fosters learning of aggressive/submissive behaviour. Young monkeys and apes play frequently with peers of varying ages, and their games include all the elements of threat, attack, and submission observed in adults (Dolhinow & Bishop, 1972; Lee, 1983).

Observation and imitation of the behaviour of others provides a pervasive context in which primates learn aggressive and submissive patterns of behaviour. From its earliest days the infant has virtually unlimited opportunities to watch others, and as it grows older it begins to observe aggressive interactions with keen interest (Hamburg & Goodall, 1974). There is clear evidence of a capacity for observational learning among non-human primates in the wild (Hamburg, 1971a). It is likely that this capacity is applied to the learning of aggressive and submissive activities.

Experimental research strengthens the evidence that non-human primates learn many aspects of aggression and submission. This learning process is both facilitated and constrained by unlearned, biological factors (Seligman & Hager, 1972; Hinde & Stevenson-Hinde, 1973). The interaction between maturation and learning in young rhesus monkeys has been elucidated by research in the University of Wisconsin laboratories (Suomi, 1979, 1982). Regardless of rearing conditions, all rhesus infants suddenly develop fear of strange situations and strange monkeys between 60 and 80 days of age. These fearful responses appear at the time when normally reared monkeys are just beginning to move beyond the mother's immediate reach, i.e. at precisely that stage of development when the infant is capable of getting into danger by itself. Fear propels the infant back into its mother's arms, presumably an adaptive response. Much later, between 6 and 8 months of age, aggressive responses appear for the first time. By this age, the normally reared infant has had several months of experience playing with peers. This play experience, and the positive attachments which the infant has formed through it, serve to moderate the expression of aggressive tendencies so that they are rarely harmful to others. At this same age, however, peer-experienced infants respond with severe aggression to a strange juvenile monkey.

Such observations suggest that a cognitive, emotional, and behavioural distinction between familiar individuals and strangers is learned early and easily in monkeys reared in social groups. This distinction underlies a great deal of the aggressive behaviour of wild monkeys and apes. Aggression toward strangers occurs in two situations: when a single individual attempts to enter a new group, and when two groups meet. Let us briefly consider each situation in turn.

In most non-human primates, members of one sex typically transfer from the natal group into a new group around adolescence; these same individuals sometimes move between troops again as full adults. Usually males are the more mobile sex, but in a few species (e.g. chimpanzees) females transfer, and in a small number of species (e.g. gorillas) both males and females may leave to join a new group (Wrangham, 1979). Individuals attempting to move into a new group often meet with fear or hostility. Pusey & Packer (1986) have recently reviewed all the field evidence of hostility to strangers trying to immigrate.

Chimpanzees are one of the few species in which females transfer to new groups. Resident females have been observed to direct aggressive behaviour toward immigrant females, threatening, chasing, and attacking them (Pusey, 1979). The new females seek protection from the adult males, who welcome them if they are sexually receptive (i.e. not lactating).

Strangers introduced to groups of captive monkeys are frequently severely attacked, mauled, and even killed, often in severe group attacks. These observations indicate that group members will kill a newcomer who is forced into proximity with no means of escape; such extremes of violence are less common in the wild, perhaps because an immigrant can choose the timing and method of approach to a new group.

The second situation in which relative strangers meet is during encounters between groups. In many species intergroup encounters are rare because groups avoid one another, often with the aid of loud calls that broadcast their locations. In other species groups may meet routinely, feed, travel, or rest near one another without aggression, and then move apart. However, in some species intergroup encounters tend to be very aggressive (Cheney, 1986).

Chimpanzee males exhibit the most sophisticated forms of intergroup violence observed in wild non-human primates (Goodall *et al.*, 1979). Therefore, it is worth emphasising here the earlier summary of inter-community aggression. Although this aggression is not based entirely or perhaps even primarily on a familiar–strange distinction, it has much that foreshadows human in-group/out-group distinctions.

Factors influencing the development of such complex and severe intergroup aggression are worthy of intense scrutiny in future research. What are the processes by which such behaviour is shaped in development? Are lementary components learned easily early in life? What tutelage shapes the behaviour in later years? What regulatory influences may serve to constrain it?

Hormonal influences on brain development may have important mediating roles (Goy, 1968; Money & Ehrhardt, 1968; Yalom, Green & Fisk, 1973). One way that this can occur is through differences in development of attention, since attention is crucial in learning processes. A hormonal influence during a sensitive period of brain development may render a certain class of stimuli more interesting to the organism at a later stage. This line of inquiry is amenable to experimental analysis in non-human primates and to a certain extent in human infants. One model is provided by an experiment in the Wisconsin laboratories (Sackett, 1966). He showed that isolated-reared rhesus macaques, exposed to various kinds of pictures, indicate certain preferences and certain distinctive reactions. One is that they tend to spend more time looking at monkey pictures than at non-monkey pictures. Another is that, within the various classes of monkey stimuli, there is a particularly powerful and emotionally disturbing effect caused by the full-face threat – a species-typical aggressive expression. The full-face threat has this effect between 2 and 4 months of age in rhesus macaques. Once an infant has responded intensely to the full-face threat, it could readily go on to learn a great deal about the conditions under which threat occurs, the conditions under which it is likely to be carried on to attack, and the actions that will tend to ameliorate the threat. How would such learning occur?

Observational learning in primate adaptation deserves further consideration here. One of the most interesting findings of primate field studies has been the recurrent theme of observational learning in a social context (Hamburg, 1971 a). In many species and diverse habitats, a behavioural sequence has been described. It begins with close observation of one animal by another. This is followed by imitation by the observing animal of the behaviour of the observed animal. The third part of the sequence is practice of the observed behaviour, especially in the play group of young animals. This sequence of observation, imitation, and practice has been described in several adaptive contexts: food-getting, tool-using, tool-making (chimpanzees), nest-building, infant care, copulation, and aggressive interactions. Overall, the young have close-range access to virtually the full range of adult behaviour (Goodall, 1986). They utilise it in learning patterns of behaviour that have been effective in adaptation. In experimental studies, it is clear that the observing animal can learn from incorrect as well as from correct responses of the animal being observed – i.e. learning from the consequences of the observed animal's mistakes (Riopelle, 1960).

The non-human primate data relate to lines of inquiry in child development. For example, experiments of Bandura and his colleagues at Stanford University on observational learning in nursery school children have shown how ready children are to learn aggressive patterns by observing models who behave aggressively (Bandura, 1973).

One fundamental line of inquiry pertains to the possibility that the human organism early in life is 'primed' to acquire certain elementary behaviour patterns with relative ease. Is there a special facility for learning along lines that have been adaptively valuable for members of the species over a very long time in the course of evolution? It is plausible that learning in such adaptively significant spheres as behaviour oriented to food, water and reproduction would have high biological priority; and aggression can serve in the implementation of these adaptive requirements. Perhaps the inherited 'wiring diagram' of the brain reflects the long-term selective advantage of facility in learning such behaviour (Hamburg, 1963). Simple preferences of the infant or young child might draw its attention to a certain class of stimuli or reward its engagement in a particular kind of activity. Once drawn in this direction early in life by an inherited preference, a great deal of complex learning could ensue, fully taking account of cultural instructions (Hamburg, 1968).

It has been an important contribution of ethological research to relate the processes of learning to the problems of survival in natural habitats and hence to the pressures of natural selection over very long time spans in the evolutionary history of a species. Ethologists have overcome the traditional dichotomy of heredity and learning. One way in which genes may operate is by facilitating an organism's ability to acquire certain patterns of behaviour in preference to others (Eibl-Eibesfeldt, 1970; Hinde & Stevenson-Hinde, 1973).

How do we acquire orientations of ethnocentrism, prejudice, dogmatism, and a susceptibility to violent 'solutions'? Are there ways to foster more constructive orientations as we gain better understanding of the factors governing the development of behaviour? The nature of parental care, experience with siblings and with peers, exposure to hatred and violence in schools and mass media, the cumulative effect of frustrating conditions, and previous experience in situations involving aggression are all important factors. So, also, in some countries, are official propaganda and the religious cultivation of stereotypes (Hinde, 1971; Groebel & Hinde, 1989).

Prejudice – the prejudgment of persons or situations – is to some extent a universal phenomenon, based in part on fundamental processes of cognitive development. Children begin to order their environment by means of their developing capacity to form categories. This process allows for rapid evaluation of the environment, determining what is familiar and unfamiliar, so that the child can make a prompt response to changing situations.

But children are not born prejudiced. Social learning builds on the basic tendency to categorise and evaluate people, groups, and situations. Prejudice is a response to the environment, reflecting the individual's need for group affiliation and for adherence to cultural and subcultural norms (Allport, 1958). The process by which affiliation to the in-group and prejudice against the out-group is formed is fundamentally similar whether the prejudice involves race, class, sex, religion, or nationality. The extent of prejudice can be affected by home, school, community, media and government, as well as by the opportunities to gain familiarity with other groups under constructive circumstances (Daniels, Gilula & Ochberg, 1970).

Recurrent major frustration is conducive to the formation of strong prejudices and to an orientation toward hateful ethnocentrism. Frustrations – disappointments, obstacles, disruptions of deep attachment – are inevitable in human life. Social conditions may ease or aggravate the sources of such frustrations, the severity of their impact, and the opportunities for coping with those that occur. In general, major frustrations of fundamental motivations tend to elicit aggressive responses: irritability, a readiness to blame others, a mood to strike out at the putative obstacles, a proneness to identify vulnerable scapegoats against whom some sort of retaliation can be mounted.

What frustrations are most powerful in eliciting severe aggressiveness? One is frustration of self-esteem or a sense of personal worth. In human history, where one has had to have a place in the organised group in order to survive, respect from others has become essential to the sense of self-esteem, and behaviour directed toward the establishment and maintenance of self-esteem has great cross-cultural generality – even though the manifestations are highly variable.

Frustrations in crucial interpersonal relations are of great importance in fostering individual aggression. The primary relationships within the group have been highly significant in the evolution of our species and have much to do with development of a sense of security in early life and a strong base from which exploration of the personal environment can proceed (Bowlby, 1969; Hinde, 1984).

Closely related is frustration of one's sense of belonging to the larger group beyond the intimate few – a group with which one closely identifies and which makes an important contribution to one's self-esteem, whether that entity is an ethnic group, a nation, a tribe, a political entity, or an occupational unit (Campbell, 1965).

But such threats may also elicit non-hateful, non-violent forms of coping. Hostile responses are not the only way to cope with recurrent major frustration. A serious frustration may lead to assertive behaviour, personal initiative, and vigorously persistent efforts toward problem-solving that may be aggressive but not hateful or destructive. Such non-destructive efforts at problem-solving may be more difficult, complicated, and tedious in the short run, but they are much more rewarding in the long run (Hamburg, Elliott & Parron, 1982).

There are several fundamental orientations that contemporary institutions – especially the family, the schools, the media and religious entities – would do well to encourage in the young in a sustained effort to foster healthy development without hatred and violence: to provide conditions for intimate and enduring interpersonal relationships and the early development of self-esteem; to establish clear guidelines for behaviour; to teach the young to internalise norms of behaviour that restrain violence and to provide them with strategies that foster preference for, and knowledge of, other modes of coping and problem-solving; to develop in the young a constructive image of the future incorporating goals, expectations and a sense of purpose that offer hope that non-hateful, non-violent means for achieving valued ends can in fact be effective; to encourage in the young interest in and respect for other groups as well as one's own.

There is a growing research literature on the effectiveness of various school- and community-based efforts to overcome prejudice and foster prosocial behaviour (Radke-Yarrow & Zahn-Waxler, 1986; Bossert, 1988; Feshbach, 1989). Education in all its forms, from family to schools to mass media, can increasingly convey the facts of a pluralistic and interdependent world, not one that is strange and hateful. Yet today's education world-wide is still considerably ethnocentric. Education everywhere could convey an accurate concept of a single species, a vast extended family sharing fundamental human similarities and a fragile planet. We must ultimately rely for survival on the give-and-take learned in childhood but now extending far beyond childhood games toward adult and even international mutual accommodation (Williams, 1977).

Even though in-group/out-group distinctions are ubiquitous in human societies, easy to learn and hard to forget, and to some extent a legacy of our evolutionary and historical experience in which such distinctions were related to survival – there is certainly the possibility that we can learn to minimise such harsh distinctions. The conditions for survival are in some respects quite different from those operating when these orientations evolved. In human development, we must now find a basis for fundamental human identification across a diversity of cultures in the face of manifest differences: we are indeed a single, interdependent, world-wide species. That is one of the central facts for modern education.

Challenge to the scientific and scholarly community

What can we do? Are the rapid and far-reaching changes of modernity essentially running out of control, beyond human capacity to overtake the events and diminish the risks of unprecedented disaster? It is possible that this is the case. There are certainly no grounds whatever for complacency. Indeed, in the present circumstances complacency may be the greatest danger. There are, in fact, ways of thinking constructively about the dilemma. If the evolutionary and historical view is essentially useful, then it should be a significant part of public education on a wider scale than anything done so far.

Evidence from research on human evolution and history provides a meaningful context within which to view contemporary predicaments. Illumination of major trends in the past experience of our species can clarify behavioural and institutional tendencies likely to be part of our heritage – social as well as biological. We can then examine how these intersect with the opportunities and dangers – indeed, the requirements for survival – in present circumstances.

445

By understanding where we as a species came from and how we got here, and how different our present circumstances are from those in which we slowly evolved, we might well be able to modify some of our old orientations that are now so dangerous – e.g. prejudice and ethnocentrism (Hamburg, 1986b). Perhaps we could widen human horizons toward a sympathetic understanding of our diverse species. This might include a growing ability to keep in mind the humanity of adversaries even in stressful circumstances. By the same token, we could strive for attachment without dehumanisation; to promote cooperative values that extend beyond one's own group.

Moreover, if the evolutionary view provides an antidote for complacency, it might help to intensify efforts on rules of prudence between nations – such as the nuclear powers have partially worked out in the nuclear era (George, Farley & Dallin, 1988). Perhaps it might increase our willingness to consider fundamental changes in attitudes and relationships involving hatred and violence, mutual accommodation, tolerance for diversity, and social justice. We might come to say, in effect 'That was then, and this is now; let us actively seek ways to adapt to unprecedented circumstances.' The widespread recognition of unprecedented dangers, but also unprecedented opportunities from science and technology, might even lead in due course to a new vision of humanity (Hamburg, 1984). Could we learn a different world view? After all, we have indeed come to accept that the world is not flat. The hardest problem is how such fundamental re-examination could occur in tightly closed societies. But even these societies are beginning to open and may well produce new opportunities for public understanding of nature, including human development and relationships.

Overall, the evolutionary and historical perspective challenges us to ask what are the high-probability carry-overs that we must change in order to survive. The more insight we have, the more we can take them into account. Can we understand how to compensate for our inherited vulnerabilities – inherited by both biological and social mechanisms? Can we draw upon inherited strengths in working out new solutions and coping with truly unprecedented circumstances?

In a world so full of hatred and violence, past and present, human conflict and its resolution is a subject that deserves the most vigorous inquiry. High standards of careful, systematic, objective inquiry must be applied to this field, involving the physical, biological, behavioural and social sciences, often acting in collaborative ways. Such crucial world problems as those involved in human aggressiveness do not come in neat packages that match traditional disciplines. In point of fact, this has not been a major subject for scientific inquiry; even now it is largely a marginal subject even in the world's great academic institutions. Nevertheless, some interesting and potentially useful approaches have emerged (Sherif & Sherif, 1966; Smith, 1971; Deutsch,

1973; de Wit & Hartup, 1974; Dahl & Wiesner, 1978; Popp & DeVore, 1979; Eichelman, Elliott & Barchas, 1981; Raiffa, 1982; Schellenberg, 1982; Dunlop, 1984; Walters & Seyfarth, 1986; Hunterford & Turner, 1987; de Waal, 1989; Rock, 1989).

Research on human aggressiveness and conflict resolution has ranged widely in recent years across a variety of disciplines, despite modest funding and inadequate institutional arrangements. Topics include:

1. Neurobiology of aggressive behaviour: cells, circuits, and chemistry mediating such behaviour.
2. Biomedical aspects of individual violence, including the role of drugs in precipitation, exacerbation, and therapy.
3. Child abuse and its effect on subsequent development.
4. The study of conflicts at various levels of organisation, such as families, communities, and nations, in the search for common factors and even principles so that discoveries at one level may illuminate issues at another level.
5. Detailed, systematic inquiry into the origin and resolution of past conflicts and ongoing efforts in relation to contemporary ones.
6. Formulation of fundamental concepts pertinent to a wide range of conflicts, such as ideas about justice.
7. Experimental research on simulated conflicts.
8. The study of various intergroup and international institutions.
9. The study of negotiations, both in real life circumstances and in simulated ones.
10. Research specifically focusing on war and peace, including ways to diminish the likelihood of nuclear war by arms control, crisis prevention, reducing the risk of accidental or inadvertent nuclear confrontation, and improvement of relations among the nuclear nations.

The needs and opportunities for major contributions in this field are immense. There is much to be overcome – the inherent complexity of the subject matter, old conceptual rigidities like the heredity–environment dichotomy, proper ethical limitations of experimental control in human research, ancient prejudices against objective inquiry on human behaviour, dogmatic social ideologies, and institutional inertia regarding any kind of major change. The study of human conflict has grown very late in the day, has recently been stimulated by deep concerns about the dangers of contemporary conflicts and belated recognition of the ubiquity of conflict in human experience. It is one of the great challenges for science policy to organise a much broader and deeper effort to understand the nature and sources of human conflict, and above all to develop more effective ways of resolving conflict short of disaster.

447

One of the most fruitful perspectives has come from research on inter-group behaviour. Social psychologists as well as anthropologists and sociologists have been interested in the human propensity to distinguish between in-groups and out-groups. Both in field studies and in experimental studies, the flow of evidence is impressive. Human beings seem readily able to learn in-group favouritism or in-group bias. People seem remarkably ready to form partisan distinctions between their own and other groups, to develop sociometric preferences for their own group, to discriminate against other groups, to accept favourable evaluations of the products and performances of the in-group, to accept unfavourable characterisations of other groups that go far beyond the objective evidence or the requirements of the situation (Colman, 1982; Brewer & Kramer, 1985). This is true not only of long-standing group commitments, but even in experimental situations where only a brief orientation is given to distinguish a newly formed group from another group in the experiment. Almost any sort of interaction within a group tends to promote in-group favouritism. Actually, it seems rather difficult to avoid this effect even if one wants to do so. In short, humans are highly susceptible to invidious in-group/out-group distinctions (Levine & Campbell, 1972). This experimental work strongly confirms the rich variety of observations from field work in many cultures over extended times and in a variety of societies. It is also consistent with the recent experimental and field research on non-human primates alluded to earlier in this paper (Cheney, 1986). That evidence indicates, in most non-human primates, strong bonds of attachment between individuals are crucial to survival and reproductive success; and protection of such bonds is a major context for aggressive behaviour. A second important context for aggression is competition for limited and highly valued resources. And finally, in most species individuals show a strong attachment to one group, and are antagonistic toward strangers from other groups.

Human societies have a pervasive tendency to make distinctions between good and bad people, between in-groups and out-groups. This sorting tendency is very widespread, readily learned, and susceptible to harsh interpretations that justify violence. Hostility between human groups is likely to arise when the groups perceive a conflict of vital interests, an unacceptable difference in status, or a difference in beliefs that jeopardises self-respect.

Many different political, social, economic, and pseudoscientific ideologies have been utilised in support of these hostile positions. The content of such intergroup hostility varies widely from time to time and from place to place, but the form is remarkably similar. Although the term ethnocentrism is employed, groups have been specified in many ways: religion, race, language, region, tribe, nation, and various political entities. The same principles seem to apply across different kinds of groups. Can human groups achieve internal cohesion, self-respect, and adaptive effectiveness without promoting hatred and violence? A deeper understanding of factors that influence ethnocentrism could have much practical value in resolving intergroup conflicts.

Concluding comment

The world-wide historical record is full of hateful and destructive activities based on religious, ethnic, national and other distinctions – often associated with deeply felt beliefs about superiority, a sense of jeopardy to group survival, or justification by supernatural powers. All that is an ancient part of the human legacy. What is new is the rapidly accelerating destructive power of weaponry: nuclear, enhanced 'conventional', chemical, biological – and the means of accurately transporting them over vast distances. Moreover, the world-wide spread of technical capability, the miniaturisation of weapons, the widely broadcast justifications for violence, and the upsurge of fanatical behaviour are occurring in ways that can readily produce large-scale conflicts of high lethality everywhere on earth. As a species, we have a rapidly growing capacity to make life miserable and disastrous. Indeed, two nations probably have the capacity to make the species extinct, and other nations may seek to acquire the same capacity.

In considering human conflict, avoidance and denial tend to substitute for careful scrutiny; authority often substitutes for evidence; blaming readily substitutes for problem-solving. The capacity for wishful thinking in these matters is enormous, as is the capacity for self-justification. But the issue must be faced soon in a way that it has never been before because the stakes have reached such an unprecedented level.

It is certainly not beyond human ingenuity to move this subject higher on the world's agenda. For instance, strong organisations covering wide sectors of science, technology, and education can take an increasingly active role in coping with this critical issue. Scientists and educators, through their most dynamic institutions, can use their considerable influence to strengthen research and education on child development, prejudice, ethnocentrism and conflict resolution. They can generate new knowledge and explore vigorously the application of such knowledge to urgent problems in contemporary society. Attitudes, emotions, beliefs, and political ideologies from our past will often hinder such efforts, but our motivation for survival is strong and our problem-solving capacities are great.

The intimate, slowly changing world of our non-human primate ancestors and of early humans is long gone. So, too, is the small and relatively simple world of more recent ancestors who lived in agrarian societies. Our contemporary world is the crowded, heterogeneous, impersonal, super-armed, rapidly changing environment shaped during the past two centuries. There is little in our very long history as a species to prepare us for this world we have suddenly made.

When we consider the profound changes in human environmental conditions within very recent evolutionary times, it seems likely that some of the mechanisms which evolved during the millions of years of mammalian, primate, and human evolution are now less useful than they once were. Since cultural change has moved much more rapidly than genetic change, the emotional response tendencies that have been built into us through their suitability for a long succession of past environments may be less suitable for the very different present environment. Similarly, cultural change is slower in some respects than others; technological change now far outpaces institutional change. And our institutional mechanisms for conflict resolution are weak in much of the world, carrying over unhelpful legacies and failing to create needed adaptations such as effective international organisations.

In adapting to these largely unprecedented conditions, it will be helpful if we can understand the nature of the human organism, the main forces that shaped it through the course of evolution, and the ways in which recent environmental changes impinge on our very old equipment – especially genes, brain and customs. The interactions of biological, psychological and social processes in the development of human aggressiveness should constitute an important frontier for science in the decades ahead (Groebel & Hinde, 1989).

Does all this mean that severe aggression and mass destruction are virtually inevitable? Certainly not! Yet the ubiquity of slaughter gives us pause. As the first draft of this paper was written in the summer of 1988, the human capacity for mass killing was once again exemplified by wrenching news from Burundi – ironically, only a few miles from the research site at Gombe where Robert Hinde and I and our dedicated colleagues shared so many positive experiences. Indeed, now as in the 1970s a large percentage of the population of Burundi has been systematically killed in tribal conflict and Burundi is by no means an isolated case (Staub, 1989). Yet also at the time of this writing, human ingenuity in conflict resolution is exemplified by remarkable improvement of US–Soviet relations with promising manifestations in several parts of the world (Nye, Allison & Carnesale, 1988; Allison, Ury & Allyn, 1989).

Will nuclear war be hard to avoid in the decades ahead, as nuclear weapons spread to many nations as well as sub-national (perhaps terrorist) groups? Certainly. Is aggressive behaviour inherited in a way that predetermines warfare or other mass destruction? No. Is it easily learned by people everywhere? Yes. Are there other factors besides aggressiveness that contribute to hatred, violence and warfare? Surely – attachment, group identification, leadership, propaganda, stress, and stereotypes, to name a few

(Hamburg, 1983). With destructive power at an utterly unprecedented level and still growing throughout most of the world, learning to regulate and control human violent tendencies will become more urgent than ever before. It is a subject of profound scientific interest to understand the conditions governing the development, expression and regulation of violent behaviour. To analyse such problems effectively will require the intimate inter-penetration of biological and psychosocial research (Haber, 1981).

The essential scientific outlook flows from some basic features of human adaptation through which our species has overcome so many vicissitudes in its long history. The evolution that is distinctively human deals centrally with the enriched capacity for learning, for communication by language, for cooperative problem-solving and for complex social organisation – as well as for advanced tool-making and tool-using. The evolution of these capacities profoundly enhanced our capabilities to adapt to a wide variety of habitats, and recently to modify our habitats extensively in ways we believe to be adaptive. Concomitantly, these capacities are available for destructive activities, intended or inadvertent. Now we are challenged as never before to find ways in which these unique capacities may be used to stop the destruction of ourselves and our life-supporting environments.

It is fitting to reflect on this profound challenge in a volume honouring a person who has done so much to break new ground in understanding behaviour and who has successfully challenged the scientific community to expand its horizons.

Acknowledgements

I am very grateful to a number of friends and colleagues who made valuable comments and suggestions that greatly helped in the preparation of this paper: Patrick Bateson, Jane Goodall, Julie Johnson, Joshua Lederberg, Anne Pusey, Patricia Rosenfield, Barbara Smuts and Sherwood Washburn.

References

Allison, G. T., Ury, W. L. & Allyn, B. J. (ed.) (1989). *Windows of Opportunity: From Cold War to Peaceful Competition in U.S.–Soviet Relations.* Cambridge, Mass.: Ballinger Publishing Co.

Allport, G. W. (1958). *The Nature of Prejudice.* New York: Doubleday.

Archer, J. (1988). *The Behavioural Biology of Aggression.* Cambridge and New York: Cambridge University Press.

Bandura, A. (1973). *Aggression: A Social Learning Analysis.* Englewood Cliffs, NJ: Prentice-Hall.

Barraclough, G. (1967). *An Introduction to Contemporary History.* Harmondsworth, Middlesex: Penguin.

Bateson, P. (1989). Is aggression instinctive? In *Aggression and War: Their Biological and Social Bases*, ed. J. Groebel and R. A. Hinde. Cambridge: Cambridge University Press.

451

Bateson, P. (1988). The biological evolution of cooperation and trust. In *Trust: Making and Breaking Cooperative Relations*, ed. D. Gambetta. Oxford: Basil Blackwell.

Bauer, H. R. (1979). Agonistic and grooming behavior in the reunion context of Gombe Stream chimpanzees. In *The Great Apes*, ed. D. A. Hamburg and E. R. McCown. Menlo Park, Calif.: Benjamin/Cummings.

Bendall, D. S. (ed.) (1983). *Evolution from Molecules to Man*. Cambridge: Cambridge University Press.

Bigelow, R. (1972). The evolution of cooperation, aggression and self-control. In *Nebraska Symposium on Motivation*. Lincoln: University of Nebraska Press.

Binford, L. R. (1983). *In Pursuit of the Past: Decoding the Archaeological Record*. New York: Thames and Hudson.

Bossert, S. T. (1988). Cooperative activities in the classroom. In *Review of Research in Education 1988–89*. ed. E. Rothkopf. Washington, DC: American Educational Research Association.

Bowlby, J. (1969). *Attachment and Loss, Vol. 1. Attachment*. New York: Basic Books.

Brewer, M. B. & Kramer, R. M. (1985). The psychology of intergroup attitudes and behavior. In *Annual Review of Psychology*, *36*, ed. M. R. Rosenzweig and L. W. Porter, pp. 219–43. Palo Alto, Calif.: Annual Reviews Inc.

Brodie, B. & Brodie, F. (1973). *From Crossbow to H-Bomb*. Bloomington: Indiana University Press.

Brown, S. (1987). *The Causes and Prevention of War*. New York: St Martin's Press.

Bygott, J. D. (1972). Cannibalism among wild chimpanzees. *Nature*, **238**, 410–11.

Bygott, J. D. (1979). Agonistic behavior, dominance, and social structure in wild chimpanzees of the Gombe National Park. In *The Great Apes*, ed. D. A. Hamburg and E. R. McCown. Menlo Park, Calif.: Benjamin/Cummings.

Campbell, D. T. (1965). Ethnocentric and other altruistic motives. In *Nebraska Symposium on Motivation*, ed. D. Levine. Lincoln: University of Nebraska Press.

Cheney, D. L. (1986). Interactions and relationships between groups. In *Primate Societies*, ed. B. B. Smuts *et al.* Chicago: University of Chicago Press.

Colman, A. (ed.) (1982). *Cooperation and Competition in Humans and Animals*. Berkshire, UK: Van Nostrand Reinhold.

Craig, G. A. & George, A. L. (1990). *Force and Statecraft: Diplomatic Problems of Our Time*, 2nd edition. Oxford: Oxford University Press.

Dahl, N. C. & Wiesner, J. B. (ed.) (1978). *World Change and World Security*. Cambridge, Mass.: MIT Press.

Daniels, D. N., Gilula, M. F. & Ochberg, F. M. (ed.) (1970). *Violence and the Struggle for Existence*. Boston, Mass.: Little, Brown.

Deutsch, M. (1973). *The Resolution of Conflict*. New Haven: Yale University Press.

DeVore, I. (1965). *Primate Behavior*. New York: Holt, Rinehart and Winston.

de Waal, F. (1989). *Peacemaking Among Primates*. Cambridge, Mass.: Harvard University Press.

de Wit, J. & Hartup, W. W. (ed.) (1974). *Determinants and Origins of Aggressive Behavior*. The Hague: Mouton.

Dolhinow, P. & Bishop, N. (1972). The development of motor skills and social relationships among primates through play. In *Primate Patterns*, ed. P. Dolhinow. New York: Holt, Rinehart and Winston.

Dunlop, J. T. (1984). *Dispute Resolution*. Dover, Del.: Auburn House Publishing Co.

Eibl-Eibesfeldt, I. (1970). *Ethology: The Biology of Behavior*. New York: Holt, Rinehart and Winston.

Eichelman, B., Elliott, G. R. & Barchas, J. D. (1981). Biochemical, pharmacological, and genetic aspects of aggression. In *Biobehavioral Aspects of Aggression*, ed. D. A. Hamburg and M. B. Trudeau. New York: Alan R. Liss.

Feshbach, N. D. (1989). Empathy training and prosocial behavior. In *Aggression and War: Their Biological and Social Bases*, ed. J. Groebel and R. Hinde. Cambridge: Cambridge University Press.

Fossey, D. (1979). Development of the Mountain Gorilla (*Gorilla gorilla beringei*): the first thirty-six months. In *The Great Apes*, Menlo Park, Calif.: Benjamin/Cummings.

Fossey, D. (1983). *Gorillas in the Mist*. Boston, Mass.: Houghton Mifflin.

Garraty, J. A. & Gay, P. (ed.) (1972). *The Columbia History of the World*. New York: Harper & Row.

George, A. L., Farley, P. J. & Dallin, A. (ed.) (1988). *U.S.–Soviet Security Cooperation: Achievements Failures Lessons*. New York: Oxford University Press.

Ghiglieri, M. P. (1984). *The Chimpanzees of Kabale Forest: A Field Study of Ecology and Social Structure*. New York: Columbia University Press.

Goldschmidt, W. (1959). *Man's Way: A Preface to the Understanding of Human Society*. Cleveland: The World Publishing Co.

Goodall, J. (1986). *The Chimpanzees of Gombe: Patterns of Behavior*. Cambridge, Mass.: Belknap Press.

Goodall, J., Bandora, A., Bergmann, E., Busse, C., Matama, H., Mpongo, E., Pierce, A. & Riss, D. (1979). Intercommunity interactions in the chimpanzee population of the Gombe National Park. In *The Great Apes*, ed. D. A. Hamburg and E. R. McCown. Menlo Park, Calif.: Benjamin/Cummings Publishing Co.

Goodall, J. & Hamburg, D. A. (1975). Chimpanzee behavior as a model for the behavior of early man: New evidence on possible origins of human behavior. In *American Handbook of Psychiatry*, *Vol. 6*, ed. D. A. Hamburg and H. Brodie. New York: Basic Books.

Goy, R. W. (1968). Organizing effects of androgen on the behavior of rhesus monkeys. In *Endocrinology and Human Behavior*, ed. R. Michael. London: Oxford University Press.

Groebel, J. & Hinde, R. A. (1989). *Aggression and War: Their Biological and Social Bases*. Cambridge: Cambridge University Press.

Haber, S. (1981). Social factors in evaluating the effects of biological manipulations on aggressive behavior in nonhuman primates. In *Biobehavioral Aspects of Aggression*, ed. D. A. Hamburg and M. B. Trudeau. New York: Alan R. Liss.

Hamburg, D. A. (1963). Emotions in the perspective of human evolution. In *Expression of the Emotions of Man*, ed. P. Knapp. New York: International Universities Press.

Hamburg, D. A. (1968). Evolution of emotional responses: Evidence from recent research on nonhuman primates. In *Animal and Human*, ed. J. Masserman. New York: Grune and Stratton.

Hamburg, D. A. (1971a). Psychobiological studies of aggressive behavior. *Nature*, **230**, 19–23.

Hamburg, D. A. (1971b). Crowding, stranger contact, and aggressive behavior. In *Stress, Society and Disease*, ed. L. Levine. New York: Oxford University Press.

Hamburg, D. A. (1974). Ethological perspectives on human aggressive behaviour. In *Ethology and Psychiatry*, ed. N. F. White. Toronto: University of Toronto Press.

Hamburg, D. A. (1983). Conflict and its resolution: biological and psychosocial perspectives. In *Biological Foundations and Human Nature*, The Katzir-Katchalsky Lecture Series. New York: Academic Press.

Hamburg, D. A. (1984). Science and technology in a world transformed. *Science*, **224**, 943–6.

Hamburg, D. A. (1986a). Understanding and preventing nuclear war: the expanding role of the scientific community. In *The Medical Implications of Nuclear War*. Washington, DC: National Academy Press.

Hamburg, D. A. (1986b). New risks of prejudice, ethnocentrism, and violence. *Science*, **231**, 533.

Hamburg, D. A., Elliott, G. R. & Parron, D. (1982). *Health and Behavior: Frontiers of Research in the Biobehavioral Sciences*. Washington, DC: National Academy Press.

Hamburg, D. A. & George, A. (1984). Nuclear crisis management. *Bulletin of the Atomic Scientists*, June/July, pp. 24–28.

Hamburg, D. A. & McCown, E. R. (ed.) (1979). *The Great Apes*. Menlo Park, Calif.: Benjamin/Cummings.

Hamburg, D. A. & Trudeau, M. B. (ed.) (1981). *Biobehavioral Aspects of Aggression*. New York: Alan R. Liss.

Hamburg, D. A. and van Lawick-Goodall, J. (1974). Factors facilitating development of aggressive behavior in chimpanzees and humans. In *Determinants and Origins of Aggressive Behavior*, ed. W. W. Hartup and J. deWit. The Hague: Mouton.

Harcourt, A. H. (1979). The social relations and group structure of wild mountain gorillas. In *The Great Apes*, ed. D. A. Hamburg and E. R. McCown. Menlo Park, Calif.: Benjamin/Cummings.

Hinde, R. A. (1971). The nature and control of aggressive behavior. *International Social Science Journal*, **23**, 48–52.

Hinde, R. A. (1974). *Biological Bases of Human Social Behaviour*. New York: McGraw-Hill.

Hinde, R. A. (1979). The nature of social structure. In *The Great Apes*, ed. D. A. Hamburg and E. R. McCown. Menlo Park, Calif.: Benjamin/Cummings.

Hinde, R. A. (1982). *Ethology: Its Nature and Relations with Other Sciences*. Oxford: Oxford University Press.

Hinde, R. A. (ed.) (1983a). *Primate Social Relationships: An Integrated Approach*. Oxford: Blackwell.

Hinde, R. A. (1983b). Ethology and child development. In *Handbook of Child Psychology*, *Vol. 2*, ed. P. H. Mussen. New York: John Wiley.

Hinde, R. A. (1984). Biological bases of the mother–child relationships. In *Frontier of Infant Psychiatry*, *Vol. 2*, ed. J. Call, E. Galensen and R. L. Tyson. New York: Basic Books.

Hinde, R. A. (1986). Can nonhuman primates help us understand human behavior? In *Primate Societies*, ed. B. B. Smuts *et al.* Chicago: University of Chicago Press.

Hinde, R. A. (1987). *Individuals, Relationships and Culture: Links between Ethology and the Social Sciences*. Cambridge: Cambridge University Press.

Hinde, R. A. & Stevenson-Hinde, J. (ed.) (1973). *Constraints on Learning: Limitations and Predispositions*. New York: Academic Press.

Howard, M. (1976). *War in European History*. Oxford: Oxford University Press.

Hunterford, F. & Turner, A. (1987). *Animal Conflict*. London: Chapman and Hall.

Konner, M. (1982). *The Tangled Wing: Biological Constraints on the Human Spirit*. New York: Harper & Row.

Lee, P. C. (1983). Play as a means for developing relationships. In *Primate Social Relationship: An Integrated Approach*, ed. R. A. Hinde. Oxford: Blackwell.

Lee, R. B. & DeVore, I. (ed.) (1968). *Man the Hunter*. Chicago: Aldine-Atherton.

Lee, R. B. & DeVore, I. (ed.) (1976). *Kalahari Hunter-Gatherers*. Cambridge, Mass.: Harvard University Press.

Lenski, G. & Lenski, J. (1987). *Human Societies*. New York: McGraw Hill.

Levine, R. & Campbell, D. (1972). *Ethnocentrism: Theories of Conflict, Ethnic Attitudes and Group Behavior*. New York: McGraw-Hill.

Marler, P. (1976). Social organization, communication, and graded signals: The chimpanzee and the gorilla. In *Growing Points in Ethology*, ed. P. P. G. Bateson and R. A. Hinde. Cambridge: Cambridge University Press.

McNeill, W. H. (1971). *A World History*, 2nd edition. New York: Oxford University Press.

McNeill, W. H. (1982). *The Pursuit of Power: Technology, Armed Force, and Society since A.D. 1000*. Chicago: University of Chicago Press.

Money, J. & Ehrhardt, A. A. (1968). Prenatal hormonal exposure: Possible effects on behavior in man. In *Endocrinology and Human Behavior*, ed. R. Michael. Oxford: Oxford University Press.

Nicolson, N. A. (1986). Infants, mothers, and other females. In *Primate Societies*, ed. B. B. Smuts *et al.* Chicago: University of Chicago Press.

Ninio J. (1983). *Molecular Approaches to Evolution*. Princeton, NJ: Princeton University Press.

Nishida, T. (1979). The social structure of chimpanzees of Mahale Mountains. In *The Great Apes*, ed. D. A. Hamburg and E. R. McCown. Menlo Park, Calif.: Benjamin/Cummings.

Nishida, T. & Hiraiwa-Hasegawa, M. (1986). Chimpanzees and bonobos: cooperative relationships among males. In *Primate Societies*, ed. B. B. Smuts *et al.* Chicago: University of Chicago Press.

Nishida, T., Hiraiwa-Hasegawa, M., Hasegawa, T. & Takahata, Y. (1985). Group extinction and female transfer in wild chimpanzees in the Mahale Mountains. *Zeitschrift für Tierpsychologie*, **67**, 284–301.

Nye, J. S., Jr, Allison, G. T. & Carnesale, A. (ed.) (1988). *Fateful Visions: Avoiding Nuclear Catastrophe*. Cambridge, Mass.: Ballinger Press.

Parkes, C. M. & Stevenson-Hinde, J. (ed.) (1982). *The Place of Attachment in Human Behavior*. New York: Basic Books.

Popp, J. L. & DeVore, I. (1979). Aggressive competition and social dominance theory: synopsis. In *The Great Apes*, ed. D. A. Hamburg and E. R. McCown. Menlo Park, Calif.: Benjamin/Cummings.

Price, T. D. & Brown, J. A. (1985). *Prehistoric Hunter-Gatherers: The Emergence of Cultural Complexity*. San Diego, Calif.: Academic Press.

Pusey, A. E. (1979). Intercommunity transfer of chimpanzees in Gombe National Park. In *The Great Apes*, ed. D. A. Hamburg and E. R. McCown. Menlo Park, Calif.: Benjamin/Cummings.

Pusey, A. E. (1983). Mother–offspring relationships in chimpanzees after weaning. *Animal Behavior*, **31**, 363–77.

Pusey, A. E. & Packer, C. (1986). Dispersal and philopatry. In *Primate Societies*, ed. B. B. Smuts *et al.* Chicago: University of Chicago Press.

Radke-Yarrow, M. & Zahn-Waxler, C. (1986). The role of familial factors in the development of prosocial behavior: Research findings and questions. In

Development of Antisocial and Prosocial Behavior, ed. D. Olweus, J. Block and M. Radke-Yarrow. San Diego, Calif.: Academic Press.

Raiffa, H. (1982). *The Art and Science of Negotiation*. Cambridge, Mass.: Belknap Press of Harvard University Press.

Riopelle, A. (1960). In *Principles of Comparative Psychology*, ed. R. Wattes, D. Rethingshater and W. Caldwell. New York: McGraw-Hill.

Robbins, K. (1985). *The First World War*. Oxford: Oxford University Press.

Rock, S. R. (1989). *Why Peace Breaks Out: Great Power Rapprochement in Historical Perspective*. Chapel Hill: University of North Carolina Press.

Sackett, G. P. (1966). Monkeys reared in isolation with pictures as visual input. Evidence for an innate releasing mechanism. *Science*, **154**, 1468.

Schellenberg, J. A. (1982). *The Science of Conflict*. New York: Oxford University Press.

Seligman, M. E. & Hager, J. L. (1972). *Biological Boundaries of Learning*. New York: Appleton-Century-Crofts.

Sherif, M. & Sherif, C. (1966). *Groups in Harmony and Tension: An Integration of Studies on Intergroup Relations*. New York: Octagon.

Simons, E. L. (1989). Human origins. *Science*, **245**, 1343–50.

Smith, C. G. (ed.) (1971). *Conflict Resolution: Contributions of the Behavioral Sciences*. Notre Dame: University of Notre Dame Press.

Smuts, B. B. (1985). *Sex and Friendship in Baboons*. New York: Aldine.

Smuts, B. B. (1986). Gender, aggression, and influence. In *Primate Societies*, ed. B. B. Smuts *et al*. Chicago: University of Chicago Press.

Smuts, B. B., Cheney, D. L., Seyfarth, R. M., Wrangham, R. W. & Struhsaker, T. T. (1986). *Primate Societies*. Chicago: University of Chicago Press.

Staub, E. (1989). *The Roots of Evil: The Origins of Genocide and Other Group Violence*. Cambridge: Cambridge University Press.

Suomi, S. L. (1979). Differential development of various social relationships by rhesus monkey infants. In *The Child in its Family*, ed. M. Lewis and A. Rosenblum. New York: Plenum Press.

Suomi, S. L. (1982). Biological foundations and development psychobiology. In *The Child: Development in a Social Context*, ed. C. Kopp and J. Krakow. London: Addison-Wesley.

Thomas, H. (1980). *An History of the World*. New York: Harper and Row.

Tutin, C. E. G., McGrew, W. C. & Baldwin, P. (1983). Social organization of savanna-dwelling chimpanzees, *Pan troglodytes verus*, at Mt. Assirik, Senegal. *Primates*, **24**, 154–73.

van Lawick-Goodall, J. (1968). The behavior of free-living chimpanzees in the Gombe stream reserve. *Animal Behavior Monographs*, **1**, 161–311.

van Lawick-Goodall, J. (1971). Some aspects of aggressive behavior in a group of free-living chimpanzees. *International Social Science Journal*, **23**, 89–97.

Walters, J. R. & Seyfarth, R. M. (1986). Conflict and cooperation. In *Primate Societies*, ed. B. B. Smuts *et al*. Chicago: University of Chicago Press.

Washburn, S. L. & Hamburg, D. A. (1965). The study of primate behavior. In *Primate Behavior: Field Studies of Monkeys and Apes*, ed. I. DeVore. New York: Holt, Rinehart and Winston.

Washburn, S. L. & Hamburg, D. A. (1968). Aggressive behavior in old world monkeys and apes. In *Primates: Studies in Adaptation and Variability*, ed. P. Jay. New York: Holt, Rinehart and Winston.

Washburn, S. L. & Harding, R. S. O. (1978). Evolution and human nature. In

American Handbook of Psychiatry, *Vol. BI*, 2nd edition, ed. D. A. Hamburg and H. K. H. Brodie. New York: Basic Books.

Washburn, S. L. & McGown, E. R. (ed.) (1978). *Human Evolution: Biosocial Perspectives, Vol. IV*. Menlo Park, Calif.: Benjamin/Cummings.

Williams, R. M. (1977). *Mutual Accommodation: Ethnic Conflict and Cooperation*. Minneapolis: University of Minnesota Press.

Wrangham, R. W. (1974). Artifical feeding of chimpanzees and baboons in their natural habitat. *Animal Behavior*, **22**, 83–94.

Wrangham, R. W. (1979). Sex differences in chimpanzee dispersion. In *The Great Apes*, ed. D. A. Hamburg and E. R. McCown. Menlo Park, Calif.: Benjamin/Cummings.

Wrangham, R. W. (1983). Social relationships in comparative perspective. In *Primate Social Relationships: An Integrated Approach*, ed. R. A. Hinde. Oxford: Blackwell.

Wrangham, R. W. (1986a). Evolution of social structure. In *Primate Societies*, ed. B. B. Smuts *et al*. Chicago: University of Chicago Press.

Wrangham, R. W. (1986b). Ecology and social relationships in two species of chimpanzee. In *Ecology and Social Evolution: Birds and Mammals*, ed. D. I. Rubenstein and R. W. Wrangham. Princeton: Princeton University Press.

Yalom, I. D., Green, R. & Fisk, N. (1973). Prenatal exposure to female hormones: Effect on psychosexual development in boys. *Archives of General Psychiatry*, **28**, 554–61.

Commentary

— 5 —

Dave Hamburg and I first met in Jane Goodall's camp at the Gombe Stream. The psychiatrist from Stanford, as he was then, seemed out of place in central Africa, and I confess that I picked up no clues about the skill, resourcefulness and courage he was to show later in extricating students who had been taken hostage across Lake Tanganyika. I refer later to the great importance to me of my contact with Jane Goodall, and the start of a relationship with Dave Hamburg was an additional bonus. For him, too, that era was an important milestone, and he has gone on to make major contributions to world peace through his work in Harvard, in Washington and with the Carnegie Foundation.

His contribution here differs from the rest of the volume. He takes as it were a bird's eye view of humanity, synthesising knowledge about the causation, development, and evolution of the behaviour of man and his close relatives in an effort to influence the future. In striding fearlessly across such a wide domain he leads where many scientists, perhaps over-anxious to test the security of the ground on which they stand, would fear to advance. The message is clear and urgent – we can use an essentially ethological approach to gain a new view on the nature of humankind and on the steps we must take if we are to preserve what humankind has won.

Hamburg does not maintain that an evolutionary and comparative approach can take us all the way. It could be suggested, for instance, that the similarities between international war and individual aggressiveness are not as important as the differences. International war is an institution, with prescribed roles for soldiers, generals, politicians and so on. The incumbents of those roles act as they do because of the rights and duties associated with their roles. Thus individual aggression plays little part in the behaviour of a soldier in a modern army. The crucial question, in my view, is how the

459

institution of war is maintained, and here we need the resources of both natural and social sciences. As Hamburg emphasises, human propensities to differentiate groups (Tajfel, 1978) and to behave aggressively play a role – for instance the propaganda used by leaders plays upon aggressive propensities – but many other historical, religious and economic issues are at least as important (Hinde, 1989, 1991). These issues must be integrated with the broad evolutionary perspective that Hamburg supplies.

References

Hinde, R. A. (1989). Towards integrating the behavioural sciences to meet the threats of violence and war. *Medicine and War*, **5**, 5–15.
Hinde, R. A. (ed.) (1991). *The Institution of War*. London: MacMillan (in press).
Tajfel, H. (1978). Contributions to *Differentiation between Social Groups*, ed. H. Tajfel. London: Academic Press.

R.A.H.

VII
Memoirs

—18—

Some personal remarks

Niko Tinbergen

When I arrived in Oxford in 1949 to take up a lectureship in Alister Hardy's Department of Zoology and Comparative Anatomy (as the Department of Zoology was then called) I was fortunate in meeting, on occasional visits to Wytham Woods, the young Robert Hinde. He was then working on his thesis on the behaviour of the Great Tit and related species, under the supervision of the late David Lack. I found it difficult to understand the flock-living tits at first, because I was so used to studying pair formation in birds that strongly defend small territories. However, I learned a lot from Robert as I followed him about while he observed his birds in the wood, dressed in his long grey RAF coat. We 'clicked' well and never lost touch afterwards. My visits to see him at Madingley were infrequent in the years after he left Oxford. But these became easier when our Department acquired a Land Rover, mainly for our field studies (and those of the late Dr E. B. Ford with whom our group had to share the vehicle). I still remember Robert's smile when, as an experienced air pilot, he watched me struggle with the controls, shortly after I had finally learned to drive the Land Rover.

I did not know exactly what Robert was up to when he was working on his now classic textbook *Animal Behaviour – a Synthesis of Ethology and Comparative Psychology*, although I realised that he was acquiring a vast knowledge of the relevant literature. However, when the book appeared, it was immediately obvious to me that his book was far more wide-ranging than my own *The Study of Instinct*, which seemed primitive by comparison. I recognised its unique importance at once. It was totally appropriate that the second edition was honoured with a multiple review in the journal *Animal Behaviour*. Apart from this book which made him the pre-eminent writer in the subject, Robert's work has always been distinguished by a happy knack

463

for quantifying and measuring behaviour, which he has taught to a large number of his own graduate students and young colleagues.

While he was still writing his great book, he was appointed to a Royal Society Research Professorship which was to be held in the Cambridge Department of Zoology. Soon the Medical Research Council began to support his work and, from then on, his distinguished career took off in earnest. He has received many honours since and no doubt more will come his way.

I was inspired by Robert to become interested in humans and especially in the behaviour of children. I do not think that without his example I would have had the persistence to continue, together with my wife, our work on the problem of early childhood autism. It was a proper acknowledgement of Robert's outstanding contribution in the field of human behaviour, that he was made an Honorary Fellow of The Royal College of Psychiatry in 1988. Personally, I owe him a great deal because he was one of those good friends who kept visiting me after I had been immobilised by a stroke which put an end to my active research in 1983.

I am glad to have been given the opportunity to contribute, however little, to this book which testifies so well to the breadth of his knowledge, his penetrating mind and his wide influence.

(Professor Tinbergen died on 21st December, 1988)

—19—
Robert Hinde in Africa

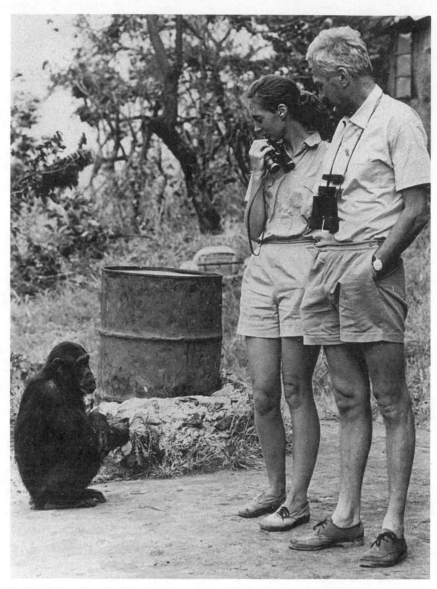

Figure 1. Robert Hinde at Gombe Stream Reserve.

—19—
Robert Hinde in Africa

Jane Goodall

Tall, ruggedly handsome, and looking distinguished despite his forest-snagged shorts and shirt, Robert Hinde watched as a female chimpanzee – Passion – stripped leaves from a twig, trimmed the end, then used her home-made tool to fish for termites from their mound nest. Carefully she inserted the tool into a subterranean tunnel that she had previously scratched open with her nails and then, after a moment, slowly pulled it out. It was bristling along half its length with termites that clung to the twig with their mandibles and helplessly waved their little legs in the air. Passion picked them off with her lips and scrunched with gusto while pushing the tool back for another catch.

Three-year-old Pom, bored now with her mother's performance, climbed to play in a tree above us. Suddenly something caught and held her attention, and she swung down to investigate. Dangling from a branch just above Robert's head, Pom gazed curiously at his hair. Brown hair and black, blonde and ginger, she knew. But a thick shock of silvery-grey hair was something new in her experience. She stretched one hand towards it, but dared not touch. For a moment she hung there, undecided. Then, quite suddenly, she stamped twice on Robert's head (quite hard, he said). As he looked up, startled, she retreated, sniffed her foot intently, then deliberately picked a handful of leaves and scrubbed the sole of her foot, again and again. Finally, the smell of this unusual contact having been wiped away to her apparent satisfaction, she swung off to continue her climbing and twirling in the upper branches.

I was delighted by that incident: it was very amusing and it also demonstrated tool-using in what was then a new context – wiping away the smell of stranger contact. But I'm not sure about Robert's reaction – I've always thought that he felt, perhaps, just a little insulted! It was his first visit

467

through seemingly impenetrable undergrowth, battling with vines and thorns and one's own exhaustion, finally one catches up with the chimps when, for a while, they have paused and the adults are feeding or grooming one another, the infants playing. Only out in the forest can one know the joy of being with the chimpanzees as they really are. 'It's not just that they are different from chimps in *zoos*' Robert told me, after describing one exhausting but wonderful follow, 'they are even different from when they are in camp. They are different creatures altogether.'

The opportunity to meet chimpanzees on their own terms in the forest, to sense something of their complex natures and vivid personalities, has impressed many eminent scientific visitors to Gombe and Robert was no exception. He wrote to say that his visit had been 'one of the most academically exciting experiences' of his life and that it would 'revolutionize and change his whole thinking about animal behaviour.'

Robert made two more visits to Gombe, one in 1970 and one in 1972. It goes without saying that all his visits had far-reaching effects upon the direction of the research there. During his first stay, for example, he instigated some major improvements in methodology. He helped to set up a mother–infant study comparable to his own study of the rhesus monkeys. The checksheet he designed, modified over time, is still in use at Gombe today. And, of course, his clear thinking and wisdom made a deep and lasting impression on many of the students who had the unique opportunity of talking to such an eminent man in the peace and quiet of Gombe. In that way alone his impact on the growing field of primatology was extended.

Robert's last visit to Gombe coincided with the death of the old chimpanzee matriarch, Flo. She was found lying dead in the Kakombe Stream. Nearby her eight and a half year old son, Flint, huddled on the bank, gazing at his mother's body. Robert was there to witness at first hand Flint's bewilderment which, quite rapidly, led to the huddled posture and staring eyes seen also in clinically depressed human patients. Soon after Robert's return to Cambridge, Flint, his immune system weakened, fell sick and died – just three and a half weeks after his mother's death. That experience had a profound effect on all of us.

I have written this piece to express my boundless admiration for Robert Hinde who will surely take his place in scientific history as one of the giants of our times. It is a token of my enormous gratitude to the man who has had the greatest direct influence on the development of my own scientific thinking. A few years ago I asked Robert when he would visit Gombe again. 'When I have retired', he replied. And so, Robert, I am expecting another visit soon.

470

Commentary
—6—

Two of the contributors have chosen to write personal messages. Though one was written by a mentor and the other by a former student, both are equally embarrassing for me because I feel that I was the principal recipient in both relationships. Niko Tinbergen arrived in Oxford when I was a DPhil student, and it was my good fortune that, not yet established in new research projects, he had time to spend with me. I was profoundly influenced by him, and what he taught me has coloured my research ever since. When he wrote for the present book shortly before his death, he had evidently forgotten that we started the book *Animal Behaviour* together as a joint project. One of my greatest regrets is that other demands forced him to forgo authorship when only one or two chapters had been drafted: it was a loss both to me and to the enterprise.

I have recently written about Niko Tinbergen in the Memoirs of Fellows of the Royal Society, but one thing that was difficult to get across was his deep enthusiasm, vitality, and enjoyment of living. His mention of Alister Hardy leads me to put on record a story about both of them. A year or two after I finished my DPhil at Oxford, I was cycling along the road from Madingley to Cambridge. I used to get tired of the cars that drove past me very fast, forcing me too close to the grass verge, and on this day I swore long and loud at a Land Rover that whizzed past. To my surprise it stopped a little way ahead, and when I caught up I was horrified to find it occupied by Alister Hardy, my recent Head of Department, and Niko Tinbergen, recently my DPhil examiner. They hardly saw me as I stopped because they were arguing vigorously with each other – Hardy, a devout Unitarian, was saying 'He was singing, I'm sure he was singing', whilst Tinbergen, convulsed with laughter, was saying 'No, he was swearing, of course he was swearing'.

Meeting Niko Tinbergen when I was a student was one lucky break for me, and meeting Jane Goodall fifteen or so years later was another. She came to Madingley as a student only because at that time no one in the country was really competent to supervise fieldwork on non-human primates. My contact with her came at a crucially important time, because it helped me to search for balance in one of the most difficult problems for the student of animal behaviour. As a DPhil student, I had been fascinated by the vicissitudes of individual Great Tits – how a particular male had two territories, lost one, expanded the other, lost his mate, found another and so on. Later, Thelma Rowell (see Chapter 10) and I learned the hard way that running a monkey colony demands attention to the idiosyncrasies of individuals. But it was my contact with Jane Goodall which brought home to me that the individuality of the chimpanzees was crucial – and if she was learning how to make moderately accurate records in order to generalise about chimpanzees, I was learning that such generalisations occluded some of the most fascinating, and biologically important, things about them. She also taught me some lessons in rigorous thinking. I remember a discussion at Gombe when the way in which each male chimpanzee would stand at the base of a different tree, blocking off the possible escape route of a treed monkey, was being cited as an example of cooperative hunting: Jane quietly pointed out that each was thereby maximising his own chances of catching the monkey.

Conclusion

Naturally I feel that I cannot adequately express my gratitude to the contributors for their chapters, or to Pat Bateson for all the work that an edited volume involves. I want also to thank the contributors, and the many others whom I know Pat Bateson would have liked to invite if it had not been for the constraints of space and balance, for the interactions we have had and the relationships we have developed over the years. I have been fortunate in my colleagues.

R.A.H.

Appendixes

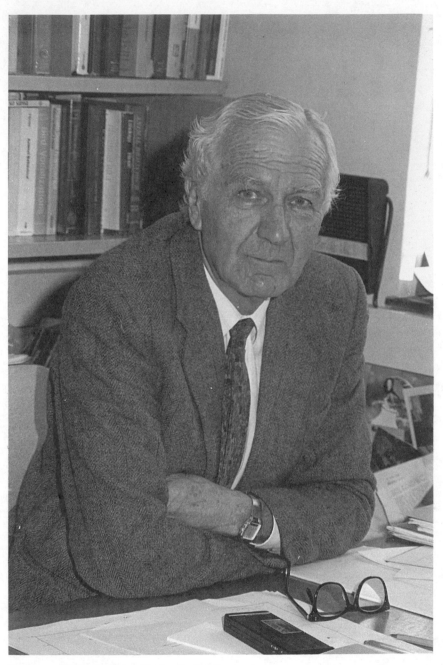

Professor Robert Hinde. Photo: L. Barden.

— Appendix 1 —
Robert Hinde's career

Born 26 October 1923 in Norwich, England

1935–40	Oundle School
1940–5	RAF Pilot, Coastal Command
1946–8	St John's College, Cambridge
1948	BA, Cambridge; BSc, London
1948–50	Research Assistant, Edward Grey Institute, Department of Zoology, Oxford University
1950	DPhil, Oxford
1950–64	Curator, Ornithological Field Station, Department of Zoology, Cambridge University (now Sub-Department of Animal Behaviour)
1951–4	Research Fellow, St John's College, Cambridge
1956–8	Steward, St John's College
1958–present	Fellow, St John's College
1958–63	Tutor, St John's College
1958	ScD, Cambridge
1961	Zoological Society's Scientific Medal
1963–89	Royal Society Research Professor
1970–89	Honorary Director, Medical Research Council Unit on the Development and Integration of Behaviour
1974	Fellow of the Royal Society (Council member 1985–7)
1974	Foreign Honorary Member of the American Academy of Arts and Sciences

1974	Docteur honoris causa dans la Faculté des Sciences Psychologiques et Pédagogiques, Université Libre, Bruxelles
1976	Honorary Fellow of the American Ornithologists' Union
1978	Honorary Foreign Associate of the National Academy of Sciences
1978	Docteur honoris causa, Université de Paris (Nanterre)
1979	Hitchcock Professor at University of California
1980	Osman Hill Medal, Primate Society of Great Britain
1980	Leonard Cammer Award, New York Psychiatric Institute, Columbia University
1981	Honorary Fellow of British Psychological Society
1983	Green Visiting Scholar, University of Texas
1986	Honorary Fellow, Balliol College, Oxford
1987	Albert Einstein Award for Psychiatry, Albert Einstein College of Medicine, New York
1987	Honorary Member, Association for the Study of Animal Behaviour
1988	Commander of the British Empire
1988	Honorary Fellow of the Royal College of Psychiatry
1988	Honorary Member of the Deutsche Ornithologische Gesellschaft
1989–present	Master, St John's College, Cambridge
1990	Croonian Lecturer, Royal Society
1990	Huxley Medal, Royal Anthropological Institute
1990	Member, Academia Europaea
1990	Honorary Fellow, Trinity College, Dublin

Publications (in addition to over 300 journal articles and chapters in books)

Own volumes

1966/70 *Animal Behaviour: A Synthesis of Ethology and Comparative Psychology.* New York: McGraw-Hill.

1974 *Biological Bases of Human Social Behaviour.* New York: McGraw-Hill.

1979 *Towards Understanding Relationships.* London: Academic Press.

1982 *Ethology: Its Nature and Relations with Other Sciences.* Oxford: Oxford University Press and Fontana Paperbacks.

1987 *Individuals, Relationships and Culture: Links between Ethology and the Social Sciences.* Cambridge: Cambridge University Press.

Appendix 1

Edited volumes

1965–83 *Advances in the Study of Behaviour, Vols 1–13* (with D. S. Lehrman & J. S. Rosenblatt). New York: Academic Press.

1969 *Bird Vocalizations*. Cambridge: Cambridge University Press.

1970 *Short-term Changes in Neural Activity and Behaviour* (with G. Horn). Cambridge: Cambridge University Press.

1972 *Non-Verbal Communication*. Cambridge: Cambridge University Press.

1973 *Constraints on Learning* (with J. Stevenson-Hinde). Cambridge: Cambridge University Press.

1976 *Growing Points in Ethology* (with P. Bateson). Cambridge: Cambridge University Press.

1983 *Primate Social Relationships*. Oxford: Blackwell Scientific Publications.

1985 *Social Relationships and Cognitive Development* (with A.-N. Perret-Clermont & J. Stevenson-Hinde). Oxford: Clarendon Press.

1987 *Essays on Violence* (with J. M. Ramirez & J. Groebel). Sevilla: Publicaciones de la Universidad de Sevilla.

1988 *Relationships within Families: Mutual Influences* (with J. Stevenson-Hinde). Oxford: Clarendon Press.

1989 *Education for Peace* (with D. A. Parry). Nottingham: Russell Press.

1989 *Aggression and War* (with J. Groebel). Cambridge: Cambridge University Press.

1991 *Cooperation and Prosocial Behaviour* (with J. Groebel). Cambridge: Cambridge University Press (in press).

1991 *The Institution of War*. London: MacMillan (in press).

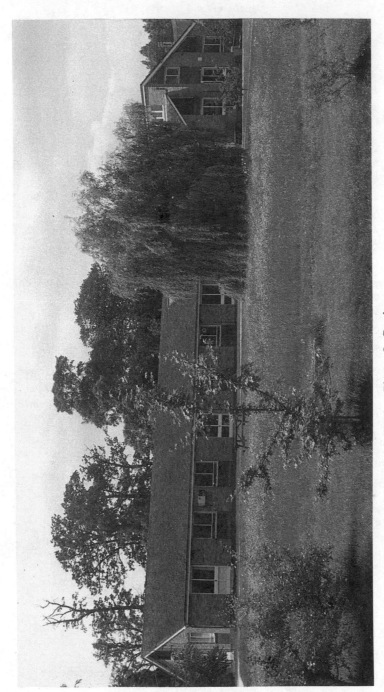

The Sub-Department of Animal Behaviour, Madingley. Photo: L. Barden.

— Appendix 2 —
The Sub-Department of Animal Behaviour at Madingley

After obtaining his doctorate at Oxford, Robert Hinde spent the rest of his working life at the laboratory in Madingley. One of the first ethological laboratories, it was established in 1950 by W. H. Thorpe, who invited Hinde to return to Cambridge to be Curator.

Bill Thorpe had been an entomologist engaged in the biological control of insects. One of his interests was in how insects that lay eggs in other species find their hosts. This led him to uncover some of the extraordinary and complex learning abilities of insects and to start work on the relations between 'instinctive' and 'learned' behaviour. After the Second World War, Thorpe's research interests turned increasingly towards birds. He was greatly excited by the theoretical ideas of Konrad Lorenz and decided that Cambridge needed a place, with plenty of aviaries and pens, to test Lorenz's theories (e.g. Thorpe, 1956, 1961). While in Oxford, Robert Hinde had been much influenced by Niko Tinbergen. Thus, the Madingley laboratory started under a strong influence from the two principal fathers of Ethology, though the work they stimulated did not always confirm their theories.

Since birds could not be housed properly in the Zoology Department, located in the centre of town, Thorpe had sought a location within cycling distance of Cambridge. He was able to obtain a site behind the Three Horseshoes Pub in Madingley village, about four miles northwest of Cambridge. Initially, the facilities consisted of an old Home Guard hut and a former blacksmith's shop, with about 70 aviaries built in large part by the Curator (Thorpe, 1962). Memories from those days are of mud, Wellington boots, and 'do-it-yourself', from building equipment to looking after animals.

In 1960, the University gave the Ornithological Field Station the status of the Sub-Department of Animal Behaviour. The change in name was appropriate, because mammals as well as birds were being studied by then. Particularly important was a rhesus monkey colony established on grants from the Medical Research Council and the Mental Health Research Fund to Robert Hinde. The Nuffield and Rockefeller Foundations provided funds for a permanent building, completed in 1962.

Over the years, much influential field work has been carried out with Madingley as the base, but after an agreement with Niko Tinbergen's group at Oxford in the 1950s, the Cambridge laboratory work focused its laboratory studies on the development

479

and integration of behaviour. Bill Thorpe founded what has become a world-wide study of bird song-learning and, with Margaret Vince and Robert Hinde, initiated studies of imprinting in birds which continue to the present day under Pat Bateson and which have led to studies of the development of mate choice. Studies of the neural and endocrine basis of behaviour started under Robert Hinde and was continued by John Hutchison; that tradition is now maintained by Barry Keverne. Analysis of parent–offspring relationships and social development has been carried out in a large number of mammals, including hamsters, gerbils, spiny mice, rats, mice, cats and, of course, rhesus monkeys. Michael Simpson took over the monkey work which had stimulated Robert Hinde to initiate studies of children's relationships. The work with children has been carried out principally by him, by Judy Dunn and by Joan Stevenson-Hinde.

Bill Thorpe retired as Director of the Sub-Department in 1969, when Hans Lissmann took over. In 1970, the Medical Research Council funded a Unit within the Sub-Department, with Robert Hinde as its Honorary Director. The principal senior members of the MRC Unit on the Development & Integration of Behaviour were: Judy Dunn, John Hutchison, Michael Simpson, and Joan Stevenson-Hinde. In 1976, Pat Bateson became Director of the Sub-Department, to be succeeded by Barry Keverne in 1988, when Bateson became head (Provost) of King's College. The installation of Robert Hinde as Master of St John's College in the following year suggests an unsuspected advantage of an ethological training at Madingley. Indeed, many others have reaped a rich harvest since their early days here, as evidenced by the following list of 'Madingley PhD's'. Much of Madingley's own development over the years is due to them.

The following obtained their doctorates from Madingley: R. J. Andrew, M. C. Appleby, R. F. W. Barnes, P. P. G. Bateson, L. Beardsall, C. M. Berman, B. C. R. Bertram, M. Bonn, D. M. Broom, R. A. Burley, J. D. Bygott, P. G. Caryl, N. R. Chalmers, D. F. Chantrey, B. Chapais, D. Cheney, J. J. Cherfas, T. H. Clutton-Brock, J. D. Colvin, J. H. Crook, D. B. Croft, N. J. Dale, S. B. Datta, S. J. J. F. Davies, E. K. DeMulder, J. Dunn, P. J. Egan (Neé Henriques), J. A. Feaver, J. C. Fentress, C. D. Fitzgibbon, D. Fossey, S. H. Francis, P. R. Green, A. H. Harcourt, D. A. Hill, S. D. Holman, C. M. Hogg, J. B. Hutchison, R. E. Hutchison, P. S. Jackson, M. C. Janus, H. G. Johnson, G. Katzir, J. Kear, R. B. Klopman, P. C. Lee, L. M. McGinnis, P. R. McGinnis, C. D. Magin, P. Marler, P. H. Martin, G. V. T. Matthews, M. Mendl, P. A. Munn, N. W. Owens, H. H. C. Plooij, J. H. Poole, R. G. W. Prescott, K. L. R. Rasmussen, M. J. Reiss, M. P. M. Richards, S. M. Richards, T. J. Roper, C. H. F. Rowell, T. E. Rowell, H. K. A. Sants, A. M. Scott, D. K. Scott, J. L. Scott, N. J. S. Scourse, R. M. Seyfarth, D. Y. Shapiro, A. E. Shouldice, M. J. A. Simpson, Y. Spencer-Booth, K. J. Stewart, R. D. Stillwell, P. J. Turner, A. Tye, S. J. Tyler, J. Van Lawick-Goodall, A. Weisler, L. E. White, A. H. Willner and R. W. Wrangham.

References

Thorpe, W. H. (1956). *Learning and Instinct in Animals*. London: Methuen.
Thorpe, W. H. (1961). *Bird-Song*. Cambridge: Cambridge University Press.
Thorpe, W. H. (1962). The Sub-Department of Animal Behaviour, University of Cambridge. *Nature*, **196**, 1043–4.

Index

Page numbers in *italics* refer to figures and illustrations.

481

Index

mechanoreceptors of canary brood patch,
   154
α-melanocyte stimulating hormone, 174
memory
   neural basis theories, 126
   neuroethological approach, 82
   retrieval, 172, 183, 184–5
   system of brain and attentional
      mechanisms, 131
memory formation
   competition, 183, 184, 185
   effects of testosterone, 183–6
   hormonal effects, 172
   OSLE role, 187
   threshold effects, 181
mental health, 302
N-methyl-D-aspartate (NMDA)
   binding, 130
   receptors, 131, 132
methyltrienolone (R1181), 156
Microtus agrestis, 89
military–industrial complex, 438
milk production, 243
mini-domes, 154
Minuchin P, 316
mobbing
   behaviour, 31
   response, 25
modal action patterns, 85
Modern Learning Theory, 411
money, 287
monogamous species, 152–3
monogamy, 230–1
   breeding success, 231, 232
   sexual dimorphism, 236
Moores J, 285
moose cow's behaviour, 195
moral understanding of children, 384
Moran J, 105
mortality, differential
   juvenile, 240–1
   in polygyny, 239–41
   population dynamics, 241
mother
   attachment relationships, 308–9
   behaviour in play, 396
   child interaction, 307–8
   facial expressions, 346
   model, 307
   over-indulgence in child, 310
   relationships, 302
mother–child
   dialogue of influences, 402
   interaction, 414
mother–child relationship, 8, 9
   behaviour prediction, 414

breakdown, 9
firstborn and birth of sibling, 382
functioning of family, 398
research situations, 396
Strange Situation method, 357, 360, 395
verbal communication, 396
mother-figure, 302, 303
mother–infant relationship, 304, 341, 358
   aggression and submission learning, 439
   firstborn child, 379–80
   hunter-gatherers, 432
   quality and stress of separation, 381
   rhesus monkeys, 379
mother–young relationship in postpartum
   period, 196–8
mothering, variation in sensitivity, 380
mothers
   adolescent, 337
   verbal communication with toddler-age
      children, 396–7
motor development in swamp sparrow, 48
motor equivalence, 84
motor neuron activity patterns, 99
motor programs, 85
   centre, 87
mountain sheep horn size, 236
multiple birth, 195
multiple independent variables, 90
mutual influences, 414–15
mutualism, 284–5
mutually interacting influences, 402–4
   clinical studies, 403
   measurement, 402
   methods of study, 402–4
   multi-child families, 403–4

Nadler R D, 203
nature/nurture controversy, 23
nervous system
   feature development, 31
   plasticity, 27
   processing, 97
   simpler networks approach, 78
nest orientation behaviour, 157
nest-building
   appearance of newborns, 193
   commitment expression, 283
   prepartum, 206
   prolactin stimulation, 194
nest-orientated behaviour
   brain oestrogen levels, 156
   oestradiol, 156
   oestrogen-sensitive mechanisms of brain,
      156
nesting behaviour, 151
network interactions, 113

496